# New Advances in COVID-19 and Pregnancy

# New Advances in COVID-19 and Pregnancy

Guest Editor

**Gaspare Cucinella**

MDPI

Basel • Beijing • Wuhan • Barcelona • Belgrade • Novi Sad • Cluj • Manchester

*Guest Editor*
Gaspare Cucinella
Department of Obstetrics and
Gynecology
University of Palermo
Palermo
Italy

*Editorial Office*
MDPI AG
Grosspeteranlage 5
4052 Basel, Switzerland

This is a reprint of the Special Issue, published open access by the journal *Journal of Clinical Medicine* (ISSN 2077-0383), freely accessible at: https://www.mdpi.com/journal/jcm/special_issues/356Z4DZY3G.

For citation purposes, cite each article independently as indicated on the article page online and as indicated below:

| |
|---|
| Lastname, A.A.; Lastname, B.B. Article Title. *Journal Name* **Year**, *Volume Number*, Page Range. |

**ISBN 978-3-7258-5911-5 (Hbk)**
**ISBN 978-3-7258-5912-2 (PDF)**
**https://doi.org/10.3390/books978-3-7258-5912-2**

# Contents

Journal of
*Clinical Medicine*

MDPI

*Article*

# Risk Factors for Severe–Critical COVID-19 in Pregnant Women

**María Guadalupe Berumen-Lechuga [1,*], Alfredo Leaños-Miranda [2], Carlos José Molina-Pérez [3], Luis Rey García-Cortes [4] and Silvia Palomo-Piñón [5]**

1 Medical Research Coordinator, Instituto Mexicano del Seguro Social, Órgano de Operación Administrativa Desconcentrada Regional Poniente, Josefa Ortiz de Domínguez S/N Colonia Centro, Toluca CP 50000, Mexico

2 Medical Research Unit in Reproductive Medicine, Instituto Mexicano del Seguro Social, Unidad Médica de Alta Especialidad, Hospital de Ginecología y Obstetricia "Luis Castelazo Ayala", Rio de la Magdalena 289, Tizapán San Ángel, Delegación Álvaro Obregón, Ciudad de México CP 01090, Mexico; alfredolm@yahoo.com

3 Clinical Coordinator, Instituto Mexicano del Seguro Social, Hospital General de Zona No. 252, Camino Flor de María y Calzada Señor del Huerto 154, Colonia San Martín, Atlacomulco CP 54050, Mexico; carlosjosem@hotmail.com

4 Medical Research Coordinator, Instituto Mexicano del Seguro Social, Órgano de Operación Administrativa Desconcentrada Regional Oriente, Calle 4 No. 25, Fraccionamiento Alce Blanco, Naucalpan CP 53370, Mexico; docluisrey@gmail.com

5 Medical Research Unit on Nephrological Diseases (External Collaborator), Instituto Mexicano del Seguro Social, UMAE Centro Médico Nacional Siglo XXI, Avenida Cuauhtémoc 330, Colonia Doctores, Ciudad de México CP 06720, Mexico; silvia-palomo@hotmail.com

* Correspondence: maria.berumen@imss.gob.mx; Tel.: +52-722-2641305

**Abstract:** Risk factors associated with severe–critical COVID-19 (coronavirus disease 2019) are based on findings in the general population. Pregnant women are at increased risk of severe–critical infection, and few reports are based on these women. A multicentric case–control study was conducted at the Mexican Institute of Social Security, State of Mexico, during the COVID-19 pandemic. We included pregnant women who were consecutively admitted to respiratory care units and were followed until 30 days after the resolution of pregnancy. A total of 758 pregnant women with a positive RT-PCR test for SARS-CoV-2 were enrolled from June 2020 to July 2021. We defined groups using the World Health Organization Severity Classification; cases were pregnant women with severe–critical COVID-19 (n = 123), and controls were subjects with non-severe COVID-19 (n = 635). Data was gathered from clinical files. A multivariate logistic regression analysis was used to adjust odds ratios and their 95% confidence intervals of factors associated with severe–critical COVID-19. Risk factors associated with severe–critical COVID-19 in pregnancy were non-vaccination (OR 10.18), blood type other than O (OR 6.29), maternal age > 35 years (OR 5.76), history of chronic hypertension (OR 5.12), gestational age at infection $\geq$ 31 weeks (OR 3.28), and multiparity (OR 2.80).

**Keywords:** COVID-19; SARS-CoV-2; coronavirus infections; pregnancy

## 1. Introduction

The coronavirus disease 2019 (COVID-19) pandemic caused a global health crisis. It is well recognized that COVID-19 in pregnant women is more frequent due to physiological changes in the immune and cardiorespiratory systems that increase the susceptibility to this infection. Pregnant women have a high frequency in the progression of COVID-19 into a severe–critical stage compared to non-pregnant women; in addition, COVID-19 is generally associated with poor fetal and maternal outcomes [1–5]. Although different in pathology and transmission, the 2015–2016 Zika virus disease epidemic shares similarities with severe acute respiratory syndrome coronavirus 2 (SARS-CoV-2), such as limited diagnostic techniques, therapeutics, and prognostic uncertainties, and both are associated with a significant risk of adverse outcomes including intrauterine transmission [6,7].

In non-pregnant subjects, many risk factors have been identified in the progression of COVID-19 into a severe stage, such as chronic hypertension, diabetes, and obesity, among others [2,8–11]. This highlights that individuals with pre-existing comorbidities related to the imbalance in expressing angiotensin-converting enzyme 2 (ACE2) (which acts as an entry receptor for SARS-CoV-2) are at high risk of developing severe disease.

Although we have gained experience about the severity, course, and treatment of disease in patients infected with SARS-CoV-2, there are scarce studies on the risk factors for severe COVID-19 in pregnancy [12]. The studies have been consistent in that maternal age (greater than 35 years) and pre-existing comorbidities (mainly chronic hypertension, pregestational diabetes, and obesity) are associated with severe–critical COVID-19 [3,13,14]. In contrast, some risk factors, such as the trimester in which the disease appeared, parity or blood group, as well as other specific disorders of pregnancy, such as pre-eclampsia or gestational diabetes, have been inconsistent [3,13,15].

Therefore, the aim of this study was to identify the risk factors for severe–critical COVID-19 in Mexican pregnant women during the pandemic caused by this virus.

## 2. Materials and Methods

A case–control study was performed. Pregnant women with a positive reverse transcription polymerase chain reaction (RT-PCR) test were consecutively admitted to the medical respiratory units in general hospitals: 71, 72, 194, and 251 of the Mexican Institute of Social Security in the State of Mexico were included from 1 June 2020 to 31 July 2021. Disease severity was defined according to the World Health Organization Classification [13]. The cases group was formed by women who developed severe–critical COVID-19 defined by the following criteria: acute respiratory distress syndrome, sepsis, septic shock, thrombosis, or other conditions that would normally require life-sustaining therapies such as mechanical ventilation (invasive or non-invasive), vasopressor therapy, or oxygen saturation < 92% on room air; severe pneumonia; or signs of severe respiratory distress such as use of accessory muscles, inability to complete full sentences, and respiratory rate > 30 breaths per minute. The control group was formed by women with non-severe COVID-19, defined as the absence of any criteria for severe or critical COVID-19. Women whose diagnosis was not confirmed by RT-PCR, pregnant minors, those at risk of losing their autonomy, and those participants with incomplete data were eliminated. All women and newborns were followed until 30 days after the resolution of pregnancy.

Data were prospectively collected from medical charts. Differences between continuous variables were determined by Student's $t$-test for unpaired data or Mann–Whitney U test for non-normally distributed variables. Differences between categorical variables were determined using the chi-squared test with Yates' continuity correction or Fisher's exact test for small samples. The association between the clinical and demographic variables reported as risk factors and the occurrence of severe–critical COVID-19 were determined. Odds ratios (ORs) and 95% confidence intervals (CIs) were calculated. Logistic regression analysis was used to adjust the ORs for maternal age > 35 years, maternal comorbidities (chronic hypertension, pregestational diabetes, and obesity), non-vaccination against COVID-19, maternal blood group, gestational age at infection, multiparity, C-reactive protein, D-dimer, and neutrophil-to-lymphocyte ratio, because these variables were significantly different among the groups studied by univariate analysis, as well as considering that this variable may distinctly affect the occurrence of severe–critical COVID-19. A 2-tailed $p < 0.05$ was considered statistically significant. SPSS version 27 statistical software was used for data analysis.

The study protocol was approved on 22 May 2020 by the National Committee of Scientific Research of the Mexican Institute of Social Security with SIRELCIS registry R-2020-785-067. Written informed consent was obtained from all participants.

## 3. Results

### 3.1. General Description of the Population Studied

A total of 1492 pregnant women were attended by the respiratory modules. Seven hundred and seventy-one (51.7%) had a positive RT-PCR test; among these patients, seven did not accept to participate, and six were eliminated due to incomplete medical charts. Therefore, 758 patients were included in the final analysis; 123 were diagnosed with severe–critical COVID-19, and 635 women had non-severe COVID-19.

#### 3.1.1. The Demographic and Clinical Characteristics Are Shown in Table 1

There was no difference between groups in terms of days to seek medical attention, smoking history during pregnancy, vaccine brand, pre-eclampsia, or gestational diabetes. In contrast, there was a significant difference in maternal age, multiparity, blood group (except AB), gestational age at infection, pulmonary involvement score on computed tomography, mechanical ventilation, vaccination, as well as in comorbidities ($p \leq 0.022$). It is important to note that only 170 pregnant women were vaccinated because recruitment began before the vaccine was approved for use in pregnancy, all of whom were in their second or third trimester.

**Table 1.** Demographic and clinical characteristics of pregnant women with and without severe–critical COVID-19.

| Variable | Cases Severe–Critical COVID-19 [n = 123] | Controls Non-Severe COVID-19 [n = 635] | *p*-Value |
|---|---|---|---|
| **Maternal age, years, median, [IQR]** | 30 [26–34] | 27 [23–31] | <0.001 * |
| **Days to seek medical attention, median, [IQR]** | 3 [2–6] | 3 [2–5] | NS * |
| **Smoking history during pregnancy, n [%]** | 6 [4.9] | 26 [4.1] | NS † |
| **Multiparity, n [%]** | 73 [59.3] | 206 [32.4] | <0.001 † |
| **Mother's blood group** | | | |
| O, n [%] | 29 [23.6] | 431 [67.9] | <0.001 † |
| A, n [%] | 79 [64.2] | 182 [28.7] | <0.001 † |
| B, n [%] | 11 [8.9] | 14 [2.2] | <0.001 † |
| AB, n [%] | 4 [3.3] | 8 [1.2] | NS ‡ |
| **Maternal comorbidities** | | | |
| Chronic Hypertension, n [%] | 12 [9.8] | 13 [2.1] | <0.001 † |
| Pregestational Diabetes, n [%] | 10 [8.1] | 15 [2.4] | 0.002 † |
| Obesity, n [%] | 15 [12.2] | 38 [6.0] | 0.022 † |
| Pre-eclampsia, n [%] | 26 [21.1] | 173 [27.2] | NS † |
| Gestational Diabetes, n [%] | 11 [9.1] | 36 [5.65] | NS † |
| **Non-vaccination, n [%]** | 117 [95.1] | 471 [74.2] | <0.001 † |
| **Gestational age at infection, median, [IQR]** | 33 [27–36] | 23 [14–32] | <0.00 * |
| **Pulmonary involvement score in computed tomography** | | | |
| Noninvolvement, n [%] | 0 [0] | 427 [67.2] | <0.001 ‡ |
| Mild, n [%] | 0 [0] | 80 [12.6] | <0.001 ‡ |
| Moderate, n [%] | 0 [0] | 128 [20.2] | <0.001 ‡ |
| Severe, n [%] | 123 [100] | 0 [0] | <0.001 ‡ |
| ° **Mechanical ventilation, n [%]** | 32 [26.0] | 4 [0.63] | <0.001 ‡ |
| °° **Vaccination, n [%]** | 9 [6.5] | 161 [25.5] | <0.001 † |
| **Vaccine brand** | | | |
| Astra Zeneca, n [%] | 3 [33.3] | 27 [16.7] | NS ‡ |
| Pfizer, n [%] | 3 [33.3] | 93 [57.9] | NS ‡ |
| Sputnik, n [%] | 2 [22.2] | 25 [15.5] | NS ‡ |
| Cansino, n [%] | 0 [0] | 5 [3.0] | NS ‡ |
| Sinovac, n [%] | 1 [11.1] | 11 [6.7] | NS ‡ |

A *p*-value < 0.05 was considered statistically significant. * U Mann–Whitney test, † chi-squared test, ‡ Fisher's exact test, ° the four pregnant women in the control group who needed mechanical ventilation had no relation with COVID-19. °° In vaccination, only 170 pregnant women received two doses because recruitment started before the vaccine authorization in pregnancy. No serious adverse events associated with vaccine administration occurred.

#### 3.1.2. The Main Clinical Signs and Symptoms and Laboratory Findings Are Shown in Table 2

No differences were found between groups except for frequency of anosmia and dysgeusia ($p \leq 0.17$). As for laboratory findings, we found differences between groups in neutrophil-to-lymphocyte ratio, C-reactive protein, and D-dimer serum concentration ($p \leq 0.032$).

**Table 2.** Main clinical manifestations and laboratory findings at admission in pregnant women with severe–critical versus non-severe COVID-19.

| Variable | Cases Severe–Critical COVID-19 [n = 123] | Controls Non-Severe COVID-19 [n = 635] | $p$-Value |
|---|---|---|---|
| **Signs and symptoms** | | | |
| Headache, n [%] | 89 [72.4] | 463 [73.0] | NS † |
| Cough, n [%] | 74 [60.2] | 355 [55.6] | NS † |
| Odynophagia, n [%] | 74 [60.2] | 359 [56.4] | NS † |
| Fever, n [%] | 71 [57.7] | 320 [50.39] | NS † |
| Myalgias, n [%] | 59 [48.0] | 282 [44.5] | NS † |
| Anosmia, n [%] | 12 [9.8] | 124 [19.6] | 0.003 † |
| Dysgeusia, n [%] | 10 [8.1] | 96 [15.1] | 0.017 † |
| **Laboratory findings** | | | |
| Leukocytes, mean ± SD | 9828 ± 3086 | 8479 ± 2357 | NS § |
| Neutrophil to lymphocyte ratio, median [IQR] | 8.72 [6.8–12.4] | 6.35 [4.1–9.2] | 0.011 * |
| Platelets [×1000], median [IQR] | 151 [111–233] | 181 [151–243] | NS * |
| Glucose [mg/dL], median [IQR] | 92 [81–124] | 81 [67–96] | NS * |
| Creatinine [mg/dL], mean ± SD | 0.96 ± 0.25 | 0.61 ± 0.16 | NS § |
| Lactic dehydrogenase [U/L], median [IQR] | 296 [189–533] | 209 [160–329] | NS * |
| D-dimer, ng/ml, median [IQR] | 1956 [1181–3435] | 1216 [518–2418] | 0.032 * |
| C-reactive protein, mg/dL, mean ± SD | 8.3 ± 6.8 | 2.1 ± 1.62 | 0.027 § |

Data are presented as count and frequency n [%], mean ± SD means standard deviation; IQR, interquartile range. A $p$-value $p < 0.05$ was considered statistically significant. † chi-squared test, § Student's $t$-test, * U Mann–Whitney.

#### 3.1.3. Maternal and Perinatal Outcomes Are Reported in Table 3

There were no differences between groups in the frequency of miscarriages or cesarean sections. All women with severe–critical COVID-19 were admitted to intensive care units, and only six women in the group of controls. The need for admission to the intensive care units in the control group was not related to respiratory causes and was not associated with the severity of COVID-19 (four patients for early postpartum hemorrhage and two patients for met severity criteria for pre-eclampsia). All maternal deaths in the cases group were due to COVID-19 complications; in contrast, in the control group, they were due to postpartum hemorrhage after cesarean section. Interestingly, there were no maternal deaths in vaccinated pregnant women.

Regarding perinatal outcomes, we found differences between groups in gestational age at delivery and infant's birth weight ($p < 0.001$). Premature delivery was more frequent in women with severe–critical COVID-19, as well as admission to the neonatal intensive care unit and perinatal deaths ($p < 0.001$). There were no differences between groups in the frequency of newborns below the 10th percentile of weight.

#### 3.1.4. Factors Associated with Severe–Critical COVID-19 during Pregnancy

The associations between risk factors and the occurrence of severe–critical COVID-19 during pregnancy are exhibited in Table 4.

We calculated the crude odds ratios (ORs) and confidence intervals at 95% (CI 95%) for those variables reported to be consistently associated with severe COVID-19 (maternal age and maternal comorbidities) and those that showed significant differences in the univariate analysis. In multivariable logistic regression analysis, variables that remained as independent risk factors associated with the occurrence of severe–critical COVID-19 during pregnancy correspond to the non-vaccination against COVID-19, maternal blood group non-O, maternal age > 35 years, gestational age at infection, chronic hypertension, and multiparity (ORs ≥ 2.80).

**Table 3.** Maternal and perinatal outcomes of pregnant women with and without severe–critical COVID-19.

| Variable | Cases Severe–Critical COVID-19 [n = 123] | Controls Non-Severe COVID-19 [n = 635] | p-Value |
|---|---|---|---|
| **Maternal outcomes** | | | |
| Miscarriage, n [%] | 3 [2.4] | 9 [1.4] | NS ‡ |
| Cesarean section, n [%] | 105 [85.3] | 555 [87.4] | NS † |
| Admission to Intensive Care Unit, n [%] | 123 [100] | 6 [0.95] | <0.001 † |
| Acute Kidney Injury, n [%] | 19 [15.2] | 6 [0.95] | <0.001 † |
| Maternal Deaths °, n [%] | 9 [7.31] | 2 [0.31] | <0.001 ‡ |
| **Perinatal Outcomes** | | | |
| Gestational age at delivery, weeks, median [IQR] | 36 [32–38] | 38 [36–39] | <0.001 * |
| Infant's birth weight, Kilograms, median [IQR] | 2.40 [1.90–2.86] | 2.88 [2.45–3.42] | <0.001 * |
| Premature delivery | | | |
| ≤28 weeks, n [%] | 9 [2.43] | 1 [0.0] | <0.001 ‡ |
| 28 to 34 weeks, n [%] | 25 [20.3] | 17 [2.67] | <0.001 † |
| >34 to <37 weeks, n [%] | 48 [39.0] | 295 [46.9] | NS † |
| Admission to Neonatal Intensive Care Unit, n [%] | 14 [11.3] | 26 [4.0] | 0.001 † |
| Birth weight < 10th percentile, n [%] | 9 [7.31] | 32 [5.0] | NS † |
| Perinatal death, n [%] | 12 [9.7] | 15 [2.4] | <0.001 † |
| 30-day hospital discharge, n [%] | 102 [82.9] | 604 [95.1] | <0.001 † |

Data are reported as median and interquartile range [IQR]; count and percentage, n [%]. A $p$-value < 0.05 was considered statistically significant. † chi-squared test, ‡ Fisher's exact test, * U Mann–Whitney's test. ° Two maternal deaths occurred in the control group; they were not related to COVID-19, and they were due to obstetric hemorrhage.

**Table 4.** Risk factors associated with the occurrence of severe–critical COVID-19 during pregnancy.

| Variable | Cases Severe–Critical COVID-19 [n = 123] | Controls Non-Severe COVID-19 [n = 635] | Crude OR [CI 95%] | Adjusted OR [CI 95%] |
|---|---|---|---|---|
| **Mother's blood type, n [%]** | | | | |
| O | 29 [23.6] | 431 [67.9] | Reference | |
| A | 79 [64.2] | 182 [28.7] | 6.45 [4.07–10.21] * | |
| B | 11 [8.9] | 14 [2.2] | 11.67 [4.86–28.00] * | |
| AB | 4 [3.3] | 9 [1.2] | 6.60 [1.91–22.74] * | |
| ° **Pregestational diabetes, n [%]** | 10 [8.1] | 15 [2.4] | 3.64 [1.59–8.30] * | NS |
| ° **Obesity, n [%]** | 15 [12.2] | 38 [6.0] | 2.18 [1.16–4.10] * | NS |
| **Multiparity, n [%]** | 73 [59.3] | 206 [32.4] | 3.04 [2.04–4.51] * | 2.80 [1.71–4.59] * |
| **Gestational age at infection ≥ 31 weeks, n [%]** | 81 [65.9] | 197 [31.0] | 4.28 [2.84–6.45] * | 3.28 [2.01–5.36] * |
| **Maternal age > 35 years, n [%]** | 39 [31.7] | 59 [9.2] | 4.53 [2.84–7.21] * | 5.76 [3.17–10.48] * |
| **Chronic hypertension, n [%]** | 12 [9.8] | 13 [2.1] | 5.17 [2.3–11.62] * | 5.12 [1.83–14.34] * |
| **Mother's blood group non-O, n [%]** | 94 [76.4] | 205 [32.2] | 6.79 [4.34–10.64] * | 6.29 [3.73–10.60] * |
| **Non vaccination against COVID-19, n [%]** | 115 [95.1] | 471 [74.2] | 5.00 [2.39–10.47] * | 10.18 [4.34–23.86] * |

Data are reported as count and frequency, n [%]. * $p$-value < 0.05 was considered statistically significant. Adjusted odds ratios by logistic regression analysis. OR means odds ratio; CI 95%, confidence interval of 95%. ° Pregestational diabetes and obesity had a significant crude OR in the univariate analysis, but not in the multivariate model.

We present a pre-vaccination analysis in Table 5, which shows that non-O blood group was the main risk factor for severe–critical COVID-19, followed by maternal age ≥ 35 years, chronic hypertension, multiparity, and gestational age at infection ≥ 31 weeks' gestation (ORs ≥ 2.50).

**Table 5.** Risk factors associated with the occurrence of severe–critical COVID-19 during pregnancy in non-vaccinated women.

| Variable | Cases Severe–Critical COVID-19 [n = 114] | Controls Non-Severe COVID-19 [n = 472] | Crude OR [CI 95%] | Adjusted OR [CI 95%] |
|---|---|---|---|---|
| **Mother's blood group non-O, n [%]** | 92 [80.7] | 120 [25.4] | 12.26 [7.37–20.41] * | 9.04 [5.02–16.28] * |
| **Maternal age > 35 years, n [%]** | 37 [32.5] | 39 [8.3] | 5.33 [3.20–8.89] * | 6.08 [3.13–11.78] * |
| **Chronic hypertension, n [%]** | 11 [9.6] | 11 [2.3] | 4.47 [1.88–10.60] * | 5.11 [1.57–16.61] * |
| **Gestational age at infection ≥ 31 weeks, n [%]** | 76 [66.7] | 135 [28.6] | 4.99 [3.22–7.73] * | 3.29 [1.93–5.59] * |
| **Multiparity, n [%]** | 65 [57.0] | 108 [22.9] | 4.47 [2.91–6.86] * | 2.50 [1.47–4.24] * |
| ° **Pregestational diabetes, n [%]** | 10 [8.8] | 12 [2.5] | 3.68 [1.55–8.76] * | NS |
| ° **Obesity, n [%]** | 15 [13.2] | 26 [5.5] | 2.59 [1.32–5.08] * | NS |

Data are reported as count and frequency, n [%]. * $p$-value < 0.05 was considered statistically significant. Adjusted odds ratios by logistic regression analysis. OR means odds ratio; CI 95%, confidence interval of 95%. ° Pregestational diabetes and obesity had a significant crude OR in the univariate analysis, but not in the multivariate model.

## 4. Discussion

In this case–control study, we identified the risk factors for the occurrence of severe–critical COVID-19 in a large sample of Mexican pregnant women with a SARS-CoV-2 infection who were admitted to the respiratory units at the Mexican Institute of Social Security at the State of Mexico. We found that during the pre-vaccination period, the frequency of severe–critical COVID-19 was 19.5%, which is similar to the previously reported frequency of 20.2% [16,17]. Interestingly, the frequency of developing severe–critical COVID-19 after vaccination decreased significantly (at 5.2%). Moreover, in the group of vaccinated pregnant women, there were no cases of maternal death, which is consistent with the large number of studies that have reported that vaccination prevents the severe form of disease and deaths caused by COVID-19 [18]. We demonstrated that gestational age at infection ≥31 weeks was an independent risk factor for severe–critical COVID-19 (OR 3.28); in this vein, similar results were reported by Kalafat E. et al. (RR 3.64) [19]. In this regard, we agree with the notion that these results appear to be related to respiratory limitation due to changes caused by pregnancy rather than immunosuppressive aspects. As previously reported, we also found that maternal age > 35 years was another independent risk factor for severe–critical disease (OR 5.76) [13,19–23].

Although few studies have attempted to associate parity with infection and severity of COVID-19, there is a controversy on this issue [13,20,24]. Our result showed that multiparity was an independent risk factor (OR 2.80), although this was probably because multiparity usually occurs in older women with more frequent comorbidities.

In this regard, a history of comorbidities have been reported as risk factors for severity of COVID-19, including hypertension due to the imbalance between the two major pathways of the renin–angiotensin–aldosterone system (RAAS), with ACE2/Ang 1-7 downregulation and ACE2/Ang II upregulation. In pregestational diabetes, due to the expression of ACE2 increased in tissues of the lung, inflammation, insulin resistance, and altered immune modulation by an increase in pro-inflammatory cytokines, and in the case of obesity also due to ACE2 overexpression in adipocytes, a pro-inflammatory state, and a reduced lung capacity, may contribute to this increased risk... However, in our study population, after multivariate analysis, only a history of chronic hypertension remained as an independent risk factor (OR 5.12), which is like previous reports [13,16,20,21].

Gestational diabetes is suggested as a risk factor like DM2 associated with overexpression of ACE2 in lung tissue and insulin resistance; however, we found no differences between groups. In relation to pre-eclampsia, endothelial dysfunction may increase the risk for severe disease as well as hypertension does, but we did not find any difference either; nonetheless, the incidence of pre-eclampsia was higher in our study population in both cases (21.1%) and controls (27.2%) compared to the 6–8% in the general population. It has been reported that COVID-19 can cause manifestations that mimic pre-eclampsia; this fact could explain why pre-eclampsia could have been overdiagnosed. In this matter, it has been previously reported that pre-eclampsia-like syndrome can be adequately differentiated using pro- and anti-angiogenic markers [2,11,25–27].

In our study, the mother's blood group of non-O was an independent risk factor associated with the occurrence of severe–critical COVID-19 during pregnancy (OR 6.29). Although there are few studies reporting this association in pregnancy, it is controversial and seems to depend on the population studied. In this vein, studies conducted in countries where there is great ethnic diversity (white, non-Hispanic black, Latin-American, and Arabic, among others) did not find differences regarding this issue. In contrast, a study that was reported on the risk of severe COVID-19 infection was 3.6 times higher in women with blood group O when they were compared with blood type non-O subjects [21,28,29]. However, our results are consistent with the findings of a recent study, also in Mexican pregnant women, suggesting that the AB blood group in pregnant women is associated with an increased risk of severity and mortality in COVID-19 [15]. In this regard, it has been reported that blood type O is associated with a lower risk of infection because anti-A and or anti-B antibodies are present in individuals with blood type O and could bind to the corresponding antigens on the viral envelope and contribute to viral neutralization [30]. The plausible explanation for this fact is that ACE2 has a similarity between 76 and 78% with the spike (S) protein receptor binding domain of SARS-CoV and SARS-CoV-2, suggesting that they may share a common receptor. ABO antigens could maximize or minimize the binding capacity of the spike protein to host cell surface receptors. Viral entry is facilitated by the interaction of subunit S1 via two domains: S1A, corresponding to the N-terminal region (which interacts with sialic-acid-containing glycoproteins and glycolipids), and S1B, corresponding to the receptor binding domain, which binds to ACE2 receptors. Another mechanism is the lower concentration and biological activity of von Willebrand factor in subjects with type O blood and longer half-life and higher circulating concentrations of von Willebrand factor and factor VIII in people with blood types other than O (A, B, or AB) since it is known that severe COVID-19 infection is associated with a hypercoagulable state [10,31,32].

Finally, we noted that non-vaccination is an important and independent factor associated with disease severity after the start of mass vaccination [13]. Specifically, studies in pregnancy are primarily designed to ensure the safety of the vaccine and to protect both the mother and the newborn from developing serious diseases [17,21]; therefore, several studies recommend vaccination, as it is safe and no serious events have been demonstrated [33,34], which is consistent with our results since in the subgroup of 170 pregnant women vaccinated we found no serious adverse reactions or complications. Nevertheless, while governments should seek and encourage mass vaccination of their populations, they should always respect the principle of autonomy, as we know that there are variables that can influence the acceptance or not acceptance of vaccination, including education, where higher levels of education have been reported to be a strong positive predictor of vaccine acceptance, as well as receiving advice from a gynecologist was reported to be independently associated with SARS-CoV-2 vaccine uptake (OR 2.55) [35,36]. Furthermore, no studies were found that estimated the risk of non-vaccination for severe–critical COVID-19 in pregnancy; our results have shown that this factor is relevant (OR 10.18).

The risk factors identified in our study may be useful for healthcare providers in identifying pregnant women at increased risk of developing severe–critical COVID-19, for advising vaccination of women planning or in early pregnancy, as well as for maintaining preventive strategies and seeking medical attention on time to reduce the transmission and complications of SARS-CoV-2 and other emerging viral pathogens capable of causing epidemics.

The strengths of our study include a large, well-defined population of women infected with SARS-CoV-2 who received the same standardized medical protocol, the recruitment and selection of the population occurred at the diagnostic confirmation (positive RT-PCR) before they were classified as case or control, and the fact that all data were collected from the medical charts which evidently avoided selection and memory bias. Further, to rule out the effects of potential confounders, the estimated ORs were adjusted for established risk factors.

We are aware of the presence of certain limitations, including lack of generalizability to pregnant women at high risk and that some laboratory tests, such as D-dimer and C-reactive protein, were not available for all participants, especially in the control group. Nonetheless, the results reported in this study are representative of the population studied.

## 5. Conclusions

Our results show that non-vaccination, the non-O blood type followed by maternal age > 35 years, chronic hypertension, gestational age at the infection $\geq$ 31 weeks, and multiparity are independent risk factors associated with the occurrence of severe–critical COVID-19 during pregnancy.

**Author Contributions:** Conceptualization, M.G.B.-L. and A.L.-M.; data curation, M.G.B.-L. and S.P.-P.; formal analysis, M.G.B.-L.; investigation, M.G.B.-L., C.J.M.-P., L.R.G.-C. and S.P.-P.; methodology, M.G.B.-L.; project administration, M.G.B.-L. and S.P.-P.; resources, M.G.B.-L. and S.P.-P.; validation, A.L.-M. and C.J.M.-P.; visualization, M.G.B.-L. and C.J.M.-P.; writing—original draft preparation, M.G.B.-L.; writing—review and editing, M.G.B.-L., A.L.-M. and C.J.M.-P. All authors have read and agreed to the published version of the manuscript.

**Funding:** This research received no external funding.

**Institutional Review Board Statement:** This study was conducted in accordance with the Declaration of Helsinki and approved by the National Committee of Scientific Research of the Mexican Institute of Social Security with SIRELCIS registry R-2020-785-067.

**Informed Consent Statement:** Informed consent was obtained from all subjects involved in this study.

**Data Availability Statement:** Data that support the findings of this study are available from the corresponding author upon reasonable request.

**Acknowledgments:** The authors thank the Programa de Maestría y Doctorado en Ciencias Médicas, Odontológicas y de la Salud at the Universidad Nacional Autónoma de México and the Consejo Nacional de Humanidades Ciencia y Tecnología (CONAHCYT) for the supporting Ph.D. studies of M.G.B.L., CVU number 519249. Additionally, we thank the participants in the medical units: head of services and personnel of the Órgano de Operación Administrativa Desconcentrada Estado de México Poniente y Oriente at the Mexican Institute of Social Security for the facilities provided to carry out this study.

**Conflicts of Interest:** The authors declare no conflict of interest.

## Abbreviations

COVID-19, coronavirus disease 2019; SARS-CoV-2, severe acute respiratory syndrome coronavirus 2; RT-PCR, reverse transcription polymerase chain reaction; OR, odds ratio; 95% CI, confidence interval at 95%; RASS, renin–angiotensin–aldosterone system; ACE2, angiotensin-converting enzyme 2; Ang 1-7, angiotensin 1-7; Ang II, angiotensin II.

## References

1. Di Mascio, D.; Khalil, A.; Saccone, G.; Rizzo, G.; Buca, D.; Liberati, M.; Vecchiet, J.; Nappi, L.; Scambia, G.; Berghella, V.; et al. Outcome of coronavirus spectrum infections (SARS, MERS, COVID-19) during pregnancy: A systematic review and meta-analysis. *Am. J. Obstet. Gynecol. MFM* **2020**, *2*, 100107. [CrossRef] [PubMed]
2. Gao, Y.D.; Ding, M.; Dong, X.; Zhang, J.J.; Kursat Azkur, A.; Azkur, D.; Gan, H.; Sun, Y.L.; Fu, W.; Li, W.; et al. Risk factors for severe and critically ill COVID-19 patients: A review. *Allergy* **2021**, *76*, 428–455. [CrossRef]
3. Panahi, L.; Amiri, M.; Pouy, S. Risks of Novel Coronavirus Disease (COVID-19) in Pregnancy; a Narrative Review. *Arch. Acad. Emerg. Med.* **2020**, *8*, e34. [PubMed]

4. Maranto, M.; Zaami, S.; Restivo, V.; Termini, D.; Gangemi, A.; Tumminello, M.; Culmone, S.; Billone, V.; Cucinella, G.; Gullo, G. Symptomatic COVID-19 in Pregnancy: Hospital Cohort Data between May 2020 and April 2021, Risk Factors and Medicolegal Implications. *Diagnostics* **2023**, *13*, 1009. [CrossRef] [PubMed]
5. Yirmiya, K.; Yakirevich-Amir, N.; Preis, H.; Lotan, A.; Atzil, S.; Reuveni, I. Women's Depressive Symptoms during the COVID-19 Pandemic: The Role of Pregnancy. *Int. J. Environ. Res. Public. Health* **2021**, *18*, 4298. [CrossRef] [PubMed]
6. McBroom, K. A Comparison of Zika Virus and COVID-19: Clinical Overview and Public Health Messaging. *J. Midwifery Womens Health* **2021**, *66*, 334–342. [CrossRef] [PubMed]
7. Gullo, G.; Scaglione, M.; Cucinella, G.; Riva, A.; Coldebella, D.; Cavaliere, A.F.; Signore, F.; Buzzaccarini, G.; Spagnol, G.; Laganà, A.S.; et al. Congenital Zika Syndrome: Genetic Avenues for Diagnosis and Therapy, Possible Management and Long-Term Outcomes. *J. Clin. Med.* **2022**, *11*, 1351. [CrossRef] [PubMed]
8. Gao, F.; Zheng, K.I.; Wang, X.B.; Sun, Q.F.; Pan, K.H.; Wang, T.Y.; Chen, Y.P.; Targher, G.; Byrne, C.D.; George, J.; et al. Obesity Is a Risk Factor for Greater COVID-19 Severity. *Diabetes Care* **2020**, *43*, e72–e74. [CrossRef]
9. Zhang, J.J.; Dong, X.; Liu, G.H.; Gao, Y.D. Risk and Protective Factors for COVID-19 Morbidity, Severity, and Mortality. *Clin. Rev. Allergy Immunol.* **2023**, *64*, 90–107. [CrossRef] [PubMed]
10. Zhang, Y.; Garner, R.; Salehi, S.; La Rocca, M.; Duncan, D. Association between ABO blood types and coronavirus disease 2019 (COVID-19), genetic associations, and underlying molecular mechanisms: A literature review of 23 studies. *Ann Hematol* **2021**, *100*, 1123–1132. [CrossRef]
11. WHO. Guidelines Approved by the Guidelines Review Committee. In *Clinical Management of COVID-19: Living Guideline*; World Health Organization: Geneva, Switzerland, 2021.
12. Thompson, J.L.; Nguyen, L.M.; Noble, K.N.; Aronoff, D.M. COVID-19-related disease severity in pregnancy. *Am. J. Reprod. Immunol.* **2020**, *84*, e13339. [CrossRef] [PubMed]
13. World Health Organization. *Clinical Management of COVID-19: Living Guideline [Internet]*; World Health Organization: Geneva, Switzerland, 2023.
14. Allotey, J.; Stallings, E.; Bonet, M.; Yap, M.; Chatterjee, S.; Kew, T.; Debenham, L.; Llavall, A.C.; Dixit, A.; Zhou, D.; et al. Clinical manifestations, risk factors, and maternal and perinatal outcomes of coronavirus disease 2019 in pregnancy: Living systematic review and meta-analysis. *BMJ* **2020**, *370*, m3320. [CrossRef]
15. Sevilla-Montoya, R.; Helguera-Reppeto, A.C.; Monroy-Muñoz, I.E.; Vargas-Pavia, T.A.; Valdés-Montoya, E.I.; Solis-Paredes, M.; Torres-Torres, J.; Velazquez-Cruz, R.; Muñoz-Medina, J.E.; Martinez-Cordero, C.; et al. Blood Type Associated with the Risk of COVID-19 Infection in Pregnant Women. *Diagnostics* **2023**, *13*, 1338. [CrossRef]
16. Samadi, P.; Alipour, Z.; Ghaedrahmati, M.; Ahangari, R. The severity of COVID-19 among pregnant women and the risk of adverse maternal outcomes. *Int. J. Gynaecol. Obstet.* **2021**, *154*, 92–99. [CrossRef] [PubMed]
17. Limaye, M.A.; Roman, A.S.; Trostle, M.E.; Venkatesh, P.; Lantigua Martinez, M.; Brubaker, S.G.; Chervenak, J.; Wei, L.S.; Sahani, P.; Grossman, T.B.; et al. Predictors of severe and critical disease in pregnant women with SARS-CoV-2. *J. Matern. Fetal Neonatal Med.* **2022**, *35*, 7536–7540. [CrossRef]
18. Zheng, C.; Shao, W.; Chen, X.; Zhang, B.; Wang, G.; Zhang, W. Real-world effectiveness of COVID-19 vaccines: A literature review and meta-analysis. *Int. J. Infect. Dis.* **2022**, *114*, 252–260. [CrossRef]
19. Kalafat, E.; Prasad, S.; Birol, P.; Tekin, A.B.; Kunt, A.; Di Fabrizio, C.; Alatas, C.; Celik, E.; Bagci, H.; Binder, J.; et al. An internally validated prediction model for critical COVID-19 infection and intensive care unit admission in symptomatic pregnant women. *Am. J. Obstet. Gynecol.* **2022**, *226*, 403.e1–403.e13. [CrossRef] [PubMed]
20. Jamieson, D.J.; Rasmussen, S.A. An update on COVID-19 and pregnancy. *Am. J. Obstet. Gynecol.* **2022**, *226*, 177–186. [CrossRef]
21. Nana, M.; Nelson-Piercy, C. COVID-19 in pregnancy. *Clin. Med.* **2021**, *21*, e446–e450. [CrossRef]
22. Kazemi Aski, S.; Norooznezhad, A.H.; Shamshirsaz, A.A.; Mostafaei, S.; Aleyasin, A.; Nabavian, S.M.; Alimohammadi, S.; Ahangari, R.; Ariana, S.; Ghotbizadeh, F.; et al. Clinical features and risk factors associated with acute respiratory distress syndrome in pregnant women diagnosed with COVID-19: A multi-center case-control study. *J. Matern. Fetal Neonatal Med.* **2022**, *35*, 4884–4888. [CrossRef]
23. Kayem, G.; Lecarpentier, E.; Deruelle, P.; Bretelle, F.; Azria, E.; Blanc, J.; Bohec, C.; Bornes, M.; Ceccaldi, P.F.; Chalet, Y.; et al. A snapshot of the Covid-19 pandemic among pregnant women in France. *J. Gynecol. Obstet. Hum. Reprod.* **2020**, *49*, 101826. [CrossRef] [PubMed]
24. Lokken, E.M.; Huebner, E.M.; Taylor, G.G.; Hendrickson, S.; Vanderhoeven, J.; Kachikis, A.; Coler, B.; Walker, C.L.; Sheng, J.S.; Al-Haddad, B.J.S.; et al. Disease severity, pregnancy outcomes, and maternal deaths among pregnant patients with severe acute respiratory syndrome coronavirus 2 infection in Washington State. *Am. J. Obstet. Gynecol.* **2021**, *225*, 77.e1–77.e14. [CrossRef]
25. Mendoza, M.; Garcia-Ruiz, I.; Maiz, N.; Rodo, C.; Garcia-Manau, P.; Serrano, B.; Lopez-Martinez, R.M.; Balcells, J.; Fernandez-Hidalgo, N.; Carreras, E.; et al. Pre-eclampsia-like syndrome induced by severe COVID-19: A prospective observational study. *BJOG* **2020**, *127*, 1374–1380. [CrossRef]
26. Tossetta, G.; Fantone, S.; Delli Muti, N.; Balercia, G.; Ciavattini, A.; Giannubilo, S.R.; Marzioni, D. Preeclampsia and severe acute respiratory syndrome coronavirus 2 infection: A systematic review. *J. Hypertens.* **2022**, *40*, 1629–1638. [CrossRef]
27. Serrano, B.; Bonacina, E.; Garcia-Ruiz, I.; Mendoza, M.; Garcia-Manau, P.; Garcia-Aguilar, P.; Gil, J.; Armengol-Alsina, M.; Fernández-Hidalgo, N.; Sulleiro, E.; et al. Confirmation of preeclampsia-like syndrome induced by severe COVID-19: An observational study. *Am. J. Obstet. Gynecol. MFM* **2023**, *5*, 100760. [CrossRef]

28. Sainz Bueno, J.A.; Cerrillos González, L.; Abascal-Saiz, A.; Rodríguez Gallego, M.V.; López Pérez, R.; Fernández Alonso, A.M.; de la Cruz Conty, M.L.; Alonso Saiz, R.; Molina Oller, M.; Santamaría Ortiz, A.; et al. Association of ABO and Rh blood groups with obstetric outcomes in SARS-CoV-2 infected pregnancies: A prospective study with a multivariate analysis. *Eur. J. Obstet. Gynecol. Reprod. Biol.* **2021**, *264*, 41–48. [CrossRef]
29. Arslan, B.; Bicer, I.G.; Sahin, T.; Vay, M.; Dilek, O.; Destegul, E. Clinical characteristics and hematological parameters associated with disease severity in COVID-19 positive pregnant women undergoing cesarean section: A single-center experience. *J. Obstet. Gynaecol. Res.* **2022**, *48*, 402–410. [CrossRef]
30. Goel, R.; Bloch, E.M.; Pirenne, F.; Al-Riyami, A.Z.; Crowe, E.; Dau, L.; Land, K.; Townsend, M.; Jecko, T.; Rahimi-Levene, N.; et al. ABO blood group and COVID-19: A review on behalf of the ISBT COVID-19 Working Group. *Vox Sang.* **2021**, *116*, 849–861. [CrossRef] [PubMed]
31. Hoiland, R.L.; Fergusson, N.A.; Mitra, A.R.; Griesdale, D.E.G.; Devine, D.V.; Stukas, S.; Cooper, J.; Thiara, S.; Foster, D.; Chen, L.Y.C.; et al. The association of ABO blood group with indices of disease severity and multiorgan dysfunction in COVID-19. *Blood Adv.* **2020**, *4*, 4981–4989. [CrossRef] [PubMed]
32. Liu, N.; Zhang, T.; Ma, L.; Zhang, H.; Wang, H.; Wei, W.; Pei, H.; Li, H. The impact of ABO blood group on COVID-19 infection risk and mortality: A systematic review and meta-analysis. *Blood Rev.* **2021**, *48*, 100785. [CrossRef]
33. Prabhu, M.; Riley, L.E. Coronavirus Disease 2019 (COVID-19) Vaccination in Pregnancy. *Obstet Gynecol* **2023**, *141*, 473–482. [CrossRef] [PubMed]
34. Zdanowski, W.; Markiewicz, A.; Zdanowska, N.; Lipińska, J.; Waśniewski, T. Tolerability of the BNT162b2 COVID-19 Vaccine during Pregnancy among Polish Healthcare Professionals. *Vaccines* **2022**, *10*, 200. [CrossRef] [PubMed]
35. Maranto, M.; Gullo, G.; Bruno, A.; Minutolo, G.; Cucinella, G.; Maiorana, A.; Casuccio, A.; Restivo, V. Factors Associated with Anti-SARS-CoV-2 Vaccine Acceptance among Pregnant Women: Data from Outpatient Women Experiencing High-Risk Pregnancy. *Vaccines* **2023**, *11*, 454. [CrossRef]
36. Montanari Vergallo, G.; Del Rio, A.; Negro, F.; Zaami, S. COVID-19 vaccine mandates: What are the current European public perspectives? *Eur. Rev. Med. Pharmacol. Sci.* **2022**, *26*, 643–652. [CrossRef] [PubMed]

Journal of
*Clinical Medicine*

MDPI

*Article*

# The Emotional Landscape of Pregnancy and Postpartum during the COVID-19 Pandemic in Italy: A Mixed-Method Analysis Using Artificial Intelligence

**Claudia Ravaldi, Laura Mosconi, Roberto Bonaiuti and Alfredo Vannacci ***

PeaRL—Perinatal Research Laboratory, CiaoLapo Foundation, Department of Neurosciences, Psychology, Drug Research and Child Health, University of Florence, 50121 Florence, Italy; claudia.ravaldi@unifi.it (C.R.); laura.mosconi@unifi.it (L.M.); roberto.bonaiuti@unifi.it (R.B.)
* Correspondence: alfredo.vannacci@unifi.it; Tel.: +39-(05)-52751857

**Abstract:** The COVID-19 pandemic affected the perinatal emotional landscape in Italy, a country that had high mortality and implemented a strict lockdown during the pandemic. This study explores the emotions and challenges of pregnant and postpartum women during the pandemic, using AI-based mixed methods. The study analyzed 1774 women from the national survey COVID-ASSESS: 1136 pregnant and 638 postpartum women. The survey had qualitative questions on emotions and feelings related to birth, communication with healthcare professionals, media, and peers and family. We used natural language processing and machine learning to classify emotions, identify themes, and extract citations from the data. Fear and anxiety replaced joy as dominant emotions during the pandemic: trust and joy decreased by 49.3% and 36.4%, respectively, while sadness and fear increased by 52.3% and 49.3%, respectively. The pandemic also induced loneliness, isolation, frustration, and anger. Women faced challenges related to birth, communication with HCPs, media, and peers and family. They also used coping strategies such as self-care, news limitation, and trying to cultivate gratitude and hope. This study provides a comprehensive exploration of the perinatal emotional landscape of Italian women during the pandemic. The findings underscore the significant psychological impact of the pandemic and also highlight women's resilience and coping strategies.

**Keywords:** COVID-19 and pregnancy; management; prevention

## 1. Introduction

In the early months of the COVID-19 pandemic, Italy was uniquely positioned as the first Western nation to be severely impacted by the virus. This period was characterized by a high degree of uncertainty and fear, as little was known about the infection and its potential effects. The rapid spread of the epidemic and the ensuing lockdown measures had a profound impact on the mental health of the population, leading to widespread psychological distress and increased mental health risks [1,2].

The societal burden of this situation was substantial. The healthcare system, already strained by the direct effects of the virus [1], faced additional pressure from the increased demand for mental health services [3]. Moreover, the economic consequences of the pandemic, including job loss and financial instability, further exacerbated mental health issues and contributed to a cycle of stress and anxiety [4].

The disruption of healthcare services afforded by the pandemic also included prenatal and postnatal care [5]. In this context, more vulnerable populations, such as pregnant and postpartum women, were particularly affected. Pregnant women with COVID-19 infection had an increased mortality rate and other adverse outcomes such as higher rates of preterm birth and pre-eclampsia [6]. Furthermore, the uncertainty and fear associated with COVID-19, combined with the isolation and social distancing measures implemented to control the spread of the virus, created additional stressors that increased the risk of developing depression and anxiety symptoms during pregnancy [7–9]. In fact, the perinatal period, by itself, is characterized by significant physiological and psychological changes and challenges, which can place women at higher risk for mental health difficulties, including depression, anxiety, and post-traumatic stress disorder (PTSD) [10–12]. Moreover, the subjective negative impact of COVID-19 has been associated with more dysfunctional coping and less emotion-focused coping [13]. The impact of COVID-19 on perinatal mental health highlights the need for additional support and resources [9,14].

Our previous research, conducted during the initial phase of the COVID-19 lockdown in Italy, provided preliminary insights into the emotional experiences of pregnant and postpartum women [15–17]. These studies found that pregnant women experienced significant psychological distress during the pandemic, including symptoms of depression, anxiety, and stress. Furthermore, exclusive breastfeeding was found to serve as an independent protective factor for women's mental health during the pandemic [17].

However, a more comprehensive analysis of the ongoing nature of the pandemic and its evolving impact is needed. The present study aims to delve deeper into the emotional landscape of pregnant and postpartum women during the first months of the pandemic, focusing on the prevalence of various emotions and the coping strategies employed. Here, we aim to build upon our previous findings and provide a more nuanced understanding of the emotional experiences of pregnant and postpartum women during this global crisis.

Understanding these emotional responses and coping mechanisms is crucial for developing effective interventions to support perinatal mental health during such crises. The present study aims to contribute to this understanding by examining, through a qualitative analysis, the emotional experiences and coping strategies of pregnant and postpartum women in Italy during the COVID-19 pandemic.

## 2. Materials and Methods

### 2.1. Survey

COVID-ASSESS is a cross-sectional study based on a survey administered during the first wave of the COVID-19 pandemic in Italy. The survey was distributed via CiaoLapo, an Italian charity for perinatal health support, using existing networks and support groups across Italy. Participants self-selected to complete the survey and participation was voluntary. The survey was launched in March 2020, and data were collected until May 2020. Each participant gave their explicit consent in an online form before enrolment. The survey was uploaded as an online tool using the Surveymonkey platform (www.surveymonkey.com) (accessed on 20 September 2023) and comprised the following sections: (A) socio-demographic information, (B) previous losses, personal and family history of psychological disorders, (C) birth expectations before and after COVID-19, (D) concerns regarding pandemic consequences, (E) postpartum health and infant feeding, (F) perception of media and health professionals' information and communication on COVID-19, and (G) psychometric evaluation tests. Methodological details, full text from the survey, and raw data have already been published [18].

This paper presents a secondary analysis of the national survey COVID-ASSESS that originally included 2448 women, of whom 1307 were pregnant and 1141 postpartum. Participants were considered eligible to be included in this post hoc analysis if they answered at least one of the qualitative questions of the survey. Full text of the survey, a general description of results, and complete raw data have already been published [18] and are freely available in an online repository [19].

### 2.2. Classification of Emotions

We employed the GPT-3.5-turbo (Generative Pre-trained Transformer) model developed by OpenAI to classify emotions in text without fine-tuning the model specifically for this task. GPT-3.5 is a state-of-the-art natural language processing model pre-trained on a large corpus of text data, primarily designed for natural language understanding and generation tasks. However, large-scale pre-training allows it to capture a wide range of linguistic features that can be useful for emotion classification [20,21].

To adapt GPT-3.5 for emotion classification without fine-tuning, we used a zero-shot learning approach. This method involves formulating the input prompt in a way that guides the model to provide the desired output, in our case, the emotion(s) associated with the text. The following steps were followed for emotion classification using GPT-3.5:

1. **Preprocessing**: any given input text was preprocessed by removing irrelevant information, text was converted to lowercase, words were tokenized, and stop words and punctuation were removed.
2. **Prompt formulation**: a prompt was formulated to include the preprocessed input text and the model was asked to identify the emotion(s) associated with it. The prompt explicitly listed the eight target emotions (anger, anticipation, joy, trust, fear, surprise, sadness, and disgust) and the model was instructed to select the most appropriate one(s). In particular, we used the Google Sheet plugin "GPT for Sheets" by Talarian (https://gptforwork.com/) (accessed on 20 September 2023), with the following prompt: "Perform sentiment analysis and input 1 or 0 separated by commas for each of the following emotions: anger, anticipation, joy, trust, fear, surprise, sadness and disgust. Example: if all are present 1, 1, 1, 1, 1, 1, 1, 1; if all are absent 0, 0, 0, 0, 0, 0, 0, 0; if only anger is present 1, 0, 0, 0, 0, 0, 0, 0, etc...".
3. **Inference**: GPT-3.5-turbo generated an output based on its pre-trained knowledge and the context provided by the prompt for each one of the 1774 rows. The output was stored as a string of comma-separated binary values in two Google sheet cells, one for 'pre-COVID emotions' and one for 'post-COVID emotions'.
4. **Post-processing**: the Google sheet document was then imported into StataBE 18 (StataCorp) and the emotion strings were converted into regular fields for each emotion coded as absent (0) or present (1), both before and after the pandemic.

We also experimented with the more recent GPT-4 model for emotion classification [22]. However, we encountered several challenges with GPT-4. First, it was more costly to run than GPT-3.5-turbo. For example, it required USD 0.03 per 1 K token, while GPT-3.5-turbo only required USD 0.002 per 1 K token. Second, it was much slower than GPT-3.5-turbo. For instance, it took an average of 30 s to process one row of data, while GPT-3.5-turbo took only 3 s. To evaluate the potential benefits of using GPT-4, we performed a sensitivity analysis on a random sample of 20 rows from our dataset. This analysis showed no significant difference in the emotion classification accuracy between GPT-3.5-turbo and GPT-4, with a concordance of 99.4%. Therefore, we decided to use GPT-3.5-turbo for our study due to its lower cost, faster speed, and comparable performance.

### 2.3. *Classification of Themes*

In order to identify and analyze the main themes present within the given text, we employed the GPT-4 language model, with a natural language processing approach. Analyses were conducted providing the text of the survey in the platform https://chat.openai.com/ (accessed on 20 September 2023) using GPT-4 as a model. Before input, all sets of answers were divided into blocks of about 1000 words, and the following steps were taken to perform the analysis using the AI model:

1. **Tokenization**. Tokenization is the process of segmenting the input text into individual units called tokens, which can be words, phrases, or punctuation marks. This is an essential pre-processing step in NLP. The GPT model tokenized the text to facilitate further analysis, as it allowed for easier identification and quantification of the most recurring words and phrases. This was achieved using the model's internal tokenization algorithms, which have been trained to recognize and separate the constituent elements of different languages, including Italian.
2. **Frequency Analysis**. After tokenization, the GPT model conducted a frequency analysis of the words and phrases in the text. This involved counting the occurrences of each token and ranking them based on their frequency. This step was crucial for deter-

mining the prominence and significance of particular words and phrases in the text, which helped in identifying the main themes. The frequency analysis was performed by leveraging the model's internal algorithms for counting and ranking tokens.

3. **Semantic Analysis**. In order to group related words and phrases into overarching themes, the GPT model performed semantic analysis. This involved leveraging its pretrained knowledge of language and understanding of semantics to identify words and phrases with similar meanings or connotations. The model used its internal algorithms to analyze the relationships between tokens, taking into account their context and meaning, and grouped them into themes that represented the broader concepts present in the text.
4. **Scoring**. The GPT model assigned a score to each theme based on the frequency of the words and phrases within the theme. Once the text was analyzed to identify words and phrases that were indicative of the themes in question, words were counted, and the proportion of words associated with each theme was calculated as a percentage of the total number of words in the text. This percentage was then mapped to a scale of 0 to 10, where a score of 0 represented no presence of the theme in the text, and a score of 10 represented extremely high prominence of the theme. This scoring system allowed for a relative comparison of the prominence of different themes within the text, based on the frequency and distribution of indicative words and phrases.
5. **Textual Citations**. To provide evidence for each identified theme, the GPT model extracted relevant textual citations in Italian from the original text. This process involved identifying sentences or phrases that exemplified the main ideas of each theme while ensuring that the citations were representative of the broader context in which the theme appeared. The model leveraged its understanding of language and context to select appropriate citations that effectively illustrated the themes and their significance within the text. Citations were manually checked for accuracy and translated into English by the authors.

### *2.4. Thematic Map*

A thematic map was created with the software Xmind (v22.11 Xmind LTD) based on four factors: the frequency of themes, the connections between themes identified by GPT-4 and explained in the Section 4, the connections underlined by literature, and the researchers' experience in qualitative data analysis.

## 3. Results

### *3.1. Characteristics of the Sample*

The study sample consisted of 1774 women, of whom 1136 (64.0%) were pregnant and 638 (36.0%) were postpartum women. The mean age of the sample was 33.6 years (SD = 4.8), and the majority of the women had a high level of education (45.3% had a first stage of tertiary education and 16.2% had a second stage of tertiary education). The pregnant women were distributed across the three trimesters of pregnancy, with 47.9% in the third trimester, 42.2% in the second trimester, and 9.9% in the first trimester. The postpartum women had babies with a mean age of 2.7 months (SD = 1.8), ranging from less than 1.4 months to more than 4 months. Most of the women were multigravidae (64.2%), and 38.0% had a history of previous pregnancy loss. Nearly half of the women (44.5%) reported having a psychopathological history, and the majority of them (51.1%) had no other children. No significant difference in baseline characteristics was present between pregnant and postpartum women. More detailed information is available in Table 1.

### *3.2. Emotions Related to Birth*

Figure 1 shows that the pandemic had a significant impact on the birth-related emotions of pregnant women. Before the pandemic, the most common emotions were trust (875 women), anticipation (735 women), and joy (703 women). During the pandemic, the most common emotions were sadness (760 people), fear (696 people), and anticipation

(449 women) (Figure 1A). In particular, the emotions that decreased the most were trust (−49.3%) and joy (−36.4%), while the emotions that increased the most were sadness (+52.3%) and fear (+49.3%) (Figure 1B).

**Table 1.** General characteristics of the sample.

| | Group | | | | | | | |
|---|---|---|---|---|---|---|---|---|
| | Pregnant | | Postpartum | | Total | | $\chi2$ | $p$ |
| | No. | % | No. | % | No. | % | | |
| **Age classes** | | | | | | | | |
| 18–25 | 15 | 1.3% | 8 | 1.3% | 23 | 1.3% | 3.075 | 0.380 |
| 25–30 | 157 | 13.8% | 74 | 11.6% | 231 | 13.0% | | |
| 30–35 | 436 | 38.4% | 268 | 42.0% | 704 | 39.7% | | |
| >35 | 528 | 46.5% | 288 | 45.1% | 816 | 46.0% | | |
| **Level of education** | | | | | | | | |
| Lower secondary education | 38 | 3.4% | 25 | 4.0% | 63 | 3.5% | 5.884 | 0.436 |
| Upper secondary education | 291 | 25.6% | 180 | 28.2% | 471 | 26.6% | | |
| Post-secondary non-tertiary education | 289 | 25.4% | 148 | 23.2% | 437 | 24.6% | | |
| First stage of tertiary education | 322 | 28.3% | 194 | 30.4% | 516 | 29.1% | | |
| Second stage of tertiary education | 196 | 17.3% | 91 | 14.3% | 287 | 16.2% | | |
| **Trimester** (pregnant only) | | | | | | | | |
| First | 113 | 9.9% | | | | | | |
| Second | 479 | 42.2% | | | | | | |
| Third | 544 | 47.9% | | | | | | |
| **Baby age** (months, postpartum only) | | | | | | | | |
| <1.4 | | | 243 | 38.1% | | | | |
| 1.5–3.9 | | | 194 | 30.4% | | | | |
| >4 | | | 201 | 31.5% | | | | |
| **Number of previous pregnancies** | | | | | | | | |
| Multigravidae | 745 | 65.6% | 394 | 61.8% | 1139 | 64.2% | 2.602 | 0.107 |
| First pregnancy | 391 | 34.4% | 244 | 38.2% | 635 | 35.8% | | |
| **Personal history** | | | | | | | | |
| Psychopathological history | 499 | 43.9% | 291 | 45.6% | 790 | 44.5% | 0.470 | 0.493 |
| **Other children (n)** | | | | | | | | |
| 0 | 565 | 49.7% | 341 | 53.4% | 906 | 51.1% | 3.493 | 0.322 |
| 1 | 500 | 44.0% | 252 | 39.5% | 752 | 42.4% | | |
| 2 | 56 | 4.9% | 36 | 5.6% | 92 | 5.2% | | |
| >2 | 15 | 1.3% | 9 | 1.4% | 24 | 1.4% | | |
| **Previous pregnancy loss** | | | | | | | | |
| No previous loss | 692 | 60.9% | 407 | 63.8% | 1099 | 62.0% | 1.435 | 0.231 |
| Previous loss | 444 | 39.1% | 231 | 36.2% | 675 | 38.0% | | |

The main concepts expressed by women regarding birth before and during the pandemic are graphically depicted in Figure 2 as word clouds. The most frequent words and relative weights used to create the word clouds are reported in Supplementary Table S1.

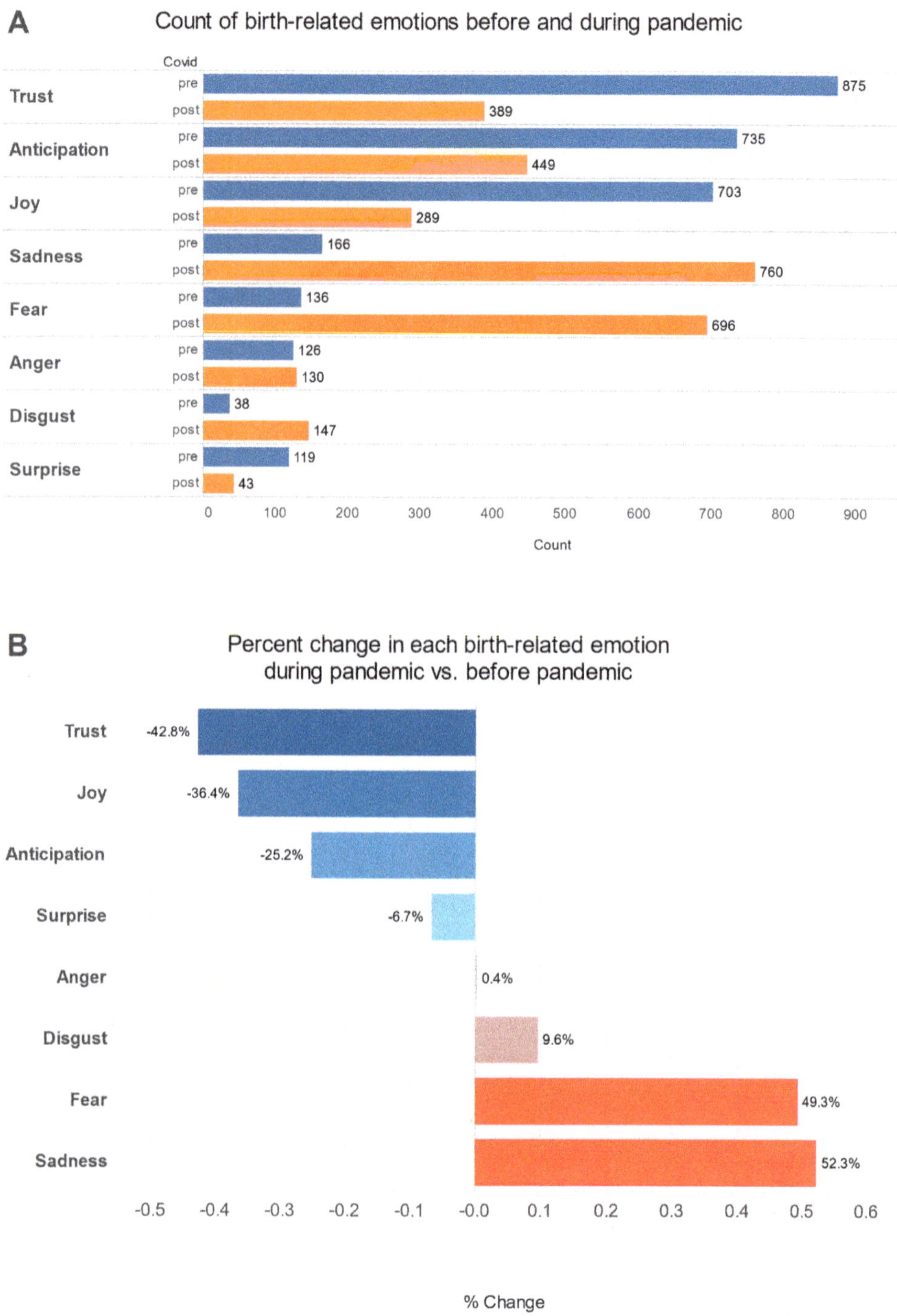


**Figure 1.** Changes in emotions before and during the pandemic. (**A**) shows women's emotions before and during the pandemic. (**B**) shows how emotions changed in percentage during the pandemic as compared to before it.

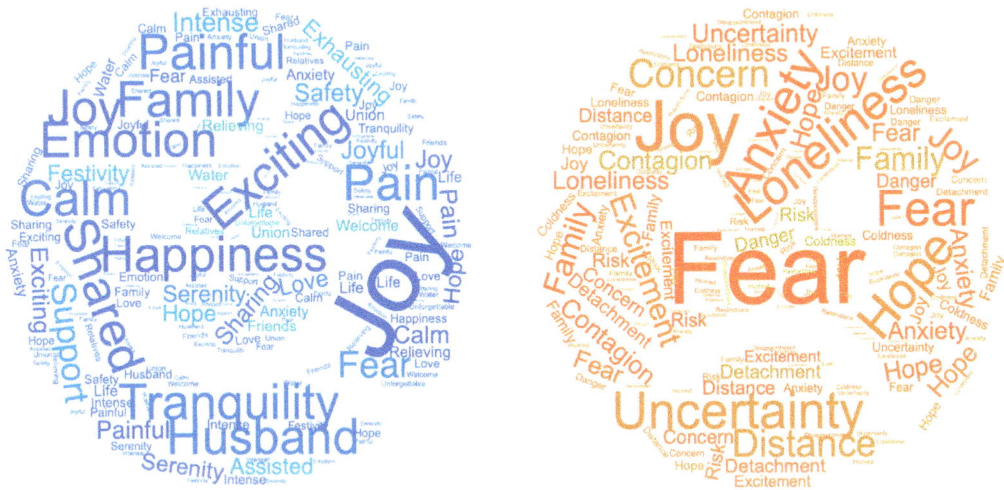


**Figure 2.** Word clouds of women's emotions before and during the pandemic.

*3.3. Communication*

The blocks of texts analyzed consisted of (a) 5434 words from phrases describing women's experiences with healthcare professionals' communication, (b) 3828 words from phrases describing women's experiences with media communication, and (c) 3767 words from phrases describing women's experiences with peers (family, friends, colleagues, etc.) during the acute phase of the pandemic. We also included a big block of 46,542 words, derived from the open-ended questions in which responders could write any reflection they wanted, without specific guidance.

A total of 59,571 words, corresponding to 341,964 characters, were analyzed. Based on the repetition of words and concepts, the themes were automatically graded by the AI on a scale from 0 to 10, with higher scores indicating greater recurrence within the text. Quotes have been provided as examples of words and phrases suggesting each theme.

A thematic map showing the synthesis of the relationships between the main themes found is shown in Figure 3.

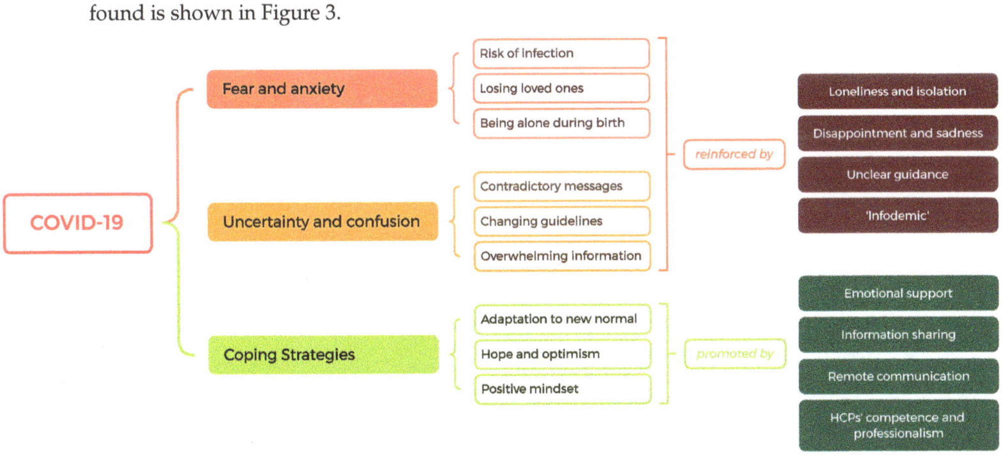


**Figure 3.** Thematic map of the main emerging themes.

3.3.1. HCPs and Communication

Five themes have emerged as prominent aspects of the communication between healthcare professionals and the public during the acute phase of the pandemic:

1. **Fear and Anxiety** (Score 8/10). Fear and anxiety were the most common emotions expressed throughout the text. Women reported feeling scared, uncertain, and panicked due to the pandemic and the information provided by healthcare professionals. This theme was prevalent across all the text. Examples of words used include the following: "fear", "anxiety", "panic", "worry", "apprehension", "tension", "dread", "terror", "anguish", and "insecurity".
2. **Uncertainty and Confusion** (Score 7/10). Many respondents described the communication from healthcare professionals as unclear, contradictory, or insufficient, leading to feelings of confusion and uncertainty. This theme was consistently present in the text. Examples of words used include the following: "uncertainty", "confusion", "disorientation", "doubt", "insecurity", "vagueness", "ambiguity", "disinformation", "hesitation", and "contradictions".
3. **Emotional Support and Reassurance** (Score 6/10). Some respondents mentioned the importance of emotional support and reassurance provided by healthcare professionals. Women reported that clear, direct, comforting and empathetic communication from their HCPs helped foster a sense of hope, even in the face of uncertainty and fear. Seeking support from HCPs was used as a coping strategy that enabled women to focus on the positive aspects of their care. Examples of terms used include the following: "emotional support", "reassurance", "comfort", "calmness", "serenity", "hope", "encouragement", "understanding", "empathy", and "positivity".
4. **Professionalism and Competence** (Score 5/10). Several individuals highlighted the professionalism and competence of healthcare workers during the pandemic. This theme recurred across the text, emphasizing the importance of skilled professionals in handling the crisis. Examples of words used include the following: "professionalism", "competence", "expertise", "prepared", "dedication", "commitment", "excellence", "skilled", "efficient", "focused", and "humanity".
5. **Distance and Detachment** (Score 4/10). The text also reflected a sense of distance and detachment, both in terms of the physical limitations imposed by the pandemic and the emotional disconnection experienced by some women in their interactions with healthcare professionals. Examples of terms used include the following: "distance", "detachment", "isolation", "separation", "limited contact", "disconnection", "remote", and "no feeling".

3.3.2. Media and Communication

Four main themes were identified describing the communication by the media during the acute phase of the pandemic:

1. **Fear and Anxiety** (Score: 10/10). The most prominent theme in the text is the sense of panic and anxiety induced by media communication during the pandemic. Respondents frequently mentioned feeling overwhelmed by the constant bombardment of alarming and sensationalist news. They reported feelings of fear, unease, and insecurity, which negatively impacted their mental health and well-being. Examples of words used include the following: "panic", "anxiety", "terror", "fear", "insecurity", "overwhelmed", "alarming", and "sensationalist news".
2. **Confusion and Contradictions** (Score: 8/10). Another significant theme is the confusion and contradictions in the media's messaging. Participants expressed frustration with the lack of clarity and consistency in the information provided, which led to uncertainty and doubt about the situation. Examples of terms used include the following: "confusion", "contradictions", "inconsistencies", "mixed messages", "unclear guidance", "ambiguity", "discrepancies", "misinformation", "divergent opinions", and "lack of clarity".

3. **Sensationalism and Alarmism** (Score: 7/10). Many respondents criticized the media's sensationalist and alarmist approach, which exacerbated feelings of panic and anxiety. They accused the media of exaggerating the situation, focusing on negative aspects, and employing a fear-based narrative to capture attention. Many women perceive a disproportionate emphasis on extreme cases, dire projections, and tragic stories while neglecting to provide context or balance with more positive or hopeful information. Such reporting practices were perceived as profit-driven, prioritizing viewer engagement and clickbait headlines over accurate and responsible journalism. As a coping strategy, women tried to limit exposure to distressing news, seeking out positive news stories. Examples of terms used include the following: "sensationalism", "alarmism", "exaggeration", "hype", "fearmongering", "over-dramatization", "catastrophizing", "scaremongering", "apocalyptic language", and "inflated claims".
4. **Misinformation and Inaccuracy** (Score: 6/10). The final theme we identified is the prevalence of misinformation and inaccuracy in media reporting. Participants mentioned issues with fake news, untrustworthy sources, and imprecise information that contributed to a chaotic and disorienting information landscape. Examples of terms used include the following: "misinformation", "inaccuracy", "false claims", "unverified reports", "disinformation", "rumors", "distorted facts", "misleading statements", "unreliable sources", and "fabricated stories".

3.3.3. Peers and Communication

Five main themes were identified describing repsondents' communication with peers (family, relatives, friends, colleagues) during the acute phase of the pandemic:

1. **Remote Communication** (Score: 8.5/10). The most recurrent theme was the reliance on remote communication methods, including phone calls, video calls, and messaging apps, as face-to-face interactions were limited. Participants often mentioned using these technologies to maintain social connections and exchange support during the pandemic. Examples of terms used include the following: "video calls", "phone calls", "messaging apps", "online platforms", "virtual meetings", "text messages", "social media", and "email".
2. **Adaptation and Coping Strategies** (Score: 7.5/10). Adjusting to the new normal and coping strategies emerged as a main theme in participants' descriptions of their experiences during the pandemic. Among the most cited strategies were seeking emotional support from family, friends, and colleagues, as well as engaging in activities to distract from stress and uncertainty. Virtual connections through video calls and social media proved invaluable for maintaining relationships and alleviating feelings of isolation. Additionally, adopting positive mindsets, focusing on self-care, and staying informed were recurring coping techniques. Examples of terms used include the following: "adaptation", "modifying", "coping", "reinventing", "emotional support", "distraction", "virtual connection", "positivity", and "helping others".
3. **Emotional Support** (Score: 7/10). Participants frequently discussed the importance of providing and receiving emotional support during this challenging period. Sharing feelings, thoughts, and concerns with their peers was a way to alleviate stress and anxiety related to the pandemic. Examples of terms used include the following: "empathy", "comfort", "reassurance", "kindness", "encouragement", "caring", "understanding", "compassion", "love", and "listening".
4. **Information Sharing** (Score: 6/10). Another significant theme was the exchange of information about the pandemic, such as updates on restrictions, health guidelines, and the availability of essential resources. Participants often highlighted how sharing information with their peers helped them stay informed and cope with the rapidly changing situation. Examples of words used include the following: "updates", "news", "facts", "details", "guidelines", "recommendations", "protocols", "procedures", "instructions", and "advice".

5. **Adaptation to the New Normal** (Score: 5.5/10). Participants also mentioned adjusting to the new normal, as the pandemic forced them to modify their communication habits and routines. This theme covered the adoption of new technologies, the struggle to maintain relationships, and the development of new ways of socializing. Examples of words used include the following: "adjusting", "adapting", "modifying", "flexibility", "changing", "coping", "reinventing", "reshaping", "reimagining", and "transforming".
6. **Fear and Anxiety** (Score: 5.5./10). Although less prevalent than in the other sections, the theme of fear and anxiety is also present in the Peers section, particularly related to the risk of infection from social interactions. Women expressed concerns about their peers' and family members' adherence to safety guidelines, which might expose them and their children to the virus. Examples of words used include the following: "scared", "worried", "anxious", "stressed", "concerned", and "nervous".

3.3.4. Open-Ended Questions

Four main themes were further identified from the open-ended questions:

1. **Fear and anxiety** (Score: 9/10). Again, this theme was the most prominent in the text, as many women express their fear and anxiety about various aspects of their situation, such as getting infected, losing their loved ones, being alone during labor, facing economic difficulties, and not knowing when the pandemic will end. Some examples of textual quotations include "I think about suicide rather than going to the hospital and risking contracting COVID", "I'm afraid I won't be able to protect my little one", "I'm scared because my childbirth would take place in less than 2 months and here we are talking about a virus that we don't know much about", and "I'm afraid that life will never go back to how it was before".
2. **Loneliness and isolation** (Score: 8/10). This theme is also very frequent in the text, as many women miss the lack of social contact and support from their family and friends, especially during a delicate moment like pregnancy or breastfeeding. Some examples of textual quotations include "I feel emotionally alone, I have no one, apart from my partner, with whom to share anxieties, fears, but also joys and progress", "I miss my family and I'm sorry that they are losing the first months of my baby", and "I miss being able to see my parents and take my son to the park".
3. **Gratitude and hope** (Score: 6/10). This theme is less frequent but still present in the text, as some women express their gratitude and hope for their situation, such as having a healthy baby or a supportive partner, or express hope for the future. Some examples of textual quotations include "I feel lucky because, unlike other colleagues, I can stay at home and not risk it", "I'm grateful to have a baby that makes us happy, me and my husband, and fills our little house with love", and "I hope that at least some women will understand how sick the world is because of globalization/pollution, too much work and how important it is to have friends and family".
4. **Disappointment and sadness** (Score: 5/10). This theme is also present in the text, as some women express their disappointment and sadness at not being able to live their pregnancy or breastfeeding as they had imagined or planned due to the restrictions and limitations imposed by the pandemic. Some examples of textual quotations include "I wish I could live this pregnancy differently....especially sharing it closely with all the women who are important to me", "I'm sad because no relative has been able to meet my son", "The fear takes away from me the enthusiasm of pregnancy", and "I miss being able to go swimming and go out with my family".

## 4. Discussion

### 4.1. Emotions Regarding Childbirth

In the context of emotions related to birth, the themes of trust, joy, sadness, and fear are particularly salient. These emotions are not isolated but are interconnected and influenced by various factors, including the communication and support received from healthcare professionals, media, and peers.

In particular, the findings of this study are in line with those of our preliminary research conducted in a sample of 200 pregnant women during the very first phase of COVID-19 lockdown in Italy in April 2020 [15]. In particular, with this further analysis, conducted on a sample more than five times larger, we can confirm that 'joy' was the most prevalent emotion expressed before COVID-19, while fear was the most prevalent during the acute phase of the COVID-19 pandemic. During the pandemic, the joy associated with the anticipation of birth and motherhood was overshadowed by fear and uncertainty. This shift in emotional landscape underscores the profound impact of external factors, such as a global health crisis, on the emotional well-being of pregnant women. As mentioned before, this resonates with the increased risk of having a maternal and neonatal adverse outcome with a SARS-CoV-2 infection [23]. Furthermore, other findings of literature underlined that unexpected complications during childbirth, including those brought about by external circumstances, can lead to negative emotions and a sense of grief [24,25].

The negative effects of the pandemic on the emotions and expectations of pregnant women in Italy also lasted beyond the first lockdown phase. These findings are consistent with a study by Smorti et al. (2022), which found that the COVID-19 social restrictions increased the risk of depression in Italian women with low-risk pregnancy compared to the previous period [26]. This study also found that women with high-risk pregnancy used hospitalization "as a resource to find a social support network with other pregnant women and to be reassured on the clinical ongoing of pregnancy" [26].

### 4.2. Communication and Open-Ended Questions: The Main EMERGING Themes

Fear and anxiety were prominent emotions expressed by women. Women felt concerned about the potential risk of infection during hospital visits, about the safety of their unborn or newborn children (fear of losing loved ones), and about being alone during childbirth. Moreover, a study conducted by Azoulay et al. (2021) reported high levels of anxiety among healthcare providers, driven by fear of infection and the pressure of managing the COVID-19 surge [27]. This shared anxiety could potentially impact the communication between HCPs and patients, further exacerbating the patients' emotions. When discussing the media, women expressed fear and anxiety stemming from the overwhelming amount of information, often contradictory and inaccurate, about the virus. This situation could be considered an infodemic characterized by uncertainty and confusion due to misinformation and inaccuracy as well as alarmism and sensationalism [28] during a disease outbreak. This is consistent with the literature, which suggests that the spread of information about COVID-19 through social media platforms has created fears that may not be entirely justified [29]. Moreover, infodemics lead to mistrust in HCPs and undermine the public health response. Regarding peers and family, fear and anxiety were also present, often related to the potential risk of infection from social interactions and to the possibility of being alone during labor and childbirth. In this sense, this theme shows a connection with the theme of loneliness and isolation.

Uncertainty and confusion were often present in the context of HCPs, tied to the rapidly evolving nature of the pandemic and the subsequent changes in healthcare protocols. This was further exacerbated by the fact that the scientific understanding of COVID-19 was a work in progress leading to repeated changes in guidelines and recommendations, often accompanied by contradictory messages and overwhelming information. This aligns with the paper of Koffman et al. (2020), who noted that uncertainty became a constant presence in daily patients' and HCPs' lives [30]. In such a situation, women may have felt without a guide (unclear guidance) during the pathway of pregnancy and childbirth.

When it came to the media, women in our study reported feeling overwhelmed by the constant stream of conflicting information (infodemic) about COVID-19. Our results align with the findings of Ruiu (2020), who noted that a lack of coordination between political and scientific levels, and between institutional claim-makers and the media, contributed to a sense of mismanagement during the early phases of the COVID-19 outbreak in Italy [31]. In terms of peers and family, as mentioned above, women expressed concern about the safety of social interactions and the potential risk of COVID-19 transmission. These feelings could be affected by the conflicting information during the first phase of the pandemic given by the media. The themes of uncertainty and confusion, linked to the misinformation and inaccuracy themes, were prominent in the experiences of the pregnant and postpartum women in our study, affecting their interactions with HCPs, media, and peers and family. This underscores the need for clear, consistent, and empathetic communication during times of crisis, as well as the importance of providing psychological support.

Regarding women's relationship with HCPs, competence and reassurance (expressed in the themes of emotional support and reassurance and professionalism and competence) were strongly linked to each other. Pregnant and postpartum women emphasized the importance of skilled and knowledgeable HCPs who are able to give clear and comforting information about COVID-19. These themes could be linked to trust or mistrust towards HCPs and the healthcare system in general. As mentioned above, mistrust also involves the media due to sensationalism and alarmism, which lead to a climate of uncertainty (uncertainty and confusion). Regarding peers and family, sharing information through remote communication technologies helped mothers cope with the situation, which rapidly changed. In this sense, social networks helped women to alleviate stress.

The theme of hope and optimism also emerged as a significant aspect of the emotional landscape in our survey. Regarding communication with HCPs, hope and optimism were often associated with clear and empathetic communication. Dimino et al. (2020) highlighted the importance of the HCPs' positive psychological state (the so-called PsyCap) characterized by hope, efficacy, resilience, and optimism to guarantee high-quality, evidence-based patient care during the COVID-19 pandemic [32]. They also emphasized the role of nurse leaders in fostering PsyCap in their staff. Finally, sharing experiences, advice, and emotional support with peers and family helped women navigate their emotional responses to the pandemic.

Disappointment and sadness emerged as themes in the open-ended questions section. Women suffered from not being able to experience pregnancy and breastfeeding as they imagined; HCPs should take into account such feelings due to the impact of a mismatch between expectations and experiences of pregnancy on mothers' psychological well-being [33]. These findings confirm the role of the pandemic in worsening mothers' mental health.

Loneliness and isolation emerged as significant themes in the experiences of pregnant and postpartum women during the COVID-19 pandemic. These feelings were reported in relation to their interactions with healthcare providers (HCPs), media, and peers and family. In the context of communication with HCPs, women reported feelings of isolation due to the necessary safety measures, such as social distancing and limited face-to-face consultations. This isolation was exacerbated by the lack of physical support systems, such as the presence of a partner or family member during prenatal visits or childbirth. These results are in line with those of Xiang et al. (2020), who noted that patients in quarantine might experience boredom, loneliness, and anger [34]. The media, while providing necessary information, may have contributed to feelings of loneliness and isolation. The constant flow of news about the pandemic, often focusing on the number of cases and deaths, could be linked to a sense of being alone. Moreover, social isolation could be the catalyst for mental health disorders, even in people without a history of psychiatric diseases [35]. These findings underlined the pivotal role of adequate psychological support for mothers during health crises. Finally, for some women, communication with peers and family could be a source of loneliness and isolation if the adaptation to the new normal communication strategies was not achieved.

Finally, the theme of coping strategies is a crucial aspect of the emotional response to the COVID-19 pandemic. Women in our study reported some strategies to manage the emotional toll of the pandemic, as reflected in their interactions with HCPs, media, and peers and family. Women reported using strategies such as seeking support from their HCPs, limiting exposure to distressing news, seeking out positive news stories, and using social media to connect with others. In their communication with peers and family, women reported the adoption of new technologies as a strategy to maintain social connections and to share information with peers and family, which was a helpful strategy to cope with the rapidly changing situation. This is consistent with the findings of Brooks et al. (2020), who noted the importance of maintaining social connections and engaging in self-care activities during periods of quarantine [36]. Moreover, hope and optimism towards aspects such as a healthy baby or a supportive partner seemed to be linked to a more optimistic outlook on the situation (positive mindset). Dispositional optimism is a significant source of coping [37] and, in this sense, further research should deepen the strategies to improve such a characteristic.

Present findings provide a deeper understanding of the complex emotional experiences of pregnant women during the acute phase of the COVID-19 pandemic. The themes of trust, joy, sadness, and fear offer valuable insights into the emotional landscape of these women, highlighting the significant impact of external factors on their emotional well-being. The role of HCPs, media, and peers in shaping these emotions underscores the importance of effective communication and support in enhancing the emotional well-being of pregnant women.

### 4.3. *Strengths and Limitations*

This study used natural language processing and machine learning methods to classify emotions, identify themes, and extract textual citations from a large national survey database. This approach has some advantages over human coding, such as speed, scalability, and consistency. AI-based coding can process large amounts of data in a relatively short time, handle complex and diverse tasks, and avoid human errors and biases [38].

However, AI-based coding also has some limitations compared to human coding, such as accuracy, interpretability, and creativity. The GPT-3.5 zero-shot learning AI-based coding used here may not yield results as accurate as a fine-tuned model or a model specifically designed for the task. It may also be difficult to explain how the AI model arrived at its results or to verify its validity. Moreover, AI-based coding lacks the human ability to generate novel and original insights from the data or to capture subtle nuances and contextual factors that influence human emotions and behaviors [39,40].

All these limitations notwithstanding, AI-automated classification of pre-COVID and post-COVID emotions in the full sample of the COVID-ASSESS survey, reported in this manuscript, is very consistent with the human-performed preliminary evaluation on the first 200 women answering the survey in April 2022 [15], suggesting satisfactory agreement between the two techniques.

## 5. Conclusions

The results of our research offer a comprehensive exploration of the emotional experiences and coping mechanisms of pregnant and postpartum women in Italy during the initial months of the COVID-19 pandemic. Our findings underscore the significant shift in the emotional landscape induced by the pandemic. Fear and anxiety emerged as dominant emotions, driven by concerns about personal health, the wellbeing of their unborn or newborn child, and the uncertainty surrounding the ongoing global crisis. This highlights the profound psychological impact of the pandemic on this specific group of people, emphasizing the need for targeted mental health support.

Crucially, our study also underscores the importance of communication during such crises. The pandemic exacerbated fear and anxiety, with misinformation and fear-mongering sometimes present in media and social networks. On the other hand, we also found that positive, supportive communication from healthcare professionals, family, and peers played a crucial role in promoting women's psychological wellbeing.

Reflecting on these findings, it is clear that the COVID-19 pandemic had a profound impact on the emotional experiences of pregnant and postpartum women. As we move forward from this global crisis, it remains crucial to prioritize the mental health of women and provide them with the necessary resources and support. Our research contributes to the discourse on mental health during significant public health crises, particularly during pregnancy and postpartum. We hope that it will inform the development of effective strategies to protect and support such important members of the population in future challenging circumstances.

**Supplementary Materials:** The following supporting information can be downloaded at https://www.mdpi.com/article/10.3390/jcm12196140/s1, Table S1: Word count and frequency of emotions before and during the pandemic.

**Author Contributions:** Conceptualization, C.R. and A.V.; methodology, C.R., L.M., R.B. and A.V.; formal analysis, A.V.; investigation, C.R. and L.M.; resources, C.R.; writing—original draft preparation, C.R. and A.V.; writing—review and editing, C.R., L.M., R.B. and A.V. All authors have read and agreed to the published version of the manuscript.

**Funding:** This research received no external funding.

**Institutional Review Board Statement:** The study was conducted in accordance with the Declaration of Helsinki and approved by the Ethics Committee of Florence University (Prot. 0064823, n. 61, 82, 03.20).

**Informed Consent Statement:** Informed consent was obtained from all subjects involved in the study.

**Data Availability Statement:** The data presented in this study are openly available in Mendeley Data at 10.17632/cn38pbwn7r.1.

**Acknowledgments:** CiaoLapo Foundation for Healthy Pregnancy and Perinatal Loss Support provided infrastructure for the realization of the study (documents, questionnaires, material, software, web platforms, open access, etc.).

**Conflicts of Interest:** The authors declare no conflict of interest.

## References


1. Remuzzi, A.; Remuzzi, G. COVID-19 and Italy: What next? *Lancet* **2020**, *395*, 1225–1228. [CrossRef] [PubMed]
2. Rossi, R.; Socci, V.; Talevi, D.; Mensi, S.; Niolu, C.; Pacitti, F.; Di Marco, A.; Rossi, A.; Siracusano, A.; Di Lorenzo, G. COVID-19 Pandemic and Lockdown Measures Impact on Mental Health Among the General Population in Italy. *Front Psychiatry* **2020**, *11*, 790. [CrossRef] [PubMed]
3. Carpiniello, B.; Vita, A. Impact of COVID-19 on the Italian Mental Health System: A Narrative Review. *Schizophr. Bull. Open* **2022**, *3*, sgac038. [CrossRef] [PubMed]
4. Lu, X.; Lin, Z. COVID-19, Economic Impact, Mental Health, and Coping Behaviors: A Conceptual Framework and Future Research Directions. *Front Psychol.* **2021**, *12*, 759974. [CrossRef] [PubMed]
5. Loughnan, S.A.; Gautam, R.; Silverio, S.A.; Boyle, F.M.; Cassidy, J.; Ellwood, D.; Homer, C.; Horey, D.; Leisher, S.H.; de Montigny, F.; et al. Multicountry study protocol of COCOON: COntinuing Care in COVID-19 Outbreak global survey of New, expectant, and bereaved parent experiences. *BMJ Open* **2022**, *12*, e061550. [CrossRef]
6. Villar, J.; Ariff, S.; Gunier, R.B.; Thiruvengadam, R.; Rauch, S.; Kholin, A.; Roggero, P.; Prefumo, F.; Do Vale, M.S.; Cardona-Perez, J.A.; et al. Maternal and neonatal morbidity and mortality among pregnant women with and without COVID-19 infection: The INTERCOVID multinational cohort study. *JAMA Pediatr.* **2021**, *175*, 817–826. [CrossRef] [PubMed]
7. Filippetti, M.L.; Clarke, A.D.F.; Rigato, S. The mental health crisis of expectant women in the UK: Effects of the COVID-19 pandemic on prenatal mental health, antenatal attachment and social support. *BMC Pregnancy Childbirth* **2022**, *22*, 68. [CrossRef]
8. Ahmad, M.; Vismara, L. The Psychological Impact of COVID-19 Pandemic on Women's Mental Health during Pregnancy: A Rapid Evidence Review. *Int. J. Environ. Res. Public Health* **2021**, *18*, 7112. [CrossRef]

9. Salehi, L.; Rahimzadeh, M.; Molaei, E.; Zaheri, H.; Saeieh, S.E. The relationship among fear and anxiety of COVID-19, pregnancy experience, and mental health disorder in pregnant women: A structural equation model. *Brain. Behav.* **2020**, *10*, e01835. [CrossRef]
10. White, T.; Matthey, S.; Boyd, K.; Barnett, B. Postnatal depression and post-traumatic stress after childbirth: Prevalence, course and co-occurrence. *J. Reprod Infant Psychol.* **2006**, *24*, 107–120. [CrossRef]
11. Czarnocka, J.; Slade, P. Prevalence and predictors of post-traumatic stress symptoms following childbirth. *Brit. J. Clin. Psychol.* **2000**, *39*, 35–51. [CrossRef] [PubMed]
12. Mental Health and Substance Use. Available online: https://www.who.int/teams/mental-health-and-substance-use/promotion-prevention/maternal-mental-health (accessed on 27 June 2023).
13. Khoury, J.E.; Atkinson, L.; Bennett, T.; Jack, S.M.; Gonzalez, A. Coping strategies mediate the associations between COVID-19 experiences and mental health outcomes in pregnancy. *Arch. Womens Ment Health* **2021**, *24*, 1007–1017. [CrossRef] [PubMed]
14. Khoury, J.E.; Atkinson, L.; Bennett, T.; Jack, S.M.; Gonzalez, A. COVID-19 and mental health during pregnancy: The importance of cognitive appraisal and social support. *J. Affect Disord.* **2021**, *282*, 1161–1169. [CrossRef] [PubMed]
15. Ravaldi, C.; Wilson, A.; Ricca, V.; Homer, C.; Vannacci, A. Pregnant women voice their concerns and birth expectations during the COVID-19 pandemic in Italy. *Women Birth* **2020**, *34*, 335–343. [CrossRef]
16. Ravaldi, C.; Ricca, V.; Wilson, A.; Homer, C.; Vannacci, A. Previous psychopathology predicted severe COVID-19 concern, anxiety, and PTSD symptoms in pregnant women during 'lockdown' in Italy. *Arch. Womens Ment. Health* **2020**, *23*, 783–786. [CrossRef]
17. Ravaldi, C.; Mosconi, L.; Wilson, A.N.; Amir, L.H.; Bonaiuti, R.; Ricca, V.; Vannacci, A. Exclusive breastfeeding and women's psychological well-being during the first wave of COVID-19 pandemic in Italy. *Front. Public Health* **2022**, *10*, 965306. [CrossRef]
18. Ravaldi, C.; Vannacci, A. The COVID-ASSESS dataset—COVID19 related anxiety and stress in prEgnancy, poSt-partum and breaStfeeding during lockdown in Italy. *Data Brief.* **2020**, *33*, 106440. [CrossRef]
19. Ravaldi, C.; Vannacci, A. COVID-ASSESS Italy—COVID19 related Anxiety and StreSs in prEgnancy, poSt-partum and breaStfeeding. *Mendeley* **2020**, V1. [CrossRef]
20. Introducing ChatGPT. Available online: https://openai.com/blog/chatgpt (accessed on 22 June 2023).
21. Wu, T.; He, S.; Liu, J.; Sun, S.; Liu, K.; Han, Q.L.; Tang, Y. A Brief Overview of ChatGPT: The History, Status Quo and Potential Future Development. *IEEE/CAA Autom. Sin.* **2023**, *10*, 1122–1136. [CrossRef]
22. GPT-4. Available online: https://openai.com/gpt-4 (accessed on 22 June 2023).
23. Di Guardo, F.; Di Grazia, F.M.; Di Gregorio, L.M.; Zambrotta, E.; Carrara, G.; Gulino, F.A.; Tuscano, A.; Palumbo, M. Poor maternal-neonatal outcomes in pregnant patients with confirmed SARS-Cov-2 infection: Analysis of 145 cases. *Arch. Gynecol. Obs.* **2021**, *303*, 1483–1488. [CrossRef]
24. Bell, A.F.; Andersson, E. The birth experience and women's postnatal depression: A systematic review. *Midwifery* **2016**, *39*, 112–123. [CrossRef]
25. Henriksen, L.; Grimsrud, E.; Schei, B.; Lukasse, M. Factors related to a negative birth experience—A mixed methods study. *Midwifery* **2017**, *51*, 33–39. [CrossRef]
26. Smorti, M.; Gemignani, A.; Bonassi, L.; Mauri, G.; Carducci, A.; Ionio, C. The impact of Covid-19 restrictions on depressive symptoms in low-risk and high-risk pregnant women: A cross-sectional study before and during pandemic. *BMC Pregnancy Childb* **2022**, *22*, 191. [CrossRef] [PubMed]
27. Azoulay, E.; Pochard, F.; Reignier, J.; Argaud, L.; Bruneel, F.; Courbon, P.; Cariou, A.; Klouche, K.; Labbé, V.; Barbier, F.; et al. Symptoms of Mental Health Disorders in Critical Care Physicians Facing the Second COVID-19 Wave: A Cross-Sectional Study. *Chest* **2021**, *160*, 944–955. [CrossRef] [PubMed]
28. Infodemic. Available online: https://www.who.int/health-topics/infodemic (accessed on 25 July 2023).
29. Sasaki, N.; Kuroda, R.; Tsuno, K.; Kawakami, N. Exposure to media and fear and worry about COVID-19. *Psychiatry Clin. Neurosci.* **2020**, *74*, 501–502. [CrossRef] [PubMed]
30. Koffman, J.; Gross, J.; Etkind, S.N.; Selman, L. Uncertainty and COVID-19: How are we to respond? *J. R. Soc. Med.* **2020**, *113*, 211–216. [CrossRef] [PubMed]
31. Ruiu, M.L. Mismanagement of COVID-19: Lessons learned from Italy. *J. Risk Res.* **2020**, *23*, 1007–1020. [CrossRef]
32. Dimino, K.; Horan, K.M.; Stephenson, C. Leading Our Frontline HEROES Through Times of Crisis with a Sense of Hope, Efficacy, Resilience, and Optimism. *Nurse Lead* **2020**, *18*, 592–596. [CrossRef]
33. Webb, R.; Ayers, S.; Bogaerts, A.; Jeličić, L.; Pawlicka, P.; Van Haeken, S.; Uddin, N.; Xuereb, R.B.; Kolesnikova, N. When birth is not as expected: A systematic review of the impact of a mismatch between expectations and experiences. *BMC Pregnancy Childb.* **2021**, *21*, 475. [CrossRef]
34. Xiang, Y.T.; Yang, Y.; Li, W.; Zhang, L.; Zhang, Q.; Cheung, T.; Ng, C.H. Timely mental health care for the 2019 novel coronavirus outbreak is urgently needed. *Lancet Psychiatry* **2020**, *7*, 228–229. [CrossRef]
35. Usher, K.; Bhullar, N.; Jackson, D. Life in the pandemic: Social isolation and mental health. *J. Clin. Nurs.* **2020**, *29*, 2756–2757. [CrossRef] [PubMed]
36. Brooks, S.K.; Webster, R.K.; Smith, L.E.; Woodland, L.; Wessely, S.; Greenberg, N.; Rubin, G.J. The psychological impact of quarantine and how to reduce it: Rapid review of the evidence. *Lancet* **2020**, *395*, 912–920. [CrossRef]

37. Niewiadomska, I.; Bień, A.; Rzońca, E.; Jurek, K. The Mediating Role of Dispositional Optimism in the Relationship between Health Locus of Control and Self-Efficacy in Pregnant Women at Risk of Preterm Delivery. *Int. J. Environ. Res. Public Health* **2022**, *19*, 6075. [CrossRef] [PubMed]
38. Jiang, F.; Jiang, Y.; Zhi, H.; Dong, Y.; Li, H.; Ma, S.; Wang, Y.; Dong, Q.; Shen, H.; Wang, Y. Artificial intelligence in healthcare: Past, present and future. *Stroke Vasc. Neurol.* **2017**, *2*, 230–243. [CrossRef]
39. Alm, C.O.; Hedges, A. Visualizing NLP in Undergraduate Students' Learning about Natural Language. *AAAI* **2021**, *35*, 15480–15488. [CrossRef]
40. Deng, J.; Lin, Y. The Benefits and Challenges of ChatGPT: An Overview. *FCIS* **2023**, *2*, 81–83. [CrossRef]

Journal of
*Clinical Medicine*

MDPI

*Article*

# Comparison of Maternal and Neonatal Outcomes between SARS-CoV-2 Variants: A Retrospective, Monocentric Study

**Giosuè Giordano Incognito [1], Rosario Emanuele Carlo Distefano [1], Giorgia Campo [1], Ferdinando Antonio Gulino [2,*], Chiara Gulisano [1], Chiara Gullotta [3], Giuseppe Gullo [4], Gaspare Cucinella [4], Attilio Tuscano [1], Maria Teresa Bruno [1] and Marco Palumbo [1]**

1 Department of General Surgery and Medical Surgical Specialties, University of Catania, 95100 Catania, Italy; giordanoincognito@gmail.com (G.G.I.); dr.rosariodistefano@gmail.com (R.E.C.D.); giorgiacampo.96@gmail.com (G.C.); chiaragulisano@hotmail.com (C.G.); attiliotuscano@gmail.com (A.T.); mt.bruno@unict.it (M.T.B.); mpalumbo@unict.it (M.P.)

2 Unit of Gynecology and Obstetrics, Department of Human Pathology of Adults and Developmental Age, University Hospital "G. Martino", 98100 Messina, Italy

3 Department of Clinical and Experimental Medicine, University of Messina, 98100 Messina, Italy; chiaragullotta96@gmail.com

4 Azienda Ospedaliera Ospedali Riuniti (AOOR) Villa Sofia Cervello, University of Palermo, 90133 Palermo, Italy; gullogiuseppe@libero.it (G.G.); gaspare.cucinella@unipa.it (G.C.)

* Correspondence: fegulino@unime.it

**Abstract:** The impact of SARS-CoV-2 variants on maternal and neonatal outcomes during pregnancy is still poorly understood, and the emergence of different variants has further complicated our understanding of the virus's effects. This retrospective, monocentric study aimed to fill this knowledge gap by analyzing the outcomes of pregnant women with acute SARS-CoV-2 infection caused by the Alpha, Delta, and Omicron variants. The study, conducted between December 2020 and March 2022 at San Marco Hospital, included 313 pregnant women with confirmed SARS-CoV-2 infection. The results showed that the Delta variant was associated with a significantly higher incidence of adverse outcomes, such as premature births, maternal intensive care unit admission, intrauterine growth restriction, and small for gestational age infants. Additionally, the Delta variant was linked to lower Apgar scores, higher maternal and fetal mortality rates, and increased levels of various biomarkers indicating more severe illness. Finally, the Delta variant also presented a greater possibility of vertical transmission. These findings underscore the complexity of understanding the impact of SARS-CoV-2 on pregnancy outcomes, especially considering the distinctive characteristics of different variants. By better understanding the specific impacts of each variant, appropriate preventive measures and management strategies can be implemented to optimize maternal and neonatal outcomes.

**Keywords:** SARS-CoV-2; COVID-19; maternal outcomes; neonatal outcomes; infection

## 1. Introduction

The SARS-CoV-2 pandemic began in China's Hubei province in December 2019, raising global health concerns due to the ease of transmission [1]. Pregnant women who contract the infection have a greater risk than non-pregnant ones of developing more severe complications, being hospitalized in the intensive care unit (ICU), and requiring mechanical ventilation [2]. They are also more likely to develop pregnancy-specific complications, such as pre-eclampsia, a premature rupture of membranes, and preterm labor [3,4]. Regarding neonatal outcomes, there was no evidence of teratogenicity of the virus when contracted in the embryonic period and no increase in the number of miscarriages was found [5]. In most cases, the virus was not transmitted vertically via the placenta; although a small percentage of placental swabs resulted positive and IgG against the viral spike protein was present in the neonatal blood. This highlights how vertical transmission is possible [6,7]. The Alpha variant was identified for the first time in September 2020. Compared to the wild-type variant, it has a higher transmissibility. It contains 17 mutations in its genome, of which 8 relate to the spike protein, leading to a greater affinity for the ACE2 receptor that the virus uses to enter cells. Furthermore, the clinical complications are also more serious than those caused by the wild-type virus [8]. The Delta variant was identified in December 2020 in India. It has a 60% higher transmission than the previous variant due to a mutation of the spike protein at the furin cleavage site. Furthermore, it has a lower sensitivity to antibodies produced by the vaccine both in vitro and in vivo [9–11]. Finally, the Omicron variant was identified in November 2021 in Africa and presents 30 new mutations of the spike protein with other mutations at the level of non-structural proteins. Transmissibility has undergone a further increase, but clinical features were less severe than in the previous variant [8]. Many features of pregnancy infection are still poorly understood; for example, further complications associated with SARS-CoV2 include gestational diabetes [12]. Thus, the aim of the study was to analyze the maternal and neonatal outcomes between the main three SARS-CoV-2 variants in pregnant women.

## 2. Materials and Methods

This is a retrospective, monocentric cohort study conducted at San Marco Hospital between December 2020 and March 2022. The study involved unvaccinated pregnant women with confirmed acute SARS-CoV-2 infection, as determined by positive time quantitative reverse transcription PCR (qRT-PCR) nasopharyngeal swabs. Female patients with physiologic pregnancies and spontaneous conception, with an age between 18 and 44 years old, were included in the study. Moreover, patients with previous/current history of obstetrics pathologies (such as preeclampsia and/or gestational diabetes) under control before the infection, as well as those with physiologic twin pregnancies, were also included in the analysis. Patients with disease that was not under control were not included, in order to eliminate any confounding bias. Accordingly, women vaccinated against SARS-CoV-2 and those with previous or obstetric pathologies that could have altered the significance of the results, monochorionic monoamniotic twin pregnancies, multiple pregnancies, assisted reproductive technology (ART) conception, and women under 18 years were excluded due to their high risk of complications.

Patients with negative qRT-PCR nasopharyngeal swabs at the time of delivery were excluded if they did not show any signs or symptoms of the disease, because they were considered and managed as physiologic pregnancies. In total, 313 pregnant women with proven acute SARS-CoV-2 infection were enrolled. Among them, 104 patients with positive qRT-PCR nasopharyngeal swabs from December 2020 and May 2021 were included in the Alpha group, 55 positive ones between July 2021 and December 2021 were included in the Delta group, and finally, 154 positive patients between January 2022 and March 2022 were enrolled in the Omicron group.

Personal, obstetric, and biochemical data were obtained from the medical records and the "Modulab" laboratory management system. The possibility of vertical transmission was assessed through SARS-CoV-2 RT-PCR placental swabs. For each of the three variant groups the following items were analyzed: the average age of the patients, the average number of pregnancies and previous types of births, the average gestational age at the time of delivery, the percentage of admissions in the II and III trimesters, deliveries in the II and III trimesters, percentage of the type of delivery, i.e., vaginal delivery (VD) or cesarean section (CS), percentage of admission to intensive care unit (ICU), maternal and neonatal death, mean of neonatal weight, mean of Apgar at 1 and 5 min, mean of the time interval between the diagnosis of SARS-CoV-2 infection and childbirth, an average of biochemical parameters recorded for the entire period of patients' hospitalization, i.e., C-reactive protein (CRP), procalcitonin (PCT), interleukin 6 (IL-6), hemoglobin (Hb), leukocytes with leukocyte formula including neutrophils and lymphocytes, D-dimer, aspartate aminotransferase (AST), and alanine aminotransferase (ALT), percentage of positive and negative placental swabs.

Continuous variables were presented as means ± standard deviations (SD). Categorical variables were summarized as percentages. A $p$-value of less than 0.05 was established as the threshold for determining statistical significance.

The study was conducted in accordance with the Declaration of Helsinki and approved by the Ethics Committee of the University of Catania (Code number 01/163 and approval date of 10 January 2022). Each woman received appropriate counseling about the purpose of the research and the guarantee of anonymous treatment of personal data, according to Italian laws guaranteeing privacy, and signed an informed consent form for data collection.

## 3. Results

### 3.1. Patient Baseline Characteristics

The average age of the patients was similar in the three groups (Alpha = 31.5 ± 4.7 years vs. Delta = 31.4 ± 5.1 years vs. Omicron = 31.7 ± 4.5 years, $p$ = 0.942), as well as the average number of previous pregnancies (1.7 (1.0–2.6) vs. 1.6 (0.9–2.4) vs. 1.5 (0.8–2.3), $p$ = 0.729), the average number of previous miscarriages (0.3 ± 0.5 vs. 0.2 ± 0.4 vs. 0.3 ± 0.5, $p$ = 0.664), the type of previous deliveries (74.4% VD and 25.6% CS vs. 73.6% VD and 26.4% CS vs. 72.2% VD and 25.8% CS, $p$ = 0.978) and the mean time interval between the diagnosis and the time of delivery (8.5 ± 3.2 days vs. 8.3 ± 3.5 days vs. 8 ± 3.1 days, $p$ = 0.863). Delta variant was associated with a lower gestational week at the time of delivery (38 ± 1.4 vs. 36 ± 1.8 vs. 37.7 ± 1.6, $p$ < 0.001) and a higher percentage of deliveries in the II trimester (2% vs. 5.8% vs. 2.4%, $p$ = 0.049). The Alpha group gave birth more frequently by means of CS (61.6%), while the lowest rate was recorded among women in the Omicron group (32.5%). 46.3% of patients in the Delta group gave birth by means of CS. Patients' baseline characteristics are illustrated in Table 1.

**Table 1.** Patients' baseline characteristics.

| | Alpha Group (n = 104) | Delta Group (n = 55) | Omicron Group (n = 154) | $p$-Value |
|---|---|---|---|---|
| Mean age (years) | 31.5 ± 4.7 | 31.4 ± 5.1 | 31.7 ± 4.5 | 0.942 |
| Mean previous pregnancies (n) | 1.7 (1.0–2.6) | 1.6 (0.9–2.4) | 1.5 (0.8–2.3) | 0.729 |
| Mean previous miscarriages (n) | 0.3 ± 0.5 | 0.2 ± 0.4 | 0.3 ± 0.5 | 0.664 |
| Type of previous deliveries (%) | VD 74.4, CS 25.6 | VD 73.6, CS 26.4 | VD 72.2, CS 25.8 | 0.978 |
| Mean gestation period (weeks) | 38 ± 1.4 | 36 ± 1.8 | 37 ± 1.6 | <0.001 |
| Interval Diagnosis–Delivery (days) | 8.5 ± 3.2 | 8.3 ± 3.5 | 8 ± 3.1 | 0.863 |
| II trimester at delivery (%) | 2.0 | 5.8 | 2.4 | 0.049 |
| III trimester at delivery (%) | 98.0 | 94.2 | 97.6 | 0.049 |
| Type of delivery (%) | VD 38.4, CS 61.6 | VD 53.7, CS 46.3 | VD 67.5, CS 32.5 | 0.003 |

Abbreviations: %: percentage; CS: cesarean section; Interval Diagnosis–Delivery: mean interval between the diagnosis of maternal COVID-19 infection and the date of delivery; n: number; VD: vaginal delivery. Continuous variables are expressed as mean ± standard deviations (SD) and categorical variables were summarized as percentages.

### 3.2. Biochemical Data

The Delta variant was correlated with higher CRP (56.93 ± 20.12 vs. 107.13 ± 40.34 vs. 59.51 ± 21.46, $p$ < 0.001), PCT (0.20 ± 0.08 vs. 6.47 ± 2.51 vs. 0.22 ± 0.09, $p$ < 0.001), IL-6 (30.21 ± 10.13 vs. 339.54 ± 100.51 vs. 24.13 ± 9.31, $p$ < 0.001), D-dimer (1257.31 ± 401.13 vs. 1594.58 ± 510.67 vs. 1279.79 ± 412.37, $p$ < 0.001), AST (54 ± 15.32 vs. 100 ± 30.13 vs. 59 ± 16.42, $p$ < 0.001) and ALT (61 ± 17.32 vs. 116 ± 33.46 vs. 65 ± 18.23, $p$ < 0.001) levels and lymphocyte rates (15.32% ± 4.51 vs. 17.57% ± 5.12 vs. 15.86% ± 4.73, $p$ = 0.032) and lower Hb levels (11.15 ± 1.51 vs. 9.79 ± 1.85 vs. 11.59 ± 1.45, $p$ < 0.001). Leukocyte levels (10.38 ± 2.13 vs. 10.89 ± 2.34 vs. 10.95 ± 2.28, $p$ = 0.572) and neutrophil rates

(74.15% ± 6.31 vs. 79.66% ± 7.24 vs. 78.55% ± 6.91, $p = 0.061$) were similar among the three groups. Biochemical data are displayed in Table 2.

**Table 2.** Biochemical data and maternal-neonatal outcomes.

| | Alpha Group (n = 104) | Delta Group (n = 55) | Omicron Group (n = 154) | *p*-Value |
|---|---|---|---|---|
| CRP (mg/L) | 56.93 ± 20.12 | 107.13 ± 40.34 | 59.51 ± 21.46 | <0.001 |
| PCT (ng/mL) | 0.20 ± 0.08 | 6.47 ± 2.51 | 0.22 ± 0.09 | <0.001 |
| IL-6 (pg/mL) | 30.21 ± 10.13 | 339.54 ± 100.51 | 24.13 ± 9.31 | <0.001 |
| Hb (g/dL) | 11.15 ± 1.51 | 9.79 ± 1.85 | 11.59 ± 1.45 | <0.001 |
| Leukocytes (n/mm$^3$) | 10.38 ± 2.13 | 10.89 ± 2.34 | 10.95 ± 2.28 | 0.572 |
| Neutrophil (%) | 74.15 ± 6.31 | 79.66 ± 7.24 | 78.55 ± 6.91 | 0.061 |
| Lymphocyte (%) | 15.32 ± 4.51 | 17.57 ± 5.12 | 15.86 ± 4.73 | 0.032 |
| D-dimer (ng/mL) | 1257.31 ± 401.13 | 1594.58 ± 510.67 | 1279.79 ± 412.37 | 0.001 |
| AST (U/L) | 54 ± 15.32 | 100 ± 30.13 | 59 ± 16.42 | <0.001 |
| ALT (U/L) | 61 ± 17.32 | 116 ± 33.46 | 65 ± 18.23 | <0.001 |
| Maternal admission to ICU (n) | 0 | 9 | 2 | 0.002 |
| Maternal mortality (%) | 0.0 | 1.8 | 0.0 | 0.049 |
| Neonatal weight (grams) | 3252 ± 412.32 | 2533 ± 513.62 | 3161 ± 402.18 | <0.001 |
| Apgar score at 1st min | 8.84 ± 1.13 | 8.18 ± 1.41 | 8.75 ± 1.19 | <0.001 |
| Apgar score at 5th min | 9.84 ± 0.67 | 9.26 ± 0.88 | 9.80 ± 0.71 | <0.001 |
| Neonatal mortality (%) | 0.0 | 5.5 | 0.0 | 0.001 |
| Vertical transmission (%) | 5.0 | 20.0 | 7.0 | <0.001 |

Abbreviations: ALT: alanine aminotransferase; AST: aspartate aminotransferase; CRP: C-reactive protein; Hb: hemoglobin; ICU: intensive care unit; IL-6: interleukin 6; n: number; %; PCT: procalcitonin. Continuous variables are expressed as mean ± standard deviations (SD) and categorical variables were summarized as percentages.

### 3.3. Maternal and Neonatal Outcomes

Nine Delta women were admitted to the ICU for worsening respiratory symptoms, while none of the Alpha group and only two Omicron patients were transferred. None of the women in the Alpha and Omicron groups died, while one Delta woman died. The Delta variant was most frequently associated with small for gestational age (SGA) newborns (with an average infant weight of 2533 ± 513.62 g vs. 3252 ± 412.32 g of the Alpha group and 3161 ± 402.18 g of the Omicron patients, $p < 0.001$) and with the lowest 1st minute and 5th minute Apgar scores ($p < 0.001$). The only three neonatal deaths were observed in the Delta group. Finally, this variant was associated with higher placental swab rates (5% vs. 20% vs. 7%, $p < 0.001$). Maternal and neonatal outcomes are reported in Table 2.

## 4. Discussion

The research and discussions prompted globally by the COVID-19 pandemic have been more extensive than any previous pandemic [13], highlighting an unprecedented global resonance and deep-rooted anxieties, especially in sensitive fields such as obstetrics.

The present study demonstrates the greater severity of the infection by the SARS-CoV-2 Delta variant compared with Alpha and Omicron variants in both pregnant women and newborns.

The Delta variant became the dominant strain in many regions around the world within a few months of its discovery, signaling its heightened transmissibility compared to earlier variants. It has been increasingly clear that the Delta variant was not only more transmissible but potentially more severe, causing higher rates of hospitalization and complications in infected individuals, including those who were pregnant with an increase in adverse maternal and fetal outcomes in pregnancies affected.

The Alpha variant was associated with the highest rate of CS. Nevertheless, this was probably related to the fact that at the beginning of the pandemic period, there was little knowledge on how to manage the infected patients and CS was preferred due to worse obstetric outcomes compared to uninfected women. Subsequently, the number of CS decreased among the Delta patients, despite worse both maternal and neonatal morbidities. With the Omicron variant, a further decrease of CS occurred thanks to a better knowledge of infection.

In order to better understand the data regarding the effect of the infection on the lab values analyzed, the authors also reviewed the current literature on their physiologic changes during pregnancy. During pregnancy, CRP values may be physiologically higher and may be related to the inflammatory processes that support the pregnancy itself, implantation, and the onset of labor. Significantly elevated or permanently elevated values should be carefully evaluated. In fact, in the middle months of gestation, quiescence of the inflammatory state and immune activation is expected. At this stage, high CRP values seem to be associated with an unfavorable evolution of gestation for both mother and fetus, due to the increased risk of pre-eclampsia, preterm delivery, and low birth weight of the newborn [14]. PCT is a biological marker of sepsis, septic shock, and severe inflammatory reactions. The finding of elevated serum PCT values is indicative of an inflammatory response to a systemic bacterial infection. It does not undergo physiological changes during pregnancy [14]. IL-6 is a protein produced by the immune system, involved in the regulation of the immune response, and its values during pregnancy are considered comparable in this case too [14]. During gestation, physiological dilution anemia can be found, linked to the fact that the total volume of blood increases by about 1.25 L, due to both the increase in plasma content and the increase in erythropoiesis in the medulla. However, the erythrocyte mass does not increase in parallel, and therefore an apparent reduction in Hb levels results. Even following both vaginal and cesarean births, hemoglobin may be reduced because of the blood losses that occur. The women will therefore have hemoglobin values of around 11 g/dl and hematocrit of around 34% [14]. Throughout pregnancy, leukocytes may reach 11,000/$mm^3$ in the first weeks and increase up to 20,000/$mm^3$ in the last trimester. However, the values increase further during labor and can even reach 30,000 leukocytes/$mm^3$. In particular, the neutrophils undergo the greatest increase because they are the first congenital line of defense that protects both the fetus and the mother. Conversely, lymphocytes undergo a physiological reduction, mainly due to hormonal changes and the increase in total body fluids that occurs during gestation, which leads to hemodilution with a slight decrease in all blood cells, especially lymphocytes [14]. With reference to D-dimer, it increases its levels during the first weeks of gestation, continuing even in the postpartum period, regardless of the type of delivery [15,16]. It can reach values above 4000 ng/mL during pregnancy in the third trimester [17]. As for the transaminases, the normal values of AST vary between 8 and 48 U/L, while for ALT they range between 7 and 55 U/L. During pregnancy, an increase in their value could be physiological because of an increase in liver activity, and hormonal changes could alter their value [14].

The Delta group was associated with worse biochemical changes than the other two variants. The almost double CRP and much higher IL-6 values indicate that the pro-inflammatory picture is much more pronounced during the infection with this variant. PCT values were much higher in this group, underlining how the probability of bacterial superinfection, which further complicates the clinical picture of patients, is greater for the Delta variant infection than for Alpha and Omicron. Higher levels of D-dimer could be correlated with an increased risk of developing thrombotic phenomena. Finally, high AST and ALT values indicate a greater likelihood that patients infected by the Delta variant have liver damage. Clinically, the laboratory values do not influence management of the pregnant patients, but these values could be an expression of a higher general serum inflammation, or, from another point of view, of reduced attention of pregnant people to SARS-CoV-2 infection, which could have determined a more severe Delta variant.

Delta women were associated with worse maternal morbidity and the only maternal death occurred in this group due to postpartum respiratory failure. A higher rate of neonatal morbidity was found in the Delta variant and the three neonatal deaths were all born prematurely by emergency CS for acute fetal distress: two were born at 28 gestational weeks weighing 1195 g and 1050 g, respectively, and the third was born at 35 gestational weeks weighing 1820 g. Finally, the study of placental swabs on both maternal and fetal sides indicates that the probability of vertical transmission is considerably higher for the Delta variant than for the other two. Some previous studies confirmed the results of our work. A retrospective cohort study conducted at the University of Alabama in Birmingham [18] states that there was a higher incidence of more severe clinical conditions in patients with the Delta variant, rather than Pre-delta and Omicron, as well as a higher admission rate to the ICU. In addition, they were more frequently subjected to pharmacological treatments, ventilatory support, or intubation and had a higher incidence of thromboembolic phenomena. There was also a higher frequency of preterm deliveries, emergency CS due to the worsening of maternal clinical conditions, and neonatal admissions to the neonatal intensive care unit. Another cohort study, conducted on 61 patients at the University of Texas Medical Branch [19], found that patients with Delta infection had a lower mean gestational age at the time of diagnosis or onset of symptoms than the previous variants and were more likely to be symptomatic. Higher morbidity in this group was also described at Parkland Hospital, particularly where vaccine acceptance is low [20]. The mortality rate of pregnant women in Brazil was double (15.6%) than it was during the former Alpha variant (7.4%) [21]. Furthermore, the intrauterine fetal mortality rate was higher in Delta patients [22]. Finally, Guan et al. confirmed that the main laboratory alterations in COVID-19 pregnant women concern proinflammatory cytokines and appear to be greatest in patients with the Delta variant [23]. Considering the Delta variant, maternal death and preterm birth <37 weeks were, respectively, 0.63% (95% CI, 0.05−1.20%), and 18.58% (95% CI, 9.52−27.65%) [24]. In a previous study of our research group [25] and in some other scientific works [26–32] Reactive C protein (CRP) serum levels were higher than the normal range, corresponding to a mean value of $56.93 \pm 49.57$ mg/L. COVID-19 infection in pregnant women seems to negatively affect both maternal and neonatal outcomes.

Our study presents several strengths in its investigation of the impacts of different SARS-CoV-2 variants on maternal and neonatal outcomes during pregnancy. One notable strength is the inclusion of a relatively large sample size, with 313 pregnant women confirmed to have SARS-CoV-2 infection. This sizable cohort provided a substantial dataset for analysis, enhancing the statistical power of the study. Another strength lies in the study's focus on physiologic pregnancies, which ensures a specific target population for analysis. By excluding individuals with uncontrolled obstetric pathologies, the authors aimed to reduce confounding biases and isolated the effects of the viral variants on pregnancy outcomes. Additionally, the study examined a range of crucial outcomes, including premature births, ICU admission, intrauterine growth restriction, and biomarker levels. By considering multiple endpoints, the study offers a comprehensive assessment of the impacts of different variants on both maternal and neonatal health. However, it is important to acknowledge the limitations of the manuscript. One significant limitation is the absence of variant typing based on molecular analysis. Instead, the study relied on the timing of maternal infection to categorize the SARS-CoV-2 variants. This approach introduces uncertainty, as the groups identified based on timing may not represent pure variant groups. It is possible that the reported findings may have been influenced by the presence of mixed variants within the identified groups, potentially impacting the accuracy of the results. Furthermore, the retrospective design of the study presents inherent limitations. The reliance on existing medical records may have introduced biases and incomplete data, leading to potential confounding factors that could impact the validity of the findings. Additionally, the single-center nature of the study may limit the generalizability of the results to a broader population. Variations in patient demographics, healthcare resources, and management protocols across different centers may affect the external validity of the findings. The study's exclusion criteria also pose limitations. While focusing on physiologic pregnancies is a strength, excluding vaccinated individuals and those with specific obstetric conditions might have introduced selection bias and limited the generalizability of the findings. The decision to exclude vaccinated people was finalized to obtain a more homogeneous sample of patients; furthermore, considering the period analyzed for infection (December 2020 to March 2022) most of the pregnant people were not vaccinated because there were no vaccinations or because most of them declined the invitation to have a vaccination. It is important to consider these limitations when interpreting the results, as they may restrict the applicability of the findings to broader populations. The limitations of our study include its retrospective design and the fact that the study did not consider symptom recurrence. In addition, the analysis of fertility and live birth outcomes was limited to our medical-assisted conception and maternity units' databases, whereas pregnancy and live birth data for patients who might have moved out of our hospital's catchment area could be missing.

## 5. Conclusions

The Delta variant is associated with more unfavorable maternal and neonatal outcomes than the Alpha and Omicron variants. In fact, this variant is associated with a higher incidence of preterm births, SGA infants, lower Apgar scores, higher maternal and fetal mortality, higher maternal admission to ICU, higher CRP levels, as well as PCT and IL-6, higher levels of lymphocytes, D-dimer, and transaminases. It is also associated with a higher rate of placental SARS-CoV-2 detection. Further research with a larger and more diverse population, encompassing multiple centers and incorporating variant typing, would help validate the results and provide a more comprehensive understanding of the effects of SARS-CoV-2 variants on maternal and neonatal health.

**Author Contributions:** Conceptualization, methodology, formal analysis, writing—original draft preparation, visualization, G.G.I., R.E.C.D., G.C. (Giorgia Campo), A.T. and F.A.G.; investigation, resources, data curation, C.G. (Chiara Gulisano); writing—review and editing, C.G. (Chiara Gulisano), C.G. (Chiara Gullotta), G.G., G.C. (Gaspare Cucinella), A.T. and M.T.B.; supervision and writing—review and editing, M.P. All authors have read and agreed to the published version of the manuscript.

**Funding:** This research received no external funding.

**Institutional Review Board Statement:** The study was conducted in accordance with the Declaration of Helsinki and approved by the Ethics Committee of the University of Catania (protocol code 01/163 and date of approval: 10 January 2022).

**Informed Consent Statement:** Informed consent was obtained from all subjects involved in the study. Written informed consent has been obtained from the patients to publish this paper.

**Data Availability Statement:** Not applicable.

**Conflicts of Interest:** The authors declare no conflict of interest.

## References

1. Yuen, K.S.; Ye, Z.W.; Fung, S.Y.; Chan, C.P.; Jin, D.Y. SARS-CoV-2 and COVID-19: The most important research questions. *Cell Biosci.* **2020**, *10*, 40. [CrossRef] [PubMed]
2. Zambrano, L.D.; Ellington, S.; Strid, P.; Galang, R.R.; Oduyebo, T.; Tong, V.T.; Woodworth, K.R.; Nahabedian, J.F., 3rd; Azziz-Baumgartner, E.; Gilboa, S.M.; et al. Update: Characteristics of Symptomatic Women of Reproductive Age with Laboratory-Confirmed SARS-CoV-2 Infection by Pregnancy Status—United States, January 22–October 3, 2020. *MMWR Morb. Mortal. Wkly. Rep.* **2020**, *69*, 1641–1647. [CrossRef] [PubMed]
3. Lai, J.; Romero, R.; Tarca, A.L.; Iliodromiti, S.; Rehal, A.; Banerjee, A.; Yu, C.; Peeva, G.; Palaniappan, V.; Tan, L.; et al. SARS-CoV-2 and the subsequent development of preeclampsia and preterm birth: Evidence of a dose-response relationship supporting causality. *Am. J. Obstet. Gynecol.* **2021**, *225*, 689–693.e1. [CrossRef] [PubMed]

4. Gullo, G.; Cucinella, G.; Tumminello, M.; Renda, B.; Donzelli, M.; Lo Bue, V.; Termini, D.; Maranto, M.; De Tommasi, O.; Tarantino, F. Convalescent plasma use in pregnant patients with COVID-19 related ARDS: A case report and literature review. *Ital. J. Gynaecol. Obs.* **2022**, *34*, 228–234. [CrossRef]
5. Baud, D.; Greub, G.; Favre, G.; Gengler, C.; Jaton, K.; Dubruc, E.; Pomar, L. Second-Trimester Miscarriage in a Pregnant Woman With SARS-CoV-2 Infection. *JAMA* **2020**, *323*, 2198–2200. [CrossRef]
6. Moreno, S.C.; To, J.; Chun, H.; Ngai, I.M. Vertical Transmission of COVID-19 to the Neonate. *Infect. Dis. Obstet. Gynecol.* **2020**, *2020*, 8460672. [CrossRef]
7. Maranto, M.; Zaami, S.; Restivo, V.; Termini, D.; Gangemi, A.; Tumminello, M.; Culmone, S.; Billone, V.; Cucinella, G.; Gullo, G. Symptomatic COVID-19 in Pregnancy: Hospital Cohort Data between May 2020 and April 2021, Risk Factors and Medicolegal Implications. *Diagnostics* **2023**, *13*, 1009. [CrossRef]
8. Aleem, A.; Akbar Samad, A.B.; Slenker, A.K. Emerging Variants of SARS-CoV-2 And Novel Therapeutics Against Coronavirus (COVID-19). In *StatPearls*; StatPearls Publishing: Treasure Island, FL, USA, 2022.
9. Galloway, S.E.; Paul, P.; MacCannell, D.R.; Johansson, M.A.; Brooks, J.T.; MacNeil, A.; Slayton, R.B.; Tong, S.; Silk, B.J.; Armstrong, G.L.; et al. Emergence of SARS-CoV-2 B.1.1.7 Lineage—United States, December 29, 2020–January 12, 2021. *MMWR Morb. Mortal. Wkly. Rep.* **2021**, *70*, 95–99. [CrossRef]
10. Male, V. SARS-CoV-2 infection and COVID-19 vaccination in pregnancy. *Nat. Rev. Immunol.* **2022**, *22*, 277–282. [CrossRef]
11. Luxi, N.; Giovanazzi, A.; Capuano, A.; Crisafulli, S.; Cutroneo, P.M.; Fantini, M.P.; Ferrajolo, C.; Moretti, U.; Poluzzi, E.; Raschi, E.; et al. COVID-19 Vaccination in Pregnancy, Paediatrics, Immunocompromised Patients, and Persons with History of Allergy or Prior SARS-CoV-2 Infection: Overview of Current Recommendations and Pre- and Post-Marketing Evidence for Vaccine Efficacy and Safety. *Drug Saf.* **2021**, *44*, 1247–1269. [CrossRef]
12. Radan, A.P.; Fluri, M.M.; Nirgianakis, K.; Mosimann, B.; Schlatter, B.; Raio, L.; Surbek, D. Gestational diabetes is associated with SARS-CoV-2 infection during pregnancy: A case-control study. *Diabetes Metab.* **2022**, *48*, 101351. [CrossRef] [PubMed]
13. Zorrilla, C.D.; García García, I.; García Fragoso, L.; De La Vega, A. Zika Virus Infection in Pregnancy: Maternal, Fetal, and Neonatal Considerations. *J. Infect. Dis.* **2017**, *216* (Suppl. S10), S891–S896. [CrossRef] [PubMed]
14. Soma-Pillay, P.; Nelson-Piercy, C.; Tolppanen, H.; Mebazaa, A. Physiological changes in pregnancy. *Cardiovasc. J. Afr.* **2016**, *27*, 89–94. [CrossRef] [PubMed]
15. Chabloz, P.; Reber, G.; Boehlen, F.; Hohlfeld, P.; de Moerloose, P. TAFI antigen and D-dimer levels during normal pregnancy and at delivery. *Br. J. Haematol.* **2001**, *115*, 150–152. [CrossRef] [PubMed]
16. Epiney, M.; Boehlen, F.; Boulvain, M.; Reber, G.; Antonelli, E.; Morales, M.; Irion, O.; De Moerloose, P. D-dimer levels during delivery and the postpartum. *J. Thromb. Haemost. JTH* **2005**, *3*, 268–271. [CrossRef] [PubMed]
17. Siennicka, A.; Kłysz, M.; Chełstowski, K.; Tabaczniuk, A.; Marcinowska, Z.; Tarnowska, P.; Kulesza, J.; Torbe, A.; Jastrzębska, M. Reference Values of D-Dimers and Fibrinogen in the Course of Physiological Pregnancy: The Potential Impact of Selected Risk Factors-A Pilot Study. *BioMed Res. Int.* **2020**, *2020*, 3192350. [CrossRef]
18. Vousden, N.; Ramakrishnan, R.; Bunch, K.; Morris, E.; Simpson, N.; Gale, C.; O'Brien, P.; Quigley, M.; Brocklehurst, P.; Kurinczuk, J.J.; et al. Impact of SARS-CoV-2 variant on the severity of maternal infection and perinatal outcomes: Data from the UK Obstetric Surveillance System national cohort. *medRxiv* **2021**. [CrossRef]
19. Wang, A.M.; Berry, M.; Moutos, C.P.; Omere, C.; Clark, S.M.; Harirah, H.M.; Jain, S.; Olson, G.L.; Pacheco, L.D.; Saade, G.R.; et al. Association of the Delta (B.1.617.2) Variant of Severe Acute Respiratory Syndrome Coronavirus 2 (SARS-CoV-2) With Pregnancy Outcomes. *Obstet. Gynecol.* **2021**, *138*, 838–841. [CrossRef]
20. Adhikari, E.H.; SoRelle, J.A.; McIntire, D.D.; Spong, C.Y. Increasing severity of COVID-19 in pregnancy with Delta (B.1.617.2) variant surge. *Am. J. Obstet. Gynecol.* **2022**, *226*, 149–151. [CrossRef]
21. Takemoto, M.L.S.; Nakamura-Pereira, M.; Menezes, M.O.; Katz, L.; Knobel, R.; Amorim, M.R.; Andreucci, C.B. Higher case fatality rate among obstetric patients with COVID-19 in the second year of pandemic in Brazil: Do new genetic variants play a role? *medRxiv* **2021**. [CrossRef]
22. Narang, K.; Enninga, E.A.L.; Gunaratne, M.D.S.K.; Ibirogba, E.R.; Trad, A.T.A.; Elrefaei, A.; Theiler, R.N.; Ruano, R.; Szymanski, L.M.; Chakraborty, R.; et al. SARS-CoV-2 Infection and COVID-19 During Pregnancy: A Multidisciplinary Review. *Mayo Clin. Proc.* **2020**, *95*, 1750–1765. [CrossRef]
23. Guan, M.; Johannesen, E.; Tang, C.Y.; Hsu, A.L.; Barnes, C.L.; Burnam, M.; McElroy, J.A.; Wan, X.F. Intrauterine Fetal Demise in the Third Trimester of Pregnancy Associated with Mild Infection With the SARS-CoV-2 Delta Variant without Protection From Vaccination. *J. Infect. Dis.* **2022**, *225*, 748–753. [CrossRef]
24. Deng, J.; Ma, Y.; Liu, Q.; Du, M.; Liu, M.; Liu, J. Association of Infection with Different SARS-CoV-2 Variants during Pregnancy with Maternal and Perinatal Outcomes: A Systematic Review and Meta-Analysis. *Int. J. Environ. Res. Public Health* **2022**, *19*, 15932. [CrossRef]
25. Di Guardo, F.; Di Grazia, F.M.; Di Gregorio, L.M.; Zambrotta, E.; Carrara, G.; Gulino, F.A.; Tuscano, A.; Palumbo, M. Poor maternal-neonatal outcomes in pregnant patients with confirmed SARS-Cov-2 infection: Analysis of 145 cases. *Arch. Gynecol. Obstet.* **2021**, *303*, 1483–1488. [CrossRef] [PubMed]
26. Skalska-Swistek, M.; Kolak, M.; Jaworowski, A.P.; Swistek, R.; Micek, A.; Huras, H. SARS-CoV-2 infection during pregnancy—Single-center retrospective study. *Ginekol. Pol.* 2023, *ahead of print*. [CrossRef] [PubMed]

27. Paixão, J.T.R.; Santos, C.J.S.E.; França, A.P.F.M.; Lima, S.S.; Laurentino, R.V.; Fonseca, R.R.S.; Vallinoto, A.C.R.; Oliveira-Filho, A.B.; Machado, L.F.A. Association of D-Dimer, C-Reactive Protein, and Ferritin with COVID-19 Severity in Pregnant Women: Important Findings of a Cross-Sectional Study in Northern Brazil. *Int. J. Environ. Res. Public Health* **2023**, *20*, 6415. [CrossRef] [PubMed]
28. Aktiz Bıçak, E.; Oğlak, S.C. Clinical characterisation and management outcome of obstetric patients following intensive care unit admission for COVID-19 pneumonia. *J. Obs. Gynaecol.* **2023**, *43*, 2218915. [CrossRef]
29. Ramezani-Jolfaie, N.; Eftekhar, E.; Dadinasab, M.; Hesarooeyeh, Z.G.; Pakdaman, P.; Razmpour, F.; Javedan, G.; Khayatian, M.; Azad, M.H.; Davoodian, P.; et al. The effect of vitamin D and magnesium supplementation on clinical symptoms and serum inflammatory and oxidative stress markers in patients with COVID-19: A structured summary of a study protocol for a randomized controlled trial. *Trials* **2023**, *24*, 87. [CrossRef]
30. Marie-Eve, B.; Elsa, B.; Josianne, C.; Yasmine, K.; Claude-Emilie, J.; Camille, C.; Dorothée, D.S.; Sylvie, G. Mediators of inflammation at the maternal-fetal interface are altered by SARS-CoV-2 infection and pandemic stress. *Am. J. Reprod. Immunol.* **2023**, *89*, e13679. [CrossRef]
31. Göklü, M.R.; Oğlak, S.C.; Gedik Özköse, Z.; Tunç, Ş.; Bolluk, G. The course of infection with the Delta variant of COVID-19 in pregnancy: Analysis of clinical, laboratory, and neonatal outcomes. *J. Turk. Ger. Gynecol. Assoc.* **2023**, *24*, 33–41. [CrossRef]
32. Hrubaru, I.; Motoc, A.; Bratosin, F.; Rosca, O.; Folescu, R.; Moise, M.L.; Neagoe, O.; Citu, I.M.; Feciche, B.; Gorun, F.; et al. Exploring Clinical and Biological Features of Premature Births among Pregnant Women with SARS-CoV-2 Infection during the Pregnancy Period. *J. Pers. Med.* **2022**, *12*, 1871. [CrossRef] [PubMed]

Journal of
*Clinical Medicine*

MDPI

*Article*

# Obstetric and Gynecological Admissions and Hospitalizations in an Italian Tertiary-Care Hospital during COVID-19 Pandemic: A Retrospective Analysis According to Restrictive Measures

**Gaetano Riemma [1,*], Pasquale De Franciscis [1], Marina Tesorone [2], Egle Coppa [1], Antonio Schiattarella [1], Valentina Billone [3], Alessandra Lopez [3], Gaspare Cucinella [3], Giuseppe Gullo [3] and Raffaela Maria Carotenuto [1]**

[1] Department of Woman, Child and General and Specialized Surgery, University of Campania "Luigi Vanvitelli", 80138 Naples, Italy; pasquale.defranciscis@unicampania.it (P.D.F.); egle.coppa@studenti.unicampania.it (E.C.); aschiattarella@gmail.com (A.S.); raffaelamaria.carotenuto@studenti.unicampania.it (R.M.C.)

[2] Local Health Services "Napoli 1 Centro", 80138 Naples, Italy; marina.tesorone@aslnapoli1centro.it

[3] Department of Obstetrics and Gynecology, Villa Sofia Cervello Hospital, University of Palermo, 90146 Palermo, Italy; valentinabillone@gmail.com (V.B.); alessandralopez91@gmail.com (A.L.); gaspare.cucinella1@gmail.com (G.C.); gullogiuseppe@libero.it (G.G.)

* Correspondence: gaetano.riemma@unicampania.it

**Abstract:** Background: The national lockdown and the different restrictions applied in 2020 during the COVID-19 pandemic brought several changes to hospitalization procedures. The aim of this study was to evaluate the patterns in access to emergency services and hospitalization in a tertiary-care obstetric and gynecological emergency department (OG-ED) throughout the restrictions applied during 2020. Methods: A single-center retrospective comparative study on data from January to December 2020 was carried out on the following timeframes: January to February 2020 (before COVID-19 pandemic), March to June 2020 (nationwide lockdown period), July to September 2020 (removal of restrictive measures), October to December 2020 (regional lockdown) and compared to the same periods of 2019. All obstetric and gynecological patients with complete medical data admitted to the OG-ED were included. Results: Overall, 4233 accesses for 2019 and 3652 for 2020 were reported, with a decreasing trend of −13.7%. Between March and June 2020 (nationwide lockdown) and 2019, the overall number of patients attending the OG-ED decreased compared to July–September and October–December differences (Δ −23.5% vs. −3.1% and −5.9%; $p = 0.001$ respectively) for 2020–2019, but this reduction was not statistically significant when compared to January–February (Δ −23.5% vs. −18.5%; $p = 0.356$). No significant differences for obstetric patients (Δ −1.8% vs. −1.0% vs. −2.3% and +1.9% respectively; $p = 0.883$) were noted. Hospitalizations showed a stable trend with an increase between October–December 2019 and 2020 (Δ +4.6%; $p = 0.001$ vs. January–February (+2.4%) and March–June (+2.6%) 2019–2020), mainly related to regional lockdowns. Conclusions: In contrast to available national studies, in our institution, the overall rate of OG-ED admissions was slightly reduced with a similar trend of decrease even before COVID-19, with an increase in admissions for serious issues, despite expectations that the suspension of elective admissions and outpatient services would have led to an increase in non-urgent hospitalizations during the COVID-19 lockdown period.

**Keywords:** COVID-19; hospital admissions; emergency care; obstetric urgency; lockdown; restrictions

## 1. Introduction

On 11 March 2020, the World Health Organization (WHO) released its 51st status report, in which the SARS-CoV-2 virus outbreak, also known as COVID-19, was classified as a pandemic [1]. Over the year 2020, to enforce social isolation and stop the spread of the SARS-CoV-2 virus, the Italian government implemented several restrictions [2].

Such restrictions were repeated in different periods according to each wave that affected Italy. In particular, the most severe lockdown was related to the wildtype SARS-CoV-2 variant and took place between March 9th and June 2020, in which a state of emergency, also known as "lockdown", was applied [3]. All non-essential activities, including office labor, commerce, sports, and leisure pursuits, as well as unrestricted movement inside and outside of the nation, were outlawed. Citizens were asked to not leave their home except for emergency reasons (e.g., urgent care needs) [3].

With the reduction in the number of infected people, such restrictions were gradually loosened to the use of masks in crowded areas between July and September 2020 [4,5]. However, with the second COVID-19 wave that took place from October 2020, with an exponential increase in infected people, Italian regions were grouped into three different epidemiological scenarios (known as yellow, orange, and red zones), with a nationwide curfew from 10 p.m. to 5 a.m., shopping malls were ordered to be closed on weekends, and distance education was used for high schools [4]. For regions in "orange zones", a ban on travel outside the municipality of residence and the closure of food services were extended, while for regions in "red zones", a ban on travel even within the municipality, the closure of stores and markets, and the use of distance education from seventh grade onward were applied [4].

During and after the lockdown, Italian hospitals significantly changed their routine by postponing all non-urgent outpatient visits and planned operations [6]. All urgent and emergent needs, including mandatory outpatient check-ups, were assured. This was carried out to relieve pressure on the intensive care units (ICUs) of hospitals that served COVID-19-positive patients and to save costs [6]. During the pandemic, ICU accessibility was crucial and lifesaving [7].

Consequently, after the initial SARS-CoV-2 infection spread to Italy, there was an abrupt and significant decline in emergency department visits. Overall, emergency department attendance drastically dropped by 41.8% from the previous year starting on 21 February [8]. Both medical and surgical wards were changed to COVID-19 units, and new supplemental sub-intensive and ICUs were established for COVID-19 patients. Elective surgery and outpatient visits were also decreased [9].

The administration of the obstetrics and gynecology emergency department (OG-ED) likewise faces open challenges regarding overcrowding and all associated complications [10]. Nearly one-third of trips to the OG-ED are for non-urgent treatments. Therefore, during the COVID-19 pandemic, the renovation of emergency services could markedly modify access and hospitalizations in large OG-EDs [11].

The aim of this study was to analyze how the restrictions used during the lockdown period and subsequent months of 2020 affected the trends of the access of emergency services and hospitalization in a tertiary-care OG-ED, compared to the corresponding periods of the previous year.

## 2. Materials and Methods

We conducted a single-center retrospective analysis on emergency medical records including a wide time window from January to December 2020 in a tertiary-care university emergency section related to the Obstetrics and Gynecology Unit, AOU Luigi Vanvitelli, Naples, Italy.

According to the Italian pandemic waves of 2020, three different timeframes were obtained:

- January to February 2020 (before COVID-19 pandemic);
- March to June 2020 (nationwide lockdown period);
- July to September 2020 (removal of restrictive measures);
- October to December 2020 (regional lockdown according to red, yellow and green zones related to each region's contagion curve) [12].

Each one of the above-mentioned time windows was compared to the corresponding period of 2019, before the spreading of COVID-19.

The Helsinki Declaration, the Committee on Publication Ethics (COPE) standards (http://publicationethics.org/, accessed on 7 October 2023), and the Reporting of studies Conducted using Observational Routinely collected health Data (RECORD) Statement are followed in the design, analysis, interpretation of data, writing, and revisions, available through the Enhancing the Quality and Transparency of Health Research (EQUATOR) network (www.equator-network.org, accessed on 7 October 2023). Given that the study was an observational one, the data obtained were anonymized to remove any information that may be used to formally identify the patients. Each participant in this study received information about the methods and provided their written agreement to enable data to be collected and analyzed for research.

The study included all the OG-ED admissions, classifying all pregnant patients as obstetric patients (from 0 to 22 gestational weeks, from 22 to 35 weeks, and from 35 weeks to term, whether single or multiparous women), as well as puerperal patients as gynecological patients. The study's findings were included for all patients who used the OG-ED.

Patients with missing data from the centralized hospitalization system, patients who left the OG-ED before the final diagnosis, or that denied consent to acquire data were therefore excluded from the analysis.

The primary outcome was the evaluation of changes in OG-ED admissions between each 2020 timeframe related to restrictive COVID-19 measures compared to the same timeframes in 2019. The secondary outcome was the evaluation of changes in terms of color code access and hospitalizations between the aforementioned timeframes. Moreover, a descriptive analysis of reasons for OG-ED access and hospitalizations was carried out to better describe the clinical scenarios.

Gynecologists, midwives, anesthetists, neonatologists, social workers, and nurses are part of the multidisciplinary team at the OG-ED. Our OG-ED operates around the clock in conjunction with the radiology and laboratory departments. Professional midwives handle the triage. The on-call doctor then assesses the patients in accordance with the codes. The following categories apply to the administration of triage codes in the hospital protocol when the patient is admitted: The yellow code means "urgency", which is the threat of impairment of a vital function of the woman or fetus at a gestational age of 23 weeks to be evaluated within 15 min; the red code means "emergency", which is the current impairment of a vital function of the woman or fetus at a gestational age of 23 weeks; the green code denotes "non-urgency", or services that may be delayed and reviewed within three hours; the white code denotes treatments that are comparable to outpatient care. The patient is discharged from the OG-ED with a discharge color when the final diagnosis has been determined, which is frequently different from the color that was allocated during triage. The color code assigned at the admission was used to evaluate the primary and secondary outcomes of the study.

Data were obtained and anonymously collected from the hospital management software for emergency access, hospitalization, and medical charts (Hero4 version 4.30, Dedalus Global S.p.A., Florence, Italy).

For each patient, the following data were collected: Month and year of the access; type of access (obstetric or gynecological); gestational age; cause of the access; OG-ED triage admission; hospitalization following OG-ED access.

Because standard clinical procedures have been followed, the study did not need approval from an institutional or ethical review body since it was classified as retrospective chart analysis of routine clinical practice.

*Statistical Analysis*

SPSS software (IBM Corp. Version 27.0, Armonk, NY, USA) was used for statistical analysis. Categorical data were analyzed by means of the chi-square test for independence, expanded Fisher exact test, and Bonferroni–Holms corrections for multiple testing for the primary and secondary outcomes, as appropriate. After the application of multiple testing corrections, a *p*-value ($p$) < 0.0125 was considered statistically significant.

## 3. Results

### 3.1. Primary Outcome: OG-ED Accesses

Overall, from January to December, 4233 accesses at the OG-ED were reported for 2019 while 3652 women were admitted in 2020, showing a decreasing trend of −13.7%

Table 1 shows that between March and June 2020, when the country was in total lockdown, the overall number of patients attending the OG-ED decreased (1124 in 2020 vs. 1477 in 2019). However, the analysis of differences among paired timeframes showed a marked reduction between March and June 2019–2020 with July–September and October–December timeframes (Δ −23.5% vs. −3.1% and −5.9%; $p = 0.001$, respectively) but not January–February 2019–2020 (Δ −23.5% vs. −18.5%; $p = 0.356$) (Table 1).

Similarly, there were no retrievable differences regarding the change in rates between obstetric and gynecological accesses among paired timeframes (Table 1).

### 3.2. Secondary Outcome: Changes in Color Code of Accesses

Table 2 summarizes data for the comparisons of OG-ED access color codes for the study period's timeframes.

While the number of green codes fell due to severe lockdown in March–June compared to other paired timeframes (Δ −12.0% vs. −8.4% and −4.1% from July–September and October–December, respectively; $p = 0.001$), a significant increase in yellow codes was observed in the same period (Δ +7.9% vs. +5.1% and +1.2% from July–September and October–December, respectively; $p = 0.001$) (Table 2). However, such trends were also seen in the January–February 2019 and 2020 timeframes (Δ −16.4%; $p = 0.001$ for green codes and +9.7%; $p = 0.001$ for yellow codes, respectively) (Table 2).

### 3.3. Descriptive Analysis of OG-ED Accesses

Gestational age at the OG-ED access with related reason for admission are reported in Table 3.

### 3.4. Hospitalizations

Table 4 shows how many patients evaluated in the OG-ED between March and December of 2019 and 2020 were hospitalized.

There was a significant increase in hospitalizations from October–December relative to March–June and July–September (Δ +4.6% vs. +2.4% and +2.5%, respectively; $p = 0.001$) 2019–2020.

They were mainly related to abdominal pain after 22 weeks, labor, non-stress tests, hypertension, diabetes, or other pregnancy complications (raised transaminases or bile acids) or syncope (Table 4).

**Table 1.** Accesses to the OG-ED: Comparison of 2019 and 2020.

| | January–February 2019 | January–February 2020 | Δ (%) | March–June 2019 | March–June 2020 | Δ (%) | July–September 2019 | July–September 2020 | Δ (%) | October–December 2019 | October–December 2020 | Δ (%) | p-Value |
|---|---|---|---|---|---|---|---|---|---|---|---|---|---|
| Accesses to OG-ED | 764 | 623 | −18.5 | 1477 | 1124 | −23.9 * | 1079 | 1046 | −3.1 | 913 | 859 | −5.9 | 0.001 |
| Obstetric accesses | 649/764 (84.9%) | 518/623 (83.1%) | −1.8 | 1258/1477 (85.2%) | 946/1124 (84.2%) | −1.0 | 922/1079 (85.4%) | 859/1046 (82.1%) | −2.3 | 759/913 (83.1%) | 730/859 (85%) | +1.9 | 0.883 |
| Gynecological accesses | 115/764 (15.1%) | 105/623 (16.9%) | +1.8 | 219/1477 (14.8%) | 178/1124 (15.8%) | +1.0 | 157/1079 (14.6%) | 187/1046 (17.9%) | +2.3 | 154/913 (16.9%) | 129/859 (15%) | −1.9 | |

* $p = 0.001$ vs. July–September and October–December.

**Table 2.** Comparison of OG-ED accesses according to triage color codes for evaluated timeframes.

| | January–February 2019 | January–February 2020 | Δ (%) | March–June 2019 | March–June 2020 | Δ (%) | July–September 2019 | July–September 2020 | Δ (%) | October–December 2019 | October–December 2020 | Δ (%) | p-Value |
|---|---|---|---|---|---|---|---|---|---|---|---|---|---|
| Color code | | | | | | | | | | | | | |
| White | 68/764 (8.9%) | 86/623 (13.8%) | +4.9 | 178/1477 (12.1%) | 145/1124 (12.9%) | +0.8 | 143/1079 (13.3%) | 159/1046 (15.2%) | +1.9 | 118/913 (12.9%) | 130/859 (15.1%) | +2.2 | 0.004 |
| Green | 658/764 (86.1%) | 434/623 (69.7%) | −16.4 | 1240/1477 (84%) | 809/1124 (72%) | −12.0 | 810/1079 (75.1%) | 698/1046 (66.7%) | −8.4 | 628/913 (68.8%) | 556/859 (64.7%) | −4.1 | 0.001 |
| Yellow | 36/764 (4.7%) | 90/623 (14.4%) | +9.7 | 53/1477 (3.5%) | 128/1124 (11.4%) | +7.9 | 91/1079 (8.4%) | 141/1046 (13.5%) | +5.1 | 129/913 (14.1%) | 131/859 (15.3%) | +1.2 | 0.001 |
| Red | 2/764 (0.3%) | 13/623 (2.1%) | +1.8 | 6/1477 (0.4%) | 42/1124 (3.7%) | +3.3 | 35/1079 (3.2%) | 48/1046 (4.6%) | +1.4 | 38/913 (4.2%) | 42/859 (4.9%) | +0.7 | 0.213 |

**Table 3.** Descriptive analysis of accesses to OG-ED between 2019 and 2020.

| | January–February 2019 | January–February 2020 | March–June 2019 | March–June 2020 | July–September 2019 | July–September 2020 | October–December 2019 | October–December 2020 |
|---|---|---|---|---|---|---|---|---|
| Gestational age at access (weeks) | | | | | | | | |
| <22 | 248/649 (38.2%) | 173/518 (33.4%) | 429/1258 (34%) | 271/946 (28.6%) | 259/922 (28.1%) | 250/859 (29.1%) | 255/759 (33.6%) | 184/730 (25.2%) |
| >22 and <35 | 91/649 (14.1%) | 66/518 (12.7%) | 187/1258 (15%) | 124/946 (13.1%) | 121/922 (13.1%) | 119/859 (13.9%) | 116/759 (15.3%) | 103/730 (14.1%) |
| >35 | 304/649 (46.8%) | 264/518 (51%) | 634/1258 (50.4%) | 540/946 (57.1%) | 524/922 (56.8%) | 482/859 (56.1%) | 377/759 (49.7%) | 436/730 (59.7%) |
| Reason | | | | | | | | |
| Hyperemesis | 11/649 (1.7%) | 11/518 (2.1%) | 15/1258 (1.2%) | 2/946 (0.2%) | 15/922 (1.6%) | 12/859 (1.4%) | 16/759 (2.1%) | 1/730 (0.1%) |
| Metrorrhagia before the 22nd gestational week | 68/649 (10.5%) | 88/518 (17.1%) | 98/1258 (7.8%) | 136/946 (14.4%) | 80/922 (8.7%) | 109/859 (12.7%) | 125/759 (16.5%) | 100/730 (13.7%) |
| Pain before the 22nd gestational week | 164/649 (25.3%) | 60/518 (11.6%) | 301/1258 (24%) | 98/946 (10.4%) | 151/922 (16.4%) | 109/859 (12.7%) | 93/759 (12.3%) | 62/730 (8.5%) |
| Metrorrhagia after the 22nd gestational week | 10/649 (1.5%) | 10/518 (1.9%) | 7/1258 (0.6%) | 25/946 (2.6%) | 20/922 (2.1%) | 24/859 (2.8%) | 31/759 (4.1%) | 16/730 (2.2%) |
| Abdominal pain after the 22nd gestational week, labor, non-stress test | 335/649 (51.6%) | 218/518 (42.1%) | 734/1258 (58.3%) | 442/946 (46.7%) | 496/922 (53.8%) | 382/859 (44.5%) | 306/759 (40.3%) | 358/730 (49%) |
| Pre-labor rupture of the membranes | 23/649 (3.5%) | 42/518 (8.1%) | 28/1258 (2.2%) | 75/946 (7.9%) | 58/922 (6.3%) | 100/859 (11.6%) | 69/759 (9.1%) | 88/730 (12%) |
| Fetal growth restriction, reduction of fetal movements, oligohydramnios, polyhydramnios | 1/649 (0.2%) | 23/518 (4.4%) | 7/1258 (0.6%) | 26/946 (2.7%) | 17/922 (1.8%) | 22/859 (2.6%) | 28/759 (3.7%) | 19/730 (2.6%) |
| Post-term pregnancy/scheduled hospitalization | 7/649 (1.1%) | 10/518 (1.9%) | 16/1258 (1.2%) | 41/946 (4.3%) | 27/922 (2.9%) | 21/859 (2.4%) | 20/759 (2.6%) | 26/730 (3.6%) |

**Table 3.** *Cont.*

| | January–February 2019 | January–February 2020 | March–June 2019 | March–June 2020 | July–September 2019 | July–September 2020 | October–December 2019 | October–December 2020 |
|---|---|---|---|---|---|---|---|---|
| Hypertension, diabetes or cholestatic/hepatic issues (raised transaminases and/or bile acids), syncope | 6/649 (0.9%) | 15/518 (2.9%) | 8/1258 (0.6%) | 49/946 (5.1%) | 10/922 (1.1%) | 38/859 (4.4%) | 16/759 (2.1%) | 32/730 (4.4%) |
| Post-discharge complications | 6/649 (0.9%) | 15/518 (2.9%) | 8/1258 (0.6%) | 11/946 (1.2%) | 18/922 (2%) | 8/859 (0.9%) | 11/759 (1.4%) | 7/730 (1%) |
| Others | 18/649 (2.8%) | 26/518 (5%) | 36/1258 (2.9%) | 43/946 (4.5%) | 30/922 (3.3%) | 34/859 (4%) | 44/759 (5.8%) | 21/730 (2.9%) |

**Table 4.** Hospital admissions from OG-ED: comparison of results for 2019 and 2020.

| | March–June 2019 | | March–June 2020 | | July–September 2019 | | July–September 2020 | | October–December 2019 | | October–December 2020 | | *p*-Value |
|---|---|---|---|---|---|---|---|---|---|---|---|---|---|
| **Hospitalization** | **Number/ Accesses** | % | **Number/ Accesses** | % | **Number/ Accesses** | % | **Number/ Accesses** | % | **Number/ Accesses** | % | **Number/ Accesses** | % | |
| | 300/1250 | 24.0 | 239/904 | 26.4 | 277/851 | 32.5 | 328/935 | 35.0 | 252/748 | 33.7 | 277/723 | 38.3 | 0.001 |
| Gestational age at hospitalization (weeks) | | | | | | | | | | | | | |
| <22 | 62/429 | 14.4 | 36/259 | 13.8 | 40/250 | 16.0 | 58/271 | 21.1 | 47/255 | 18.4 | 40/184 | 21.7 | |
| >22 and <35 | 17/187 | 9 | 14/121 | 11.6 | 18/119 | 15.1 | 18/124 | 14.5 | 12/116 | 10.3 | 18/103 | 17.4 | 0.519 |
| >35 | 221/634 | 35 | 189/524 | 36.1 | 219/482 | 45.4 | 252/540 | 46.6 | 193/377 | 51.2 | 219/436 | 50.2 | |
| Reason for obstetric hospitalization | | | | | | | | | | | | | |
| Metrorrhagia before the 22 GW | 25/98 | 25.5 | 23/80 | 28.7 | 31/109 | 28.4 | 43/136 | 31.6 | 35/125 | 28.0 | 31/100 | 31.0 | |
| Pain before the 22 GW | 32/301 | 10.6 | 7/151 | 4.6 | 2/109 | 1.2 | 3/98 | 3.0 | 6/93 | 6.4 | 2/62 | 3.2 | |
| Metrorrhagia after the 22 GW | 2/7 | 28.6 | 3/20 | 15.0 | 1/24 | 4.2 | 1/25 | 4.0 | 6/31 | 19.3 | 1/16 | 6.2 | <0.001 |
| Abdominal pain after the 22 GW, labor, non-stress test | 194/734 | 26.4 | 119/496 | 24.0 | 121/382 | 31.7 | 139/442 | 31.4 | 107/306 | 34.9 | 121/358 | 33.8 | |

**Table 4.** *Cont.*

| | March–June 2019 | | March–June 2020 | | July–September 2019 | | July–September 2020 | | October–December 2019 | | October–December 2020 | | *p*-Value |
|---|---|---|---|---|---|---|---|---|---|---|---|---|---|
| **Hospitalization** | Number/ Accesses | % | Number/ Accesses | % | Number/ Accesses | % | Number/ Accesses | % | Number/ Accesses | % | Number/ Accesses | % | |
| Fetal growth restriction, reduction of fetal moves, oligohydramnios, polyhydramnios | 1/7 | 14.3 | 6/17 | 35.3 | 12/22 | 54.5 | 14/26 | 53.8 | 8/28 | 28.6 | 12/19 | 63.1 | <0.001 |
| Hypertension, diabetes or cholestatic/hepatic issues (raised transaminases and/or bile acids), syncope | 5/8 | 62.5 | 9/10 | 90.0 | 18/38 | 47.4 | 24/49 | 49.0 | 11/21 | 52.4 | 18/32 | 56.2 | |
| Reason for gynecological hospitalization | | | | | | | | | | | | | |
| Pelvic abdominal pain (also scheduled admissions for cysts, prolapse, renal colic, ovarian carcinoma, myoma) | 12/137 | 8.7 | 8/70 | 11.4 | 12/60 | 20.0 | 14/68 | 20.6 | 6/48 | 12.5 | 12/58 | 20.7 | 0.001 |
| Menometrorrhagia (including cervical and endometrial cancer) | 4/33 | 12.1 | 7/41 | 17.1 | 12/66 | 18.2 | 10/57 | 17.5 | 9/48 | 18.8 | 12/48 | 25.0 | |

GW: gestational weeks.

## 4. Discussion

During the lockdown period (March to June 2020), most hospital facilities were overwhelmed by COVID-19 cases, making them inaccessible to non-COVID patients, including pregnant women, due to health restrictions imposed by the government, resulting in a decrease in OG-ED accesses of about 13% [13,14]. Although the suspension of elective admissions and outpatient services for high-risk pregnancies was expected to result in an increase in hospitalizations during the COVID-19 period [15,16], this retrospective study showed that the overall rate of emergency admissions slightly decreased in the evaluated timeframes [17] but had a declining trend that may have already been present in the pre-COVID-19 era [18].

To date, four studies have reported the influence of COVID-19 on OG-ED accesses in Italy [11,19–21]. All of them reported in favor of a significant impact on admissions and hospitalizations which could have deeply reduced the quality of health in pregnant and non-pregnant women. However, our study showed a non-significant decrease when, for the first time, a side-by-side comparison based on the different subtypes of restrictions between two consecutive years with and without COVID-19 restrictions was made.

The study from Carbone et al. [21] reported data from the same Italian region as our research. They reported a significant reduction of both admissions and hospitalizations in each month of 2020 compared to 2019. Conversely, we reported that only the lockdown period (March to June 2020) was deemed to have a substantial impact on OG-ED admissions, while hospitalizations remained mainly untouched. The use of different admission policies could be one of the most compelling explanations. Differently from our institution, the hospital of Carbone et al. [21] was a referral center for COVID-19-positive pregnancies, which might also explain the different rates of admissions and hospitalizations.

Amadori et al. [11] reported a reduction of more than the half for accesses from 2019 to 2020, which was similar to Grandi et al.'s [20] study results, which showed that there was a reduction in accesses and hospitalizations when comparing the timeframes 1–30 November 2019 and 11 March–9 April 2020. Similar results were also reported by Dell'Utri et al. [19] for the timeframes 23 February–23 June 2019 and 2020.

Conversely, we reported that the same trends of an overall decrease in OG-ED admissions and changes concerning the reduction of non-serious cases and the increase in those with higher priority were present even before the inclusion of the restraint measures due to COVID-19. In some situations, the reduction of cases marked as green codes was even greater than when the national lockdown was applied; in fact, we recorded a 16.4% reduction between January and February 2019–2020 compared to 12.0% of the March–June period of the same two years. This condition was also noted for the increase in yellow codes, with a greater increase even before the implementation of the restrictive measures.

Multiple explanations could be attributed to these findings. Firstly, one reason may the increased fear of contagion related to media reports that may have played a conditioning role on public health even before the restrictions [22]. On the contrary, analyzing the data on admissions and hospitalizations in 2019 more deeply, our and other hospitals might show a decreasing trend that was already present, so the impact of restrictive measures on the total cost computation related to hospitalizations would be even less than what was expected. Therefore, this evidence needs further retrospective analyses to overcome previous limitations.

During the lockdown, we also noted increased gynecological hospitalizations resulting from pelvic abdominal pain, particularly acute adnexal pathologies, and oncological emergencies. This strengthens the evidence that the reduced outpatient and regular activities of Italian hospitals increased the need for urgent admissions and hospitalizations and that pain, rather than blood loss, is still reported as the most unpleasant and worrying symptom that pushes women to seek emergency care [23,24].

From July to September 2020, we could not observe changes in obstetric patients' accesses. This was partially expected because during this period there was a reopening, albeit partial, of facilities and outpatient clinics, so that patients were freer both in terms of travel and access to services [25]. This suggests that while the national closure caused a large proportion of people to minimize travel for fear of infection, the introduction of regional lockdowns did not have a negative impact on hospital access, probably due to greater awareness of the nature and mode of infection [26–28].

Interestingly, hypertension and obstetrics women with gestational diabetes or cholestatic and hepatic issues were all increased in 2020 compared to 2019. With this finding, in accordance with Carbone et al. [21] and La Verde et al. [12], it was reasonable to suppose that the lifestyle restrictions of the lockdown would have raised the likelihood of the emergence of such issues. Indeed, a decrease in physical activity, an increase in house rest, an associated rise in maternal weight, as well as stress and worry, might all be potential contributors to the rise in blood pressure [29–32].

However, this study has several limitations. Possible flaws in the recording of data might have influenced the retrospective collection of patient data. In the computerized records, the final diagnoses were heterogeneously categorized, therefore their inclusion in a specific subcategory could be biased by the operator's decisional process. Similarly, all the biases in its retrospective design (including selection bias) should be considered while reading the results. Concerning the admission to the OG-ED, although the triage midwives' characterization of the primary complaint was often uniform, it is also conceivable that they had a varied interpretation of the patients' concerns. It appears plausible to assume that this minor scenario may occur again in additional, related epidemiological scenarios [9].

Nonetheless, there are several points of strength that could be attributed to our analysis. First, the introduction of a dedicated pathway with universal antigen screening tests and the strict scheduling of maternity admissions with prior SARS-CoV-2 molecular swabs have helped to ensure trust and safety, preventing a reduction in emergency services in our emergency department and outpatient facilities. Moreover, the exclusion of patients with missing data was useful to avoid confounding.

## 5. Conclusions

Our study did not show a marked reduction in the number of OG-ED admissions due to COVID-19, showing that OG-ED accesses were decreasing even before the application of national restrictions. Obstetric care seemed less affected by the pandemic, highlighting the importance of antenatal care and screening at all stages. However, there were differences between the pandemic and pre-pandemic periods in terms of presenting to the OG-ED. Although the suspension of elective admissions and outpatient services for high-risk pregnancies was expected to result in an increase of hospitalizations during the COVID-19 lockdown period, the only significant trend of increased hospitalizations was seen during the regional lockdown period (October–December 2020), probably due to reasons not related to the COVID-19 emergency.

**Author Contributions:** Conceptualization, G.R. and P.D.F.; methodology, A.S.; formal analysis, E.C.; investigation, E.C. and A.L.; data curation, R.M.C.; writing—original draft preparation, G.R. and R.M.C.; writing—review and editing, V.B., G.G., M.T., A.S. and P.D.F.; supervision, P.D.F. and G.C. All authors have read and agreed to the published version of the manuscript.

**Funding:** This research received no external funding.

**Institutional Review Board Statement:** Ethical review and approval were waived for this study because normal clinical practices in accordance with the Declaration of Helsinki were followed.

**Informed Consent Statement:** Written informed consent for data acquisition, anonymization, assessment, and publication was obtained from all the included study subjects who were admitted to the OG-ED.

**Data Availability Statement:** Data and material are available from the corresponding author upon reasonable request.

**Conflicts of Interest:** The authors declare no conflict of interest.

## References


1. Porto, E.D.; Naticchioni, P.; Scrutinio, V. Lockdown, essential sectors, and COVID-19: Lessons from Italy. *J. Health Econ.* **2022**, *81*, 102572. [CrossRef] [PubMed]
2. Sebastiani, G.; Palu, G. COVID-19 and School Activities in Italy. *Viruses* **2020**, *12*, 1339. [CrossRef] [PubMed]
3. Bressy, S.; Zingarelli, E.M. COVID-19 and primary care in Italy: One year later. *J. Prim. Health Care* **2022**, *14*, 96–98. [CrossRef] [PubMed]
4. Chiesa, R.; Kahlberg, A.; Rinaldi, E.; Mascia, D. Emergency management of the COVID-19 pandemic in a vascular surgery department of a large metropolitan hospital in Italy. Preparation, escalation, de-escalation, and normal activity. *J. Card. Surg.* **2021**, *36*, 1632–1636. [CrossRef]
5. Eichenberg, C.; Grossfurthner, M.; Kietaibl, S.; Riboli, G.; Borlimi, R.; Holocher-Benetka, S. Emotional distress in the early stages of the COVID-19 related lockdowns depending on the severity of the pandemic and emergency measures: A comparative online-survey in Germany, Austria and Italy. *BMC Psychiatry* **2021**, *21*, 509. [CrossRef]
6. Giorgi, P.D.; Gallazzi, E.; Capitani, P.; D'Aliberti, G.A.; Bove, F.; Chiara, O.; Peretti, G.; Schiro, G.R. How we managed elective, urgent, and emergency orthopedic surgery during the COVID-19 pandemic: The Milan metropolitan area experience. *Bone Jt. Open* **2020**, *1*, 93–97. [CrossRef]
7. Vitale, S.G.; Carugno, J.; Riemma, G.; Farkas, Z.; Krasznai, Z.; Bacsko, G.; Lampe, R.; Torok, P. The role of hysteroscopy during COVID-19 outbreak: Safeguarding lives and saving resources. *Int. J. Gynaecol. Obstet.* **2020**, *150*, 256–258. [CrossRef]
8. Bongiovanni, M.; Arienti, R.; Bini, F.; Bodini, B.D.; Corbetta, E.; Gianturco, L. Differences between the waves in Northern Italy: How the characteristics and the outcome of COVID-19 infected patients admitted to the emergency room have changed. *J. Infect.* **2021**, *83*, e32–e33. [CrossRef]
9. Capanna, F.; Haydar, A.; McCarey, C.; Bernini Carri, E.; Bartha Rasero, J.; Tsibizova, V.; Helmer, H.; Makatsarya, A.; Di Renzo, G.C. Preparing an obstetric unit in the heart of the epidemic strike of COVID-19: Quick reorganization tips. *J. Matern. Fetal Neonatal Med.* **2022**, *35*, 1412–1418. [CrossRef]
10. Villar, J.; Ariff, S.; Gunier, R.B.; Thiruvengadam, R.; Rauch, S.; Kholin, A.; Roggero, P.; Prefumo, F.; do Vale, M.S.; Cardona-Perez, J.A.; et al. Maternal and Neonatal Morbidity and Mortality Among Pregnant Women with and without COVID-19 Infection: The INTERCOVID Multinational Cohort Study. *JAMA Pediatr.* **2021**, *175*, 817–826. [CrossRef]
11. Amadori, R.; Buscemi, R.; Desando, A.; Grillo, F.; Remorgida, V.; Surico, D. Obstetrics and Gynecology Emergency Department Activity during Lockdown in a Teaching Hospital, Hub Center, for COVID-19. *Obstet. Gynecol. Int.* **2022**, *2022*, 7557628. [CrossRef] [PubMed]
12. La Verde, M.; Torella, M.; Riemma, G.; Narciso, G.; Iavarone, I.; Gliubizzi, L.; Palma, M.; Morlando, M.; Colacurci, N.; De Franciscis, P. Incidence of gestational diabetes mellitus before and after the COVID-19 lockdown: A retrospective cohort study. *J. Obstet. Gynaecol. Res.* **2022**, *48*, 1126–1131. [CrossRef] [PubMed]
13. Athiel, Y.; Civadier, M.S.; Luton, D.; Ceccaldi, P.F.; Bourret, A.; Sroussi, J.; Mandelbrot, L.; Ville, Y.; Nizard, J.; Sibony, O.; et al. Impact of the outbreak of SARS-CoV-2 infection on urgent gynecological care. *J. Gynecol. Obstet. Hum. Reprod.* **2020**, *49*, 101841. [CrossRef]
14. Wolf, T.G.; Schulze, R.K.W.; Ramos-Gomez, F.; Campus, G. Effectiveness of Telemedicine and Teledentistry after the COVID-19 Pandemic. *Int. J. Environ. Res. Public Health* **2022**, *19*, 13857. [CrossRef] [PubMed]
15. Ciarleglio, F.A.; Rigoni, M.; Mereu, L.; Tommaso, C.; Carrara, A.; Malossini, G.; Tateo, S.; Tirone, G.; Bjerklund Johansen, T.E.; Benetollo, P.P.; et al. The negative effects of COVID-19 and national lockdown on emergency surgery morbidity due to delayed access. *World J. Emerg. Surg.* **2021**, *16*, 37. [CrossRef]
16. Dashraath, P.; Wong, J.L.J.; Lim, M.X.K.; Lim, L.M.; Li, S.; Biswas, A.; Choolani, M.; Mattar, C.; Su, L.L. Coronavirus disease 2019 (COVID-19) pandemic and pregnancy. *Am. J. Obstet. Gynecol.* **2020**, *222*, 521–531. [CrossRef] [PubMed]
17. Maranto, M.; Zaami, S.; Restivo, V.; Termini, D.; Gangemi, A.; Tumminello, M.; Culmone, S.; Billone, V.; Cucinella, G.; Gullo, G. Symptomatic COVID-19 in Pregnancy: Hospital Cohort Data between May 2020 and April 2021, Risk Factors and Medicolegal Implications. *Diagnostics* **2023**, *13*, 1009. [CrossRef] [PubMed]
18. Santi, L.; Golinelli, D.; Tampieri, A.; Farina, G.; Greco, M.; Rosa, S.; Beleffi, M.; Biavati, B.; Campinoti, F.; Guerrini, S.; et al. Non-COVID-19 patients in times of pandemic: Emergency department visits, hospitalizations and cause-specific mortality in Northern Italy. *PLoS ONE* **2021**, *16*, e0248995. [CrossRef]
19. Dell'Utri, C.; Manzoni, E.; Cipriani, S.; Spizzico, C.; Dell'Acqua, A.; Barbara, G.; Parazzini, F.; Kustermann, A. Effects of SARS CoV-2 epidemic on the obstetrical and gynecological emergency service accesses. What happened and what shall we expect now? *Eur. J. Obstet. Gynecol. Reprod. Biol.* **2020**, *254*, 64–68. [CrossRef]
20. Grandi, G.; Del Savio, M.C.; Caroli, M.; Capobianco, G.; Dessole, F.; Tupponi, G.; Petrillo, M.; Succu, C.; Paoletti, A.M.; Facchinetti, F. The impact of COVID-19 lockdown on admission to gynecological emergency departments: Results from a multicenter Italian study. *Int. J. Gynaecol. Obstet.* **2020**, *151*, 39–42. [CrossRef]
21. Carbone, L.; Raffone, A.; Travaglino, A.; Sarno, L.; Conforti, A.; Gabrielli, O.; De Vivo, V.; De Rosa, M.; Migliorini, S.; Saccone, G.; et al. Obstetric A&E unit admission and hospitalization for obstetrical management during COVID-19 pandemic in a third-level hospital of southern Italy. *Arch. Gynecol. Obstet.* **2022**, *305*, 859–867. [CrossRef] [PubMed]

22. Meller, F.O.; Schafer, A.A.; Quadra, M.R.; Demenech, L.M.; Paludo, S.D.S.; da Silva, P.A.; Neiva-Silva, L.; Dumith, S.C. Fear of COVID-19 and health-related outcomes: Results from two Brazilian population-based studies. *Psychiatry Res.* **2022**, *313*, 114596. [CrossRef] [PubMed]
23. Alfieri, N.; Manodoro, S.; Marconi, A.M. COVID-19 does not stop obstetrics: What we need to change to go on safely birthing. The experience of a University Obstetrics and Gynecology Department in Milan. *J. Perinat. Med.* **2020**, *48*, 997–1000. [CrossRef] [PubMed]
24. Fumagalli, S.; Borrelli, S.; Ornaghi, S.; Vergani, P.; Nespoli, A. Midwives' experiences of providing maternity care to women and families during the COVID-19 pandemic in Northern Italy. *Women Birth* **2023**, *36*, e57–e64. [CrossRef]
25. Miralles, O.; Sanchez-Rodriguez, D.; Marco, E.; Annweiler, C.; Baztan, A.; Betancor, E.; Cambra, A.; Cesari, M.; Fontecha, B.J.; Gasowski, J.; et al. Unmet needs, health policies, and actions during the COVID-19 pandemic: A report from six European countries. *Eur. Geriatr. Med.* **2021**, *12*, 193–204. [CrossRef]
26. Geremia, S.; Valente, E.P.; Mariani, I.; Dalena, P.; Lazzerini, M. Women's suggestions on how to improve the quality of maternal and newborn care during the COVID-19 pandemic in Italy: A co-occurrence network analysis. *J. Glob. Health* **2023**, *13*, 06013. [CrossRef]
27. McElfish, P.A.; Willis, D.E.; Shah, S.K.; Bryant-Moore, K.; Rojo, M.O.; Selig, J.P. Sociodemographic Determinants of COVID-19 Vaccine Hesitancy, Fear of Infection, and Protection Self-Efficacy. *J. Prim. Care Community Health* **2021**, *12*, 21501327211040746. [CrossRef]
28. Heiat, M.; Heiat, F.; Halaji, M.; Ranjbar, R.; Tavangar Marvasti, Z.; Yaali-Jahromi, E.; Azizi, M.M.; Morteza Hosseini, S.; Badri, T. Phobia and Fear of COVID-19: Origins, complications and management, a narrative review. *Ann. Ig. Med. Prev. Comunità* **2021**, *33*, 360–370. [CrossRef]
29. Hori, N.; Shiraishi, M.; Harada, R.; Kurashima, Y. Association of Lifestyle Changes Due to the COVID-19 Pandemic with Nutrient Intake and Physical Activity Levels during Pregnancy in Japan. *Nutrients* **2021**, *13*, 3799. [CrossRef]
30. Gow, M.L.; Rossiter, C.; Roberts, L.; Henderson, M.J.; Yang, L.; Roche, J.; Hayes, E.; Canty, A.; Denney-Wilson, E.; Henry, A. COVID-19, lifestyle behaviors and mental health: A mixed methods study of women 6 months following a hypertensive pregnancy. *Front. Public Health* **2022**, *10*, 1000371. [CrossRef]
31. Scott, J.; Hauspurg, A.; Davis, E.M.; Bryan, S.; Catov, J.M. Maternal Mental Health, COVID-19-Related Distress, and Disruptions in Lifestyle Behaviors among Postpartum Mothers with a Previous Hypertensive Disorder of Pregnancy. *J. Cardiovasc. Nurs.* 2023, *ahead of print*. [CrossRef]
32. Roggio, F.; Trovato, B.; Ravalli, S.; Di Rosa, M.; Maugeri, G.; Bianco, A.; Palma, A.; Musumeci, G. One Year of COVID-19 Pandemic in Italy: Effect of Sedentary Behavior on Physical Activity Levels and Musculoskeletal Pain among University Students. *Int. J. Environ. Res. Public Health* **2021**, *18*, 8680. [CrossRef] [PubMed]

Journal of
*Clinical Medicine*

MDPI

*Article*

# The Importance of Vaccination, Variants and Time Point of SARS-CoV-2 Infection in Pregnancy for Stillbirth and Preterm Birth Risk: An Analysis of the CRONOS Register Study

**Antonella Iannaccone [1,*], Alexandra Gellhaus [1], Beatrix Reisch [1], Mark Dzietko [2], Boerge Schmidt [3], Laven Mavarani [3], Katrina Kraft [4], Kristin Andresen [5], Rainer Kimmig [1], Ulrich Pecks [6] and Ekkehard Schleußner [7]**

[1] Department of Obstetrics and Gynecology, University Hospital, University of Duisburg-Essen, 45147 Essen, Germany; alexandra.gellhaus@uk-essen.de (A.G.); beatrix.reisch@uk-essen.de (B.R.); rainer.kimmig@uk-essen.de (R.K.)
[2] Department of Pediatrics, University Hospital Essen, University of Duisburg-Essen, 45147 Essen, Germany; mark.dzietko@uk-essen.de
[3] Institute for Medical Informatics, Biometry and Epidemiology, University of Duisburg-Essen, 45147 Essen, Germany; boerge.schmidt@uk-essen.de (B.S.)
[4] Department of Obstetrics and Gynecology, University Hospital of Lübeck, 23562 Lübeck, Germany; katrina.kraft@uksh.de
[5] Department of Obstetrics and Gynecology, University Hospital of Kiel, 24105 Kiel, Germany; kristin.andresen@uksh.de
[6] Department of Obstetrics and Gynecology, University Hospital of Würzburg, 97080 Würzburg, Germany; pecks_u@ukw.de
[7] Department of Obstetrics, Jena University Hospital, 07747 Jena, Germany; ekkehard.schleussner@med.uni-jena.de
* Correspondence: antonella.iannaccone@uk-essen.de; Tel.: +49-201-7233574

**Abstract: Background:** The risk of preterm birth (PTB) and stillbirth increases after a SARS-CoV-2 infection during gestation. We aimed to estimate the risk depending on gestational age at infection (early <28 + 0 and late ≥28 weeks of gestation, WoG), virus variants, severity of infection, and vaccination. **Methods:** PTB was divided into early PTB (<32 + 0) and late PTB (32 + 0–36 + 6 WoG). The prospective register COVID-19 Related Obstetrics and Neonatal Outcome Study (CRONOS) included 8032 pregnant women with a confirmed SARS-CoV-2 infection from 3 April 2020 to 31 December 2022, in Germany and Austria. **Results:** Stillbirth and early preterm births rates were higher during the Alpha (1.56% and 3.13%) and Delta (1.56% and 3.44%) waves than during the Omicron wave (0.53% and 1.39%). Early SARS-CoV-2 infection increased the risk for stillbirth (aRR 5.76, 95% CI 3.07–10.83) and early PTB before 32 + 0 (aRR, 6.07, 95% CI 3.65–10.09). Hospital admission increased the risks further, especially in the case of ICU admission. Vaccination against SARS-CoV-2 significantly reduced the risk of stillbirth (aRR 0.32, 95% CI 0.16–0.83). **Conclusions:** This multicentric prospective study shows an increased risk of stillbirth and preterm birth after infection early in pregnancy and therefore the importance of obstetrical surveillance thereafter. Vaccination offers effective protection.

**Keywords:** vaccination; preterm birth; stillbirth; COVID -19; SARS-CoV-2; alpha; delta; omicron; wild-type

## 1. Introduction

Since the outbreak of the SARS-CoV-2 (severe acute respiratory syndrome coronavirus 2) pandemic in 2020, questions about the risk of infection during pregnancy have arisen. Overall, the pandemic situation had a tremendously negative impact on maternal and neonatal health [1].

Pregnancy is a physiological state that predisposes women to respiratory complications from viral infection [2,3].

SARS-CoV and MERS-CoV (*Middle East respiratory syndrome-related coronavirus*) were responsible for severe complications during pregnancy [4]. SARS-CoV-2 belongs to the same β-coronavirus subgroup, and it has a genome similarity of about 80% and 50% with SARS-CoV and MERS-CoV, respectively [5].

COVID-19 (coronavirus disease 2019), the disease induced by the SARS-CoV-2 infection, caused more severe respiratory complications in pregnant than in non-pregnant women, with a two to three times higher risk of being admitted to an intensive care unit, needing invasive ventilation and extracorporeal membrane oxygenation (ECMO) or even of dying [6]. The risk increases with ongoing pregnancy and is highest at around 32 weeks of gestation [7], most probably due to physiological changes in pregnancy leading to restricted pulmonary residual capacity and alterations in immune defense [8].

Several studies showed that risk of adverse perinatal outcome increases after maternal SARS-CoV-2 infection [9,10].

The gestational week at the time of infection appears to be an important determining factor [11].

In particular, studies have shown that the risk of preterm birth (PTB) and stillbirth increased after an infection in the first half of pregnancy [12], and that the severity of the disease does not play an important role [11]. Yet, hospitalization seems to be important in determining the respiratory [10] but also obstetrical [12] risks.

Stillbirth definitions vary between countries around the globe and differ especially between high- and low-income countries around the world [13]. The American College of Obstetricians and Gynecologists (ACOG) defines stillbirth as delivery of fetus which shows no signs of life, e.g., absence of breathing, heart beats, pulsations in umbilical cord are absent, no voluntary movement of muscle. The suggested requirement is to report fetal deaths at 20 weeks or more of gestation (if the gestational age is known) or a weight greater than or equal to 350 g, if the gestational age is not known. The cut-off of 350 g is the 50th percentile for weight at 20 weeks' gestation [14]. Regarding preterm births (PTB), these are those that occur at under 37 weeks' gestational age; however, the low-gestational age cutoff, or that used to distinguish preterm birth from spontaneous abortion, varies by location [15]. PTB is further subdivided on the basis of gestational age (GA): extremely preterm (<28 weeks), very preterm (28–<32 weeks) and moderate or late preterm (32–<37 completed weeks of gestation) [16]. Preterm births account for 75% of perinatal mortality and more than half the long-term morbidity [15].

Different virus variants circulated in Germany and epidemiological data on variant dominance are available from the German Surveillance System of the Robert Koch Institute (https://edoc.rki.de/bitstream/handle/176904/9483/EB-10-2022-Phaseneinteilung.pdf, accessed on 30 January 2024). Recent data suggest an increased rate of stillbirth during the Delta period [17]. PTB rates were significantly lower during the Omicron period [18]. An epidemiological study revealed recently that the risk of preterm birth is lower when the vaccination rate is higher [19].

The main aim of this study is to compare the PTB and stillbirth risk depending on the time point of infection, dominant virus variant, severity of disease requiring hospitalization, and vaccination status.

## 2. Materials and Methods

### 2.1. Study Design and Setting

From 3 April 2020 to 31 December 2022, the data of 8032 women with acute or previous SARS-CoV-2 infection (positive PCR or antigen test) at any time during their pregnancy and who, regardless of indication, were cared for in one of the participating obstetric departments were collected in the multicentric and prospective register COVID-19 Related Obstetrics and Neonatal Outcome Study (CRONOS). CRONOS is an observational study established by the German Society of Perinatal Medicine (DGPM) to rapidly provide data to counsel women with SARS-CoV-2-infection during pregnancy. Information on the study is available at www.dgpm-online.org and the German Clinical Trials Register

(DRKS00021208). All German maternity hospitals were invited to participate in the study. Obstetrical Units covering almost 1/3 of the deliveries in Germany as well as the Kepler University Hospital in Linz, Austria, participated and included cases. Methodology and study results were published recently [7,20–25]. Approval of the Institutional Ethics Board was obtained for the study (University Hospital Schleswig-Holstein in Kiel, file number D 451/20) and for each study site separately.

### 2.2. Data Capture and Study Variables

After obtaining informed consent from patients, information on the demographic characteristics, medical and obstetrical history, infection-specific symptoms and/or treatments, obstetrical and neonatal outcomes of the current pregnancy were entered by each participating hospital in the cloud-based electronic data capture platform of the service provider castoredc.com (Amsterdam, The Netherlands). The virus variant was calculated based on information and epidemiological data on variant dominance from the German Surveillance System of the Robert Koch Institute (https://edoc.rki.de/bitstream/handle/176904/9483/EB-10-2022-Phaseneinteilung.pdf, accessed on 30 January 2024). From the first recorded cases (27 January 2020) until the end of the second wave on the 28th of February 2021, the wild-type virus circulated in Germany. During the third wave, from the 1 March 2021 until the end of the summer plateau on the 1 August 2021, the variant of concern (VOC) was Alpha. From the 2nd of August, the new VOC Delta took over, causing the fourth wave until the 26 December 2021. From the 27th of December 2021 the VOC was Omicron.

#### Endpoints

The primary endpoints were stillbirth after 20 weeks of gestation WoG and PTB (livebirth before completed 37 WoG). Those were further classified as early PTB (<32 + 0 (WoG)) or late PTB (from 32 + 0) and. The timing of exposure was dichotomized into early (<28 + 0 weeks of gestation) and late (third trimester $\geq$ 28 weeks) infections.

### 2.3. Statistical Analysis

To evaluate the impact of the time point of infection in pregnancy, of vaccination against SARS-CoV-2, and of dominant virus variant on the endpoints, we conducted a stepwise statistical analysis strategy.

1. A descriptive analysis of baseline characteristics of the population: categorical variables are presented as absolute and relative frequencies (*N*/%); continuous baseline variables were shown as mean and standard deviation (mean ± SD) for each group (Table 1).

**Table 1.** Baseline and pregnancy characteristics of the study participants.

| | Mean/*N* | SD/% | Missing |
|---|---|---|---|
| Maternal age (years) | 31.1 | 5.4 | 37 |
| BMI at inclusion (kg/m$^2$) | 29.1 | 5.8 | 2282 |
| Week of gestation at birth | 38.2 | 3.3 | 735 |
| PTB | 835 | 11.4 | 735 |
| History of PTB | 138 | 1.7% | 17 |
| IVF | 292 | 4.1% | 959 |
| Multiple pregnancy | 237 | 3% | 76 |
| Smoking during pregnancy | 333 | 4.1% | 240 |
| Any symptoms | 6025 | 81.6% | 644 |
| Vaccine against SARS-CoV-2 | 2156 | 26.8% | 702 |
| Hospital admission | 5585 | 71.9% | 265 |
| Hospital admission for COVID-19 | 828 | 10.7% | 264 |
| Hospital admission for obstetric reasons | 3756 | 48.3% | 264 |
| ICU admission | 223 | 2.9% | 267 |

2. A descriptive bivariate analysis to assess the proportion of stillbirth, early (<32 + 0), and late (32 + 0–36 + 6) PTB, depending on the time point of infection, virus variant, and vaccination status (Table 2).

**Table 2.** Descriptive bivariate analysis of stillbirth, early preterm and late preterm birth depending on time point of infection, virus variant and vaccination status.

| | | | Stillbirth (N = 70, 0.87%) | | Early PTB (N = 165, 2.05%) | | Late PTB (N = 670, 8.34%) | |
|---|---|---|---|---|---|---|---|---|
| | N | % | N | % | N | % | N | % |
| **Early infection** | 3119 | 38.8% | 46 | 1.47% | 113 | 3.62% | 212 | 6.80% |
| **Late infection** | 4913 | 61.2% | 24 | 0.49% | 52 | 1.05% | 458 | 9.32% |
| **Wild-type** | 2334 | 29.1% | 16 | 0.69% | 41 | 1.76% | 217 | 9.30% |
| **Alpha** | 766 | 9.5% | 12 | 1.56% | 24 | 3.13% | 72 | 9.40% |
| **Delta** | 1542 | 19.2% | 24 | 1.56% | 53 | 3.44% | 132 | 8.56% |
| **Omicron** | 3390 | 42.2% | 18 | 0.53% | 47 | 1.39% | 249 | 7.35% |
| **Vaccine** | 2156 | 26.8% | 11 | 0.51% | 27 | 1.25% | 141 | 6.54% |
| **No vaccine** | 5174 | 64.4% | 54 | 1.04% | 138 | 2.66% | 488 | 9.43% |

3. Finally, multivariate log-binomial models for calculating adjusted relative risk (aRR) and corresponding 95% confidence intervals (95% CI) were used to correct the risk for maternal characteristics and common risk factors.

Statistical analyses were performed using Statistical Package for Social Sciences (SPSS; version 29; IBM Corp, Armonk, NY, USA) for Windows (Microsoft, Redmond, WA, USA). Missed values are dropped by default in SPSS for log-binomial models; therefore, sample sizes may differ in the statistical analyses. Inferential statistics were used in a descriptive manner. Thus, no significance levels were determined, and no adjustment for multiplicity was applied. However, $p$ values < 0.05 were considered to be statistically significant.

## 3. Results

### 3.1. Descriptive Statistics

The baseline maternal demographic and clinical characteristics of the 8032 infected pregnant women are presented in Table 1.

The mean maternal age was 31.11 ± 5.35 years and the mean gestational week at delivery was 38.15 ± 3.31.

The mean BMI was 29.06 ± 5.83 kg/m$^2$. The study population included 3% twin pregnancies and 4.1% pregnancies were induced by medically assisted reproduction. In 1.7% of women, a history of preterm birth was indicated.

Of the pregnant women, 4.3% smoked during the pregnancy.

Some 71.9% of the women were inpatients at the time of the infection, with 10.7% admitted for symptoms related to COVID-19 and 48.35% for obstetrics complication or delivery. Of the patients, 2.9% were admitted to the intensive care units (ICU).

Most women were infected with SARS-CoV-2 during the Omicron dominant phase (3390, 42.2%). During the 3 months of Alpha as VOC, the registered number of infections was 766 (9.5%). During the period of 5 months when Delta was prevalent, there were 1542 (19.2%) recorded infections during pregnancy. During the first 13 months of the pandemic, 2334 cases of infection were reported in which only the wild-type virus was detected.

In the population studied, 26.8% women were vaccinated against SARS-CoV-2 at the time of infection.

Of the women analyzed, 3119 (38.8%) acquired the infection early in pregnancy and 4913 (61.2%) in the third trimester.

### 3.2. Rate of Stillbirth, Early and Late PTB

Seventy patients (0.87%) suffered a stillbirth after 20 + 0 week of gestation (WoG), but rates vary depending on the time point of infection in pregnancy, virus variant, and vaccination status (Table 2).

Depending on the time point of infection, the stillbirth rate was higher after an early infection compared with an infection in the third trimester: 1.47% (46/70) versus 0.49% (24/70).

The rate of stillbirth was higher during the Alpha and Delta periods: 1.56% in both periods (12/766 and 24/1542), almost three times higher than during the wild-type and Omicron periods: 0.69% (16/2334) and 0.53% (18/3390, Table 2).

Further, in the vaccinated women, the stillbirth rate was almost half compared to the unvaccinated group: 0.51% (11/2156) versus 1.04% (54/5174).

Eight hundred and thirty-five pregnant women (10.39%) had a preterm birth: 165 (2.05%) deliveries were early preterm and 670 (8.43%) occurred after 32 + 0 WoG (Table 2)

In the case of early infection, the rate of PTB before 32 + 0 WoG was higher: 3.63% (113/3119) versus 1.05% (52/4913) after a late infection. In cases of late infection, the rate of late PTB was higher: 9.32% (458/4913) compared to 6.80% (212/3119) after early infection (Table 2).

Regarding the virus types, the rate of early PTB was higher among pregnant women infected during the Alpha and Delta period: 3.13% (24/766) and 3.44% (53/1542) versus 1.76% (41/2334) and 1.39% (47/3390) during the wild-type and Omicron periods. The rate of late PTB was lowest during the Omicron period with 7.35% (249/3390). During the wild-type, Alpha, and Delta waves, the rates of late PTB were 9.30% (217/2334), 9.40% (72/766), and 8.56% (132/1542) (Table 2).

In cases where vaccinations had been given, the rate of early PTB almost halved: 2.66% (138/5174) in the unvaccinated population versus 1.25% (27/2156) among vaccinated pregnant individuals. Also, the rate of late PTB was lower in the vaccinated population: 6.54% (141/2156) versus 9.43% (488/5147) in the unvaccinated population.

### 3.3. Adjusted Relative Risks of Stillbirth and Preterm Delivery

Having any symptoms, independent of the severity, reduced the risk of stillbirth (adjusted relative risk—aRR 0.16, 95% CI 0.26–1.125) and early PTB (aRR 0.35, 95% CI 0.20–0.61), but had no influence on the aRR for late PTB (aRR 0.99, 95% CI 0.77–1.27, Table 3). Inpatients admitted for symptoms related to the SARS-CoV-2 infection, had increased risks, with an aRR of 2.86 for stillbirth (95% CI 1.08–8.02) and 1.49 for early PTB (95% CI 1.14–5.47). The aRR for late PTB was 1.71 in the case of symptomatic disease with hospital admission (95% CI 1.25–2.51). Hospital admission for obstetrical reasons increased the aRR for stillbirth by 5.50 times (95% CI 2.90–10.41), for early PTB 4.40 times (95% CI 2.80–6.90), and for late PTB 2.06 times (95% CI 1.70–2.51, Table 3).

The admission to an intensive care unit (ICU) increased the adjusted relative risk of stillbirth 3.44 times (95% CI 1.04–11.38), the adjusted relative risk of early PTB was 11.66 (95% CI 5.22–26.05), for late PTB 1.98 (95% CI 1.31–3.00, Table 3).

Being infected during the Alpha or Delta periods, compared with other variants, increased the adjusted relative risk of stillbirth (aRR 1.76, 95% CI 0.99–3.08) and early PTB (aRR 1.45, 95% CI 0.96–2.18). The risk of late PTB was not increased (aRR 0.89, 95% CI 0.72–1.10, Table 3).

Regarding the timepoint of infection, the relative risks of stillbirth and early PTB were higher after an infection early in pregnancy: aRR 5.76, 95% CI 3.07–10.83 and aRR 6.07, 95% CI 3.65–10.09. The risk of late PTB is not increased after an infection early in pregnancy (aRR 0.79, 95% CI 0.62–1.01, Table 3).

**Table 3.** Multivariate log-bin model regarding the adjusted relative risk (aRR) of stillbirth, early and late PTB depending on symptomatic infection, hospital admission due to SARS-CoV 2 infection, for obstetrical reasons, ICU admission, being infected with Alpha or Delta variants compared to other virus types, early infection compared to late infection and being vaccinated. Significant *p*-values are marked in bold. The 95% lower and upper confidence intervals (CI) are indicated. RR adjusted for maternal age, BMI, multiples and history of miscarriage/preterm delivery.

| Outcome | Parameter | Symptomatic | CoV Admission | Ob Admission | ICU Admission | Alpha Delta vs. Others | Early vs. Late | Vaccine |
|---|---|---|---|---|---|---|---|---|
| **Stillbirth** | aRR | 0.16 | **2.86** | **5.50** | **3.44** | 1.76 | **5.76** | **0.32** |
| | 95% CI | 0.26–1.25 | **1.08–8.02** | **2.90–10.1** | **1.04–11.38** | 0.99–3.08 | **3.07–10.83** | **0.16–0.83** |
| | *p*-Value | 0.573 | **0.035** | **<0.001** | **0.043** | 0.055 | **<0.001** | **0.019** |
| **Early PTB** | aRR | **0.35** | **2.49** | **4.40** | **11.66** | 1.45 | **6.07** | 0.65 |
| | 95% CI | **0.20–0.61** | **1.14–4.47** | **2.80–6.91** | **5.22–26.05** | 0.96–2.18 | **3.65–10.09** | 0.38–1.11 |
| | *p*-Value | **<0.001** | **0.023** | **<0.001** | **<0.001** | 0.077 | **<0.001** | 0.112 |
| **Late PTB** | aRR | 0.99 | **1.71** | **2.06** | **1.98** | 0.89 | 0.79 | **0.73** |
| | 95% CI | 0.77–1.27 | **1.25–2.51** | **1.70–2.51** | **1.31–3.00** | 0.72–1.10 | 0.62–1.01 | **0.58–0.92** |
| | *p*-Value | 0.924 | **<0.001** | **<0.001** | **<0.001** | 0.269 | 0.065 | **0.008** |

Being vaccinated against SARS-CoV 2 reduced the risk of stillbirth (aRR 0.32 CI 0.11–0.92, $p = 0.035$). The risks of early and late preterm birth were also lower: aRR 0.65 (95% CI 0.38–1.11) and aRR 0.73 (95% CI 0.58–0.92, Table 3).

## 4. Discussion

### 4.1. Principal Findings

The rate of early preterm delivery and stillbirth was higher after infection before the third trimester and during the Alpha and Delta periods of SARS-CoV-2 infections. The rate of stillbirth and early PTB were lower in the vaccinated population. SARS-CoV-2 infection early in pregnancy and infection during the Alpha and Delta periods increased the risk for stillbirth and early preterm birth. Having symptoms independent of the severity reduced the risk for PTB, especially for early PTB. Hospital admission for COVID-19-related symptoms as a surrogate of a more severe course of COVID-19 disease increased the risks. Vaccination against SARS-CoV-2 significantly reduced the risks, especially for stillbirth. It is known that the risk of stillbirth after a SARS-CoV-2 infection in pregnancy is increased [26]. A recent meta-analysis estimated that the odds ratio of stillbirth in COVID-19 compared to non-COVID-19 pregnant women was 1.89 [27]. In 2022, we reported the increased risk especially after early infection in a smaller cohort based on our CRONOS register data [12]. Since the rate and risk of stillbirth is dependent on gestational age, it is not possible to exclude that not only the infection, but gestational age itself affected our results. Pregnant individuals may have presented in hospital due to the diagnosis of intrauterine demise and have had an early infection detected through hospital screening. In a retrospective study from 2010, the stillbirth rate was higher early in gestation, but the risk increased late in gestation, especially at 42 weeks [28]. The hypothesis is that the infection produced an inflammation in the maternal body affecting the fetus correlated with an adverse outcome increasing the risk of stillbirth and preterm birth.

Pregnant women with COVID-19 versus without COVID-19 are more likely to deliver preterm and could have an increased risk of maternal death and of being admitted to the intensive care unit [29]. Pregnant women especially early in the second trimester seem to be more susceptibly and tend to have a worse outcome after infection in this period [18]. In 2022, Piekos et al. [11] analyzed the risk of maternal and pregnancy complications depending on the time point of infection in 882 infected pregnant women compared with 889 matched control pregnant women. An infection in the first and second trimester increased the risk of stillbirth and early PTB. They also found that gestational week at infection could predict the week of gestation at delivery, but the severity of the infection was not correlated with gestational age at delivery. In our first analysis of a smaller cohort from CRONOS, which included 1149 pregnant women [12], and in this study including

8032 infections in pregnancy, the admission to hospital as a surrogate for the severity of infection increased the risk for stillbirth and preterm birth. In the case of admission to an ICU, the risk increase was even higher. Differently applied statistical models, but also the population size, could be explanations for the different results, since the number of infected women was lower in the cohort of Piekos and colleagues [11].

The prevalence of congenital malformations in SARS-CoV-2-infected women did not increase in the CRONOS register compared to the known European prevalence [30]. In countries where the Zika Virus is endemic, the clinical differentiation between the two entities with similar symptoms is difficult and represents an issue due to the late diagnosis of congenital Zika syndrome, which includes microcephaly and neurodevelopmental delay [31].

The Delta and the Alpha variants showed increased transmissibility shortly after being discovered compared to earlier variants. It soon became clear that the Delta variant was not only more transmissible but potentially more severe, leading to higher rates of hospitalization and complications in pregnant women, resulting in an increase in adverse maternal and fetal outcomes in affected pregnancies [32].

The study of Favre [17] examined the period before and after Delta. In this analysis, the higher risk for maternal health but also the increased risk for obstetrical complications especially preterm birth and stillbirth during Delta is evident. During the Delta period, the stillbirth rate was 2.8%, higher than the one observed in our study. The reason for this could be the smaller examined population with n = 1402, n = 262, and n = 391 for pre-Delta, Delta, and post-Delta, respectively.

Depending on different virus variants, different PTB rates were described at an academic center in New York (US) [18]: 9.9% during Omicron compared with a peak in PTB rate of 20.3% during the original period, which is of course much higher than the 11.06% PTB rate registered during the wild-type period in our study. The German preterm birth rate is 9%, stable in recent years [33] whereas the PTB birth rate in the US is higher, at 10.38% in 2022, with a higher rate among black non-Hispanic women (14.59%) [34]. The reason in this case could also be the different size of the studied populations, since in the study, 8983 women were analyzed but only 638 were infected.

Regarding vaccination, the main body of research evaluates the safety of vaccination against SARS-CoV-2 in pregnancy [35,36]. The role of vaccination and its effect on obstetrical outcomes has not yet been intensively examined. One recent study showed that the risk increase for PTB after infection was lower when the vaccination rate in the population was higher [19]. Our data support not only the safety of vaccination against SARS-CoV-2 in pregnancy, they underline the importance of vaccination by lowering the risk for adverse outcomes like stillbirth and preterm birth in the vaccinated population.

### 4.2. Clinical Implications

Our data provide a valid instrument for consulting pregnant women on the modulation of risk after SARS-CoV-2 infection during pregnancy and the role of vaccination. Overall, obstetrical complications seemed to be lower during the Omicron wave. However, an infection early in pregnancy has been shown to increase the risks of the analyzed obstetrical complications. Therefore, intensive obstetrical surveillance after an early pregnancy infection is still mandatory. Vaccination offers effective protection against the risk of stillbirth and preterm birth (PTB), and women should be encouraged to receive immunization against SARS-CoV-2 infection. Vaccination during pregnancy is a delicate topic that arouses a lot of skepticism in patients. The pandemic is a case in point. Since the results of the vaccination studies, including pregnant individuals, were available later than those regarding other populations, immunization in pregnancy started later. An earlier analysis of this important group could have prevented many complications making it a current and exemplary issue, an important lesson for the future.

### 4.3. Research Implications

The reasons for the susceptibility of the studied pregnancy complications after an early infection need further evaluation. The placenta may play a crucial role. Different molecular pathways could be modulated at this stage, potentially contributing to the elevated risk of placental dysfunction, which correlates with the increased risk of medically induced preterm birth. We also hypothesize that infections in the late second trimester could trigger an escalation of inflammation, possibly accounting for most cases of spontaneous preterm birth. Given the multifactorial nature of preterm birth and the often unexplained reasons for stillbirth, confirming this hypothesis will be challenging. Detailed and extensive biomolecular placental research could provide answers, but clinical examination and matching cases with a control group may also yield valuable insights.

### 4.4. Strengths and Limitations

We present one of the largest cohorts of infected women from high-income countries such as Germany and Austria, offering detailed insights into their symptoms, pregnancy outcomes, and medical histories. Our study meticulously examines the impact of vaccination, reaffirming its crucial role in preventing the elevated risks of stillbirth and early preterm birth. The recruited infected pregnant women primarily originated from obstetrical hospitals, predominantly tertiary care centers. As a result, most cases involved hospitalized and often high-risk individuals. We acknowledge that future studies should include an uninfected group for a comprehensive comparison. Additionally, we did not differentiate between spontaneous and medically indicated preterm deliveries, recognizing that both may be influenced by the infection. In the case of stillbirth, we did not categorize by specific causes, considering any delivery involving an unviable fetus as a stillbirth.

## 5. Conclusions

Our analysis reaffirms the critical need for obstetric surveillance following a SARS-CoV-2 infection in early pregnancy. The heightened risks of preterm birth and stillbirth are substantiated in this study. The presence of mild symptoms appears to have little relevance, while severe symptomatic cases necessitating treatment and hospitalization emerge as significant risk factors for preterm birth and stillbirth. Moreover, this analysis provides further support for the presumed protective effect of vaccination, particularly in preventing stillbirth.

**Author Contributions:** A.I. designed and conducted the analyses reported in this study and wrote the manuscript. B.S. and L.M. contributed significantly to the design of these analyses. E.S. and U.P. contributed significantly by discussing the results and their interpretations and by revising earlier drafts. A.G., B.R. and M.D. contributed to the final draft of this manuscript. U.P. is one of the principal investigators of the CRONOS Network. K.K., K.A. and R.K. contributed to the interpretation of results, revised the paper draft. All authors have read and agreed to the published version of the manuscript.

**Funding:** The CRONOS Network received funding from CAU/UKSH, DGPM, Krumme-Stiftung Kiel and the German Society of Diabetes. We acknowledge support from the Open Access Publication Fund of the University of Duisburg-Essen.

**Institutional Review Board Statement:** Approval of the Institutional Ethics Board was obtained for the study (University Hospital Schleswig-Holstein in Kiel, file number D 451/20, approve date: 31 March 2020) and for each study site separately.

**Informed Consent Statement:** Written informed consent was obtained from all subjects involved in the study.

**Data Availability Statement:** Data are contained within the article.

**Acknowledgments:** We are grateful to all women who agreed to be registered for this study. We thank the whole CRONOS Network.

**Conflicts of Interest:** All authors declare that the research was conducted without any commercial or financial relationship that could be construed as potential conflicts of interest.

## References


1. Chmielewska, B.; Barratt, I.; Townsend, R.; Kalafat, E.; van der Meulen, J.; Gurol-Urganci, I.; O'Brien, P.; Morris, E.; Draycott, T.; Thangaratinam, S.; et al. Effects of the COVID-19 pandemic on maternal and perinatal outcomes: A systematic review and meta-analysis. *Lancet Glob. Health* **2021**, *9*, e759–e772. [CrossRef]
2. Maranto, M.; Zaami, S.; Restivo, V.; Termini, D.; Gangemi, A.; Tumminello, M.; Culmone, S.; Billone, V.; Cucinella, G.; Gullo, G. Symptomatic COVID-19 in Pregnancy: Hospital Cohort Data between May 2020 and April 2021, Risk Factors and Medicolegal Implications. *Diagnostics* **2023**, *13*, 1009. [CrossRef]
3. Siston, A.M.; Rasmussen, S.A.; Honein, M.A.; Fry, A.M.; Seib, K.; Callaghan, W.M.; Louie, J.; Doyle, T.J.; Crockett, M.; Lynfield, R.; et al. Pandemic 2009 influenza A(H1N1) virus illness among pregnant women in the United States. *JAMA* **2010**, *303*, 1517–1525. [CrossRef] [PubMed]
4. Poon, L.C.; Yang, H.; Lee, J.C.S.; Copel, J.A.; Leung, T.Y.; Zhang, Y.; Chen, D.; Prefumo, F. ISUOG Interim Guidance on 2019 novel coronavirus infection during pregnancy and puerperium: Information for healthcare professionals. *Ultrasound Obstet. Gynecol.* **2020**, *55*, 700–708. [CrossRef] [PubMed]
5. Lu, R.; Zhao, X.; Li, J.; Niu, P.; Yang, B.; Wu, H.; Wang, W.; Song, H.; Huang, B.; Zhu, N.; et al. Genomic characterisation and epidemiology of 2019 novel coronavirus: Implications for virus origins and receptor binding. *Lancet* **2020**, *395*, 565–574. [CrossRef] [PubMed]
6. Zambrano, L.D.; Ellington, S.; Strid, P.; Galang, R.R.; Oduyebo, T.; Tong, V.T.; Woodworth, K.R.; Nahabedian, J.F., 3rd; Azziz-Baumgartner, E.; Gilboa, S.M.; et al. Update: Characteristics of Symptomatic Women of Reproductive Age with Laboratory-Confirmed SARS-CoV-2 Infection by Pregnancy Status-United States, January 22–October 3, 2020. *MMWR Morb. Mortal. Wkly. Rep.* **2020**, *69*, 1641–1647. [CrossRef] [PubMed]
7. Pecks, U.; Mand, N.; Kolben, T.; Rüdiger, M.; Oppelt, P.; Zöllkau, J.; Dempfle, A. SARS-CoV-2 Infection During Pregnancy. *Dtsch. Arztebl. Int.* **2022**, *119*, 588–594. [CrossRef] [PubMed]
8. Nassikas, N.; Malhamé, I.; Miller, M.; Bourjeily, G. Pulmonary Considerations for Pregnant Women. *Clin. Chest Med.* **2021**, *42*, 483–496. [CrossRef] [PubMed]
9. Epelboin, S.; Labrosse, J.; De Mouzon, J.; Fauque, P.; Gervoise-Boyer, M.-J.; Levy, R.; Sermondade, N.; Hesters, L.; Bergère, M.; Devienne, C.; et al. Obstetrical outcomes and maternal morbidities associated with COVID-19 in pregnant women in France: A national retrospective cohort study. *PLoS Med.* **2021**, *18*, e1003857. [CrossRef] [PubMed]
10. Ferrara, A.; Hedderson, M.M.; Zhu, Y.; Avalos, L.A.; Kuzniewicz, M.W.; Myers, L.C.; Ngo, A.L.; Gunderson, E.P.; Ritchie, J.L.; Quesenberry, C.P.; et al. Perinatal Complications in Individuals in California With or Without SARS-CoV-2 Infection During Pregnancy. *JAMA Intern. Med.* **2022**, *182*, 503–512. [CrossRef]
11. Piekos, S.N.; Roper, R.T.; Hwang, Y.M.; Sorensen, T.; Price, N.D.; Hood, L.; Hadlock, J.J. The effect of maternal SARS-CoV-2 infection timing on birth outcomes: A retrospective multicentre cohort study. *Lancet Digit. Health* **2022**, *4*, e95–e104. [CrossRef] [PubMed]
12. Iannaccone, A.; Mand, N.; Schmidt, B.; Rüdiger, M.; Reisch, B.; Pecks, U.; Schleussner, E. Is the risk of still and preterm birth affected by the timing of symptomatic SARS-CoV-2 infection during pregnancy? Data from the COVID-19 Related Obstetrics and Neonatal Outcome Study Network, Germany. *Am. J. Obstet. Gynecol.* **2022**, *228*, 351–352.e2. [CrossRef] [PubMed]
13. Kelly, K.; Meaney, S.; Leitao, S.; O'Donoghue, K. A review of stillbirth definitions: A rationale for change. *Eur. J. Obstet. Gynecol. Reprod. Biol.* **2021**, *256*, 235–245. [CrossRef] [PubMed]
14. ACOG. ACOG Practice Bulletin No. 102: Management of stillbirth. *Obstet. Gynecol.* **2009**, *113*, 748–761. [CrossRef]
15. Goldenberg, R.L.; Culhane, J.F.; Iams, J.D.; Romero, R. Epidemiology and causes of preterm birth. *Lancet* **2008**, *371*, 75–84. [CrossRef] [PubMed]
16. Quinn, J.A.; Munoz, F.M.; Gonik, B.; Frau, L.; Cutland, C.; Mallett-Moore, T.; Kissou, A.; Wittke, F.; Das, M.; Nunes, T.; et al. Preterm birth: Case definition & guidelines for data collection, analysis, and presentation of immunisation safety data. *Vaccine* **2016**, *34*, 6047–6056. [CrossRef]
17. Favre, G.; Maisonneuve, E.; Pomar, L.; Daire, C.; Poncelet, C.; Quibel, T.; Monod, C.; Martinez de Tejada, B.; Schäffer, L.; Papadia, A.; et al. Maternal and perinatal outcomes following pre-Delta, Delta, and Omicron SARS-CoV-2 variants infection among unvaccinated pregnant women in France and Switzerland: A prospective cohort study using the COVI-PREG registry. *Lancet Reg. Health Eur.* **2023**, *26*, 100569. [CrossRef]
18. Seaton, C.L.; Cohen, A.; Henninger, E.M.; Gendlina, I.; Hou, W.; Bernstein, P.S.; Duong, T.Q. Coronavirus Disease 2019 (COVID-19) Perinatal Outcomes Across the Pandemic at an Academic Medical Center in New York City. *Obstet. Gynecol.* **2023**, *141*, 144–151. [CrossRef]
19. Torche, F.; Nobles, J. Vaccination, immunity, and the changing impact of COVID-19 on infant health. *Proc. Natl. Acad. Sci. USA* **2023**, *120*, e2311573120. [CrossRef]
20. Kleinwechter, H.J.; Weber, K.S.; Mingers, N.; Ramsauer, B.; Schaefer-Graf, U.M.; Groten, T.; Kuschel, B.; Backes, C.; Banz-Jansen, C.; Berghaeuser, M.A.; et al. Gestational diabetes mellitus and COVID-19: Results from the COVID-19-Related Obstetric and Neonatal Outcome Study (CRONOS). *Am. J. Obstet. Gynecol.* **2022**, *227*, 631.e1–631.e19. [CrossRef]
21. Sitter, M.; Pecks, U.; Rüdiger, M.; Friedrich, S.; Fill Malfertheiner, S.; Hein, A.; Königbauer, J.T.; Becke-Jakob, K.; Zöllkau, J.; Ramsauer, B.; et al. Pregnant and Postpartum Women Requiring Intensive Care Treatment for COVID-19-First Data from the CRONOS-Registry. *J. Clin. Med.* **2022**, *11*, 701. [CrossRef] [PubMed]

22. Pecks, U.; Kuschel, B.; Mense, L.; Oppelt, P.; Rüdiger, M. Pregnancy and SARS-CoV-2 Infection in Germany-the CRONOS Registry. *Dtsch. Arztebl. Int.* **2020**, *117*, 841–842. [CrossRef] [PubMed]
23. Mand, N.; Iannaccone, A.; Longardt, A.C.; Hutten, M.; Mense, L.; Oppelt, P.; Maier, R.F.; Pecks, U.; Rüdiger, M. Neonatal outcome following maternal infection with SARS-CoV-2 in Germany: COVID-19-Related Obstetric and Neonatal Outcome Study (CRONOS). *Arch. Dis. Child. Fetal Neonatal Ed.* **2021**, *107*, 454–456. [CrossRef] [PubMed]
24. Weschenfelder, F.; Zöllkau, J.; Schohe, A.; Pecks, U.; Groten, T.; Schaefer-Graf, U.; On Behalf Of, C.-N. Obesity during Pregnancy and SARS-CoV-2/COVID-19-Case Series of the Registry Study "COVID-19 Related Obstetric and Neonatal Outcome Study" (CRONOS-Network). *J. Clin. Med.* **2023**, *12*, 2089. [CrossRef] [PubMed]
25. Ziert, Y.; Abou-Dakn, M.; Backes, C.; Banz-Jansen, C.; Bock, N.; Bohlmann, M.; Engelbrecht, C.; Gruber, T.M.; Iannaccone, A.; Jegen, M.; et al. Maternal and neonatal outcomes of pregnancies with COVID-19 after medically assisted reproduction: Results from the prospective COVID-19-Related Obstetrical and Neonatal Outcome Study. *Am. J. Obstet. Gynecol.* **2022**, *227*, 495.e1–495.e11. [CrossRef] [PubMed]
26. Gurol-Urganci, I.; Jardine, J.E.; Carroll, F.; Draycott, T.; Dunn, G.; Fremeaux, A.; Harris, T.; Hawdon, J.; Morris, E.; Muller, P.; et al. Maternal and perinatal outcomes of pregnant women with SARS-CoV-2 infection at the time of birth in England: National cohort study. *Am. J. Obstet. Gynecol.* **2021**, *225*, 521.e1–522.e11. [CrossRef] [PubMed]
27. Mohan, M.; Appiah-Sakyi, K.; Oliparambil, A.; Pullattayil, A.K.; Lindow, S.W.; Ahmed, B.; Konje, J.C. A Meta-Analysis of the Global Stillbirth Rates during the COVID-19 Pandemic. *J. Clin. Med.* **2023**, *12*, 7219. [CrossRef]
28. Heuser, C.; Manuck, T.; Hossain, S.; Silver, R.; Varner, M. Non-anomalous stillbirth by gestational age: Trends differ based on method of epidemiologic calculation. *J. Matern. Fetal Neonatal Med.* **2010**, *23*, 720–724. [CrossRef]
29. Allotey, J.; Stallings, E.; Bonet, M.; Yap, M.; Chatterjee, S.; Kew, T.; Debenham, L.; Llavall, A.C.; Dixit, A.; Zhou, D.; et al. Clinical manifestations, risk factors, and maternal and perinatal outcomes of coronavirus disease 2019 in pregnancy: Living systematic review and meta-analysis. *BMJ* **2020**, *370*, m3320. [CrossRef]
30. Hofbauer, A.; Schneider, H.; Kehl, S.; Reutter, H.; Pecks, U.; Andresen, K.; Morhart, P. SARS-CoV-2 Infection in Pregnancy and Incidence of Congenital Malformations-is there a Correlation? Analysis of 8032 Pregnancies from the CRONOS Registry. *Z. Geburtshilfe Neonatol.* **2024**, *228*, 65–73. [CrossRef]
31. Gullo, G.; Scaglione, M.; Cucinella, G.; Riva, A.; Coldebella, D.; Cavaliere, A.F.; Signore, F.; Buzzaccarini, G.; Spagnol, G.; Laganà, A.S.; et al. Congenital Zika Syndrome: Genetic Avenues for Diagnosis and Therapy, Possible Management and Long-Term Outcomes. *J. Clin. Med.* **2022**, *11*, 1351. [CrossRef] [PubMed]
32. Incognito, G.G.; Distefano, R.E.C.; Campo, G.; Gulino, F.A.; Gulisano, C.; Gullotta, C.; Gullo, G.; Cucinella, G.; Tuscano, A.; Bruno, M.T.; et al. Comparison of Maternal and Neonatal Outcomes between SARS-CoV-2 Variants: A Retrospective, Monocentric Study. *J. Clin. Med.* **2023**, *12*, 6329. [CrossRef] [PubMed]
33. Berger, R.; Rath, W.; Abele, H.; Garnier, Y.; Kuon, R.-J.; Maul, H. Reducing the Risk of Preterm Birth by Ambulatory Risk Factor Management. *Dtsch. Arztebl. Int.* **2019**, *116*, 858–864. [CrossRef] [PubMed]
34. Martin, J.A.; Hamilton, B.E.; Osterman, M.J.K. Births in the United States, 2022. *NCHS Data Brief* **2023**, 1–8.
35. Ellington, S.; Olson, C.K. Safety of mRNA COVID-19 vaccines during pregnancy. *Lancet Infect. Dis.* **2022**, *22*, 1514–1515. [CrossRef]
36. Magnus, M.C.; Örtqvist, A.K.; Dahlqwist, E.; Ljung, R.; Skår, F.; Oakley, L.; Macsali, F.; Pasternak, B.; Gjessing, H.K.; Håberg, S.E.; et al. Association of SARS-CoV-2 Vaccination During Pregnancy With Pregnancy Outcomes. *JAMA* **2022**, *327*, 1469–1477. [CrossRef]

Journal of
*Clinical Medicine*

MDPI

*Article*

# Personality Traits and Depression in Infertile Couples during the COVID-19

**Sofia Burgio [1,*], Concetta Polizzi [2], Marianna Alesi [2], Antonio Perino [1], Gaspare Cucinella [1], Yulia Kotlik [1], Alessandra Lopez [1], Alessandra Vassiliadis [3] and Giuseppe Gullo [1]**

1 Department of Obstetrics and Gynaecology, IVF UNIT, Villa Sofia—V. Cervello Hospital, University of Palermo, 90128 Palermo, Italy
2 Department of Psychology, Educational Science and Human Movement, University of Palermo, 90128 Palermo, Italy
3 Department of Health Promotion, Mother and Child Care, Internal Medicine and Medical Specialties, University of Palermo, 90128 Palermo, Italy
* Correspondence: sofiaburgio4@gmail.com

**Abstract: Background/Objectives**: The study presented in this paper seeks to examine how personality traits and depressive symptoms, influenced by the fear of COVID-19, interact in infertile couples, who are on the verge of commencing treatments with assisted reproductive technology (ART). The purpose of this observational study was to explore the relationship between personality traits in infertile couples and the occurrence of depressive symptoms, taking into account the mediating effect of COVID-19 fear. **Methods**: The study sample consisted of 108 women and 71 men (N = 179), all of whom had received an infertility diagnosis and expressed a desire to begin ART treatment at a Sicilian ART center; they were subsequently recruited. The Personality Inventory (PI), Beck Depression Inventory (BDI) and Fear of COVID (FCV-19S) were used for data collection. **Results**: The FCV-19S demonstrates a significant positive correlation with both neuroticism ($r = 0.25$, $p = 0.001$) and agreeableness ($r = 0.19$, $p = 0.012$). In addition, there is a significant correlation between FCV-19S ($r = 0.67$, $p < 0.001$) and depression symptoms. The mediation analysis reveals that neuroticism is a predictor of fear of COVID-19 ($\beta = 1.77$, $p = 0.001$) and depression ($\beta = 0.22$, $p = 0.002$). Additionally, the fear of COVID-19 significantly influences ($\beta = 0.12$, $p < 0.001$) depression. **Conclusions**: This study found that neuroticism and agreeableness are positively linked to the fear of COVID-19, and women displayed notable mild mood disorders. Neuroticism predicted both depression and fear of COVID-19, while fear of COVID-19 predicted depressive symptoms. However, the total efficacy of the mediation model was not significant, thereby suggesting that the variables do not fully explain this model.

**Keywords:** infertility; personality traits; depression; COVID-19; assisted reproductive technology (ART)

## 1. Introduction

Many consider that assisted reproduction technology (ART) treatments represent the most significant scientific advancement in the search for solutions to address infertility and the difficulties of spontaneous conception in achieving desired parenthood. Previously considered as uncommon and atypical conditions, these issues are now increasingly prevalent due to the advancing age of mothers [1] and various environmental factors.

It is worth noting that, from 2013 to 2021, there was an exponential increase in the number of couples undergoing first, second, and third level ART techniques (from 71,741 couples in 2013 to 86,090 in 2021), and that Sicily has a high percentage of currently active ART centers [2] (Activities of the Italian National ART Registry—2021).

Infertility is identified as the inability to achieve pregnancy after one year of attempting through frequent and unprotected sexual intercourse, or as the inability of an individual or couple to conceive [3]. This condition, which affects 10 to 15% of couples worldwide, with half of the cases attributed to the male factor [4], represents a significant public health issue, both in terms of increasingly concerning low birth rates and costs [3,5]. The number of couples in Italy experiencing difficulties in natural conception has doubled since 1996, reaching a proportion of one in five [6].

From a psychological perspective, infertility is particularly burdensome for both men and women. It deeply affects individual and couple well-being [7]. Symptoms related to depression and anxiety are the most frequent reactions to infertility and the beginning of an ART journey [8]. The high prevalence of depressive and/or anxiety disorders raises the possibility that certain personality traits may predispose individuals to the development of depression and anxiety in response to the condition of infertility, in addition to the emotional burden of treatments to achieve a pregnancy [9].

A longitudinal study conducted in Italy has highlighted that 17.9% of the women involved in such treatments exhibited depressive symptoms, while 14.7% displayed symptoms of anxiety. However, depressive symptoms affected 6.9% of men and symptoms of anxiety affected 4.5% of cases [10]. Depression, compared to anxiety, therefore, seems to be more prevalent among infertile couples. Furthermore, a survey of 43 women has revealed that certain beliefs regarding motherhood and the desire for 'perfectionism', perceived as a personality trait, are associated with lower levels of fertility-related quality of life [11].

According to the Big Five theory of personality traits, Costa and McCrae [12] have proposed the following taxonomy, which is based on five major factors: extraversion, neuroticism, agreeableness, conscientiousness, and openness to experience. Various studies have demonstrated that there are personality differences in determining reproductive behavior [13,14].

Neuroticism reflects a general tendency to experience negative emotions, such as anxiety, and to become easily distressed. Neuroticism has been associated with difficulties in social relationships, such as lower relational quality and interpersonal negativity in marriage [15,16]. Furthermore, neuroticism has been linked to intentions of procreation. In a sample of young German adults, individuals with high neuroticism displayed greater decisional ambivalence regarding the idea of becoming a parent [17]. Such decisional ambivalence can lead to postponing parenthood, in addition to having fewer children [14] and, therefore, to seeking ART, also due to advanced maternal age.

In light of this review of studies in the literature, it is of great interest to understand which relationships might exist between such personality traits and depressive symptoms, in a social context mediated by the presence of the COVID-19 pandemic.

In the context of the latter [18], the main scientific and professional societies regarding the field of fertility [19,20] have advised postponing a pregnancy [21] insofar as monitoring an ART journey requires continuous checks, which are not only gynecological but also hormonal. With a rationale of containing the pandemic emergency, with measures such as social distancing and lockdown, it was preferable to advise delaying taking all unnecessary risks. Moreover, ART services are often located in facilities not immediately adapted to respecting safety guidelines issued by governments around the world in containing the pandemic.

Personality traits can have a significant impact on how individuals perceive threats and react to crises like pandemics [22]. Individuals with tendencies towards neuroticism, anxiety, emotional instability, and lack of security have shown an increase in stress levels and negative emotional reactions [23]. Caci and colleagues [24] observed that individuals with a high degree of neuroticism exhibited greater fears related to the effects of COVID-19 in everyday life, tending to experience boredom more easily and to indulge in negative thoughts and fantasies.

Precisely because neuroticism is identified, according to the Big Five model [12], as the primary trait influencing the management of fear, people with a high level of neurotic traits may be more susceptible to perceiving danger, an intense emotional response, and pay greater attention to threats, with a reduced capacity to deal with stressful situations [25].

Although the stress related to fertility can be considered comparable to that generated by the pandemic [26,27], the emotional impact of the pandemic on infertile patients is significant [28].

In light of what has been presented, the purpose of this observational study is to investigate personality factors in infertile couples and their relationship with the presence of any depressive symptoms, considering the role of fear of COVID-19 as a mediating variable.

This study, therefore, has the following hypotheses:

- To verify the existence of significant correlations between personality factors, depression, and fear of COVID;
- To verify the relationship between personality traits and depression, taking into account the role that a fear of COVID-19 may have played in mediating such an association, in infertile men and women who were about to commence a medically assisted reproduction (MAR) journey.

## 2. Materials and Methods

### 2.1. Participants

A total of 108 women and 71 men (N = 179), who had received an infertility diagnosis and expressed a desire to start ART treatment at a Sicilian ART center, were recruited. The study was conducted over the course of one year from July 2021 to July 2022, and the inclusion criteria were to have received an infertility diagnosis and an understanding of Italian for the administration of psychometric tests. Some cases were excluded where questionnaires were incomplete.

The sample characteristics (see Table 1) confirmed that the study participants were mostly couples from a middle–low socioeconomic and cultural background. Indeed, the assisted reproduction center, where the participants were recruited, is located in an area particularly at risk of socioeconomic disadvantage. The center, therefore, serves as the only clinic offering ART services at reduced costs compared to other centers.

**Table 1.** Descriptive characteristics of the sample (N = 179).

| Variables | Women | | Men | |
|---|---|---|---|---|
| | Mean | SD | Mean | SD |
| Age: | 34.6 | 5.65 | 37.3 | 5.93 |
| Nationality: | | | | |
| Italian | 75.9% | | 77.5% | |
| Other | 24.1% | | 22.5% | |
| | 96.3% | | 97.2% | |
| | 3.7% | | 2.8% | |
| Relationship status: | | | | |
| Married | 75.9% | | 77.5% | |
| Cohabiting | 24.1% | | 22.5% | |
| Educational level: | | | | |
| Elementary school | 5.6% | | 1.4% | |
| Middle school | 35.1% | | 31% | |
| Vocational diploma | 9.3% | | 25.4% | |
| High school diploma | 24.1% | | 28.2% | |
| Bachelor's degree | 21.3% | | 11.3% | |
| PhD/Specialization | 4.6% | | 2.8% | |
| Job type: | | | | |
| Homemaker | 39.2% | | 1.4% | |
| Student | 2.8% | | | |
| Factory worker | 0.9% | | 18.6% | |
| Office worker | 32.7% | | 34.3% | |

**Table 1.** *Cont.*

| Variables | Women | Men |
|---|---|---|
| Executive | 2.8% | 1.4% |
| Craftsman/woman | | 7.1% |
| Merchant | 0.9% | 2.9% |
| Freelancer | 0.9% | 17.1% |
| Teacher | 4.7% | 1.4% |
| Unemployed | 10.3% | 15.7% |
| Seeking initial employment | 4.7% | |
| Presence of children: | | |
| No | 85% | 85.5% |
| 1 | 14% | 13% |
| 2 | | 1.4% |
| 3 or >3 | 0.9% | |
| Miscarriages: | | |
| No | 72.9% | |
| Yes, spontaneous | 24.3% | |
| Yes, voluntary termination of pregnancy | 2.8% | |
| First attempt at ART: | | |
| Yes | 72.9% | 69.5% |
| No | 27.1% | 30.5% |
| Presence of other Pathologies: | | |
| No | 71.3% | 84.6% |
| Yes, organic type | 23.1% | 12.3% |
| Yes, psychological type | 0.9% | |
| Healthy carrier | 4.6% | 3.1% |
| Healthy diet: | | |
| Yes | 83.3% | 78.3% |
| No | 16.7% | 21.7% |
| Sport: | | |
| Yes | 22.2% | 40.6% |
| No | 77.8% | 59.4% |
| Smoking: | | |
| Yes | 29.6% | 40.6% |
| No | 70.4% | 59.4% |
| Alcohol: | | |
| Yes | 4.6% | 5.8% |
| No | 95.4% | 94.2% |
| Taking medication: | | |
| Yes | 22.2% | 18.8% |
| No | 77.8% | 81.2% |
| Social support network: | | |
| Limited | 54.2% | 42.6% |
| Wide | 45.8% | 57.4% |
| Support system for ART journey: | | |
| Family | 62.9% | 53% |
| Friends | 3.7% | 4.5% |
| Both | 33.3% | 42.4% |

Fear of COVID-19 is significantly and positively correlated with neuroticism (r = 0.25, $p$ = 0.001), as well as with agreeableness (r = 0.19, $p$ = 0.012). Furthermore, fear of COVID-19 (r = 0.67, $p$ < 0.001) is significantly correlated with depressive symptoms.

### 2.2. Procedures and Instruments

The survey sample was recruited during the first gynecological visit, following a clinical interview in which couples were invited to participate in the research, and where informed consent to the study was provided and read. Participation was voluntary and anonymous, and the administration time of the psychometric tools lasted for approximately 20 min.

The research journey included the use of the following measures:

- A socio-demographic form, constructed ad hoc, in which the following data were collected: sex, age, nationality, relationship status, educational level, profession type (where relevant), number of children, incidence of previous miscarriages, information relating to whether it was the first attempt at ART, presence of previous pathologies, healthy eating habits, engaging in physical and sports activities, smoking habit, alcohol consumption, use of pharmacotherapy, and the presence of a social support network.
- Personality Inventory (PI) [29], a self-reporting questionnaire consisting of 20 items to assess personality factors, according to the Big Five model [12]. The questionnaire has five subscales which investigate the relative personality factors: extraversion, defined as a search for aggregation, assertiveness, positive emotionality, and a search for excitement; conscientiousness, defined as a sense of duty and self-discipline; openness regarding experiences and intellectual curiosity; agreeableness, defined as trusting in others and the ability to cooperate; and neuroticism, defined as a tendency to be emotionally unstable. Each item had a 5-point Likert scale with scores ranging from 1 = strongly disagree to 5 = strongly agree. Regarding psychometric properties, the tool demonstrated reliable internal consistency ($\alpha > 0.70$).
- Beck Depression Inventory II (BDI) [30] is a self-reporting questionnaire consisting of 21 items; its aim is to measure the cognitive, motivational, affective, and behavioral symptoms of depression. Each item has a score ranging from 0 to 3, and the higher the BDI score, the more profound the degree of depression is. Regarding psychometric properties, the tool demonstrated reliable internal consistency ($\alpha > 0.80$).
- A fear of COVID-19 (FCV-19S) [31] is a seven-item scale which assesses the fear of COVID-19. The seven items are rated on a 5-point Likert scale from 1 (strongly disagree) to 5 (strongly agree), with scores ranging from 7 to 35. The higher the score, the greater the fear of COVID-19. Regarding psychometric properties, the FCV-19S also demonstrated reliable internal consistency ($\alpha > 0.80$).

### 2.3. Statistical Analyses

Preliminary analyses (means, SDs, and percentages) were calculated for the various socio-demographic variables. The variables being studied were investigated by performing Pearson correlations among personality factors, depression, and fear of COVID-19. An independent samples *t*-test was conducted to investigate the difference between the mean values of men and women for the depression variable. Finally, a mediation model was constructed in order to investigate the relationship between personality traits and depression, exploring the mediating role of the COVID-19 fear variable. Confidence intervals were reported, and bootstrapping was used to estimate these intervals. The significance of the indirect effect is indicated if the interval between the upper and lower confidence limits does not contain zero [32]. All analyses were performed using the SPSS statistical software version 28 (IBM SPSS Statistics).

## 3. Results

The results demonstrated that the average age of the women in the study was 34.6 (SD = 5.65), while that for men was 37.3 (SD = 5.93). The majority of women (96.3%) and men (97.2%) were Italian. The most prevalent relationship status was 'marriage' for women (75.9%) and men (77.5%). Regarding education level, 35.3% of women and 31% of men had completed lower secondary education. Approximately 38.3% of the women were housewives, while the majority of men were employed (34.3%). Additionally, 85% of the women did not already have children, similar to the majority of men (85.5%).

In total, 72.9% of the women reported having had no previous miscarriages, in addition to not having any psychological or organic pathological conditions apart from infertility; this statement was shared by 71.3% of the women and the majority of men reported the same characteristic (84.6%).

Although most women (83.3%) and men (78.3%) claimed to follow a healthy diet, the majority of them did not engage in any sports or physical activity (77.8% of women and 59.4% of men). Similarly, a regular smoking habit (70.4%), alcohol consumption (95.4%), and medication (77.8%) were absent among women. Men displayed similar habits, with 59.4% stating that they were non-smokers, 94.2% confirming they did not regularly consume alcohol, and 81.2% did not regularly use medication.

While the majority of women described their social network as "limited" (54.2%), most men referred to having an extensive social network (57.4%). Finally, both women (62.9%) and men (53%) reported having their family as the main reference point regarding support and emotional backing in starting their ART journey.

Descriptive statistics are reported in Table 1 above.

The results of the correlations are shown in Table 2 below.

**Table 2.** Correlations between personality factors, depression (BDI), and fear of COVID-19 (FCV-19S) in infertile couples.

| Variables | 1 | 2 | 3 | 4 | 5 | 6 | 7 |
|---|---|---|---|---|---|---|---|
| 1. Neuroticism | - | | | | | | |
| 2. Conscientiousness | −0.071 | - | | | | | |
| 3. Openness | −0.051 | 0.107 | - | | | | |
| 4. Extroversion | −0.035 | 0.059 | 0.152 | - | | | |
| 5. Agreeableness | 0.102 | 0.035 | 0.021 | −0.011 | - | | |
| 6. BDI | −0.004 | −0.009 | 0.043 | 0.016 | −0.004 | - | |
| 7. FCV-19S | 0.252 ** | 0.050 | 0.141 | 0.072 | 0.188 * | 0.666 ** | - |
| M | 8.78 | 15.06 | 12.4 | 12.9 | 13.1 | 9.63 | 13.7 |
| SD | 3.07 | 2.23 | 2.46 | 1.80 | 2.40 | 5.27 | 6.41 |
| Skewness | 0.91 | −0.81 | 0.23 | 0.20 | −0.14 | −0.66 | 1.13 |
| Kurtosis | 1.09 | 1.55 | 0.37 | 1.9 | 0.38 | −0.60 | 1.07 |

* $p < 0.05$; ** $p < 0.01$.

Additionally, the independent samples *t*-test indicated a difference regarding the depression variable [t (1177) = 15.75, $p < 0.001$].

Descriptive analyses highlighted BDI scores greater than 10, that is, the cut-off point for identifying a mild mood disorder in women (M = 12.8; SD = 1.6) but not in men (M = 4.6; SD = 5).

Based on the results obtained from the correlations, and from the literature, mediation models were developed in which the relationships between personality factors, fear of COVID-19, and depressive symptoms were analyzed.

The mediation hypothesis was examined by testing the significance of the indirect effect of fear of COVID-19 on depressive symptoms.

The results of the mediation analyses performed with Hayes' procedure [33] are presented in Figure 1 below.

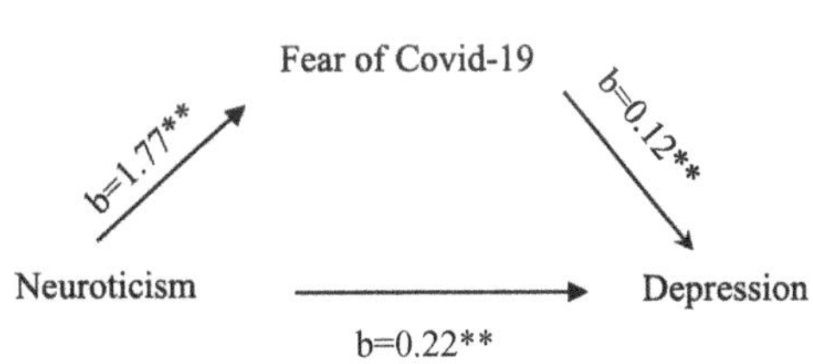


**Figure 1.** Mediation model.

The results demonstrated that neuroticism predicted a fear of COVID-19 ($\beta$ = 1.77, ** $p = 0.001$), as well as depression ($\beta$ = 0.22, ** $p = 0.002$). The mediator, fear of COVID-19, also significantly predicted ($\beta$ = 0.12, ** $p < 0.001$) the depression variable. In conclusion, the mediation test indicated that neuroticism directly influenced depression ($p = 0.002$), and the effect of the mediator, fear of COVID-19, was also significant (SE = 0.016, 95% CI = [0.02, 0.08]). However, no total effect of the model was found to be significant ($p = 0.96$).

## 4. Discussion

The results of the observational study have demonstrated that a fear of COVID-19 is significantly correlated with neuroticism and the personality trait of agreeableness. The correlation between fear of COVID-19 and neuroticism aligns with the literature in the field, which indicates that this personality trait is more closely associated with the presence of anxiety disorders, depression, and generally a lower level of satisfaction with one's quality of life [34–36]. Other studies that have examined different variables and sample characteristics have reported strong associations between neuroticism and various mental health problems, thereby highlighting how this personality trait is a significant risk factor, even in non-pregnant populations [37]. Indeed, as is known, personality traits are predictors of significant health outcomes as they also affect physical illnesses and influence an individual's mental health [38]. Thus, as supported by other studies in the literature, having a personality with high levels of neuroticism increases the fear of COVID-19 [39], and this was also detected in a predictive sense. On the other hand, the correlation between fear of COVID-19 and agreeableness is inconsistent with studies in the literature [40,41], which suggests that this personality trait corresponds to a greater acceptance of the changes imposed by COVID-19, in addition to the presence of less dysfunctional behaviors.

It could be hypothesized that, in the sample examined, being willing and open to meeting others (a characteristic typical of individuals who report high levels of agreeableness) may increase the perception of a greater fear of social contact, which is so central in the organization of their personality. Furthermore, results from other recent studies have suggested that individuals with high levels of agreeableness (in particular) have tended to comply more with government rules and recommendations to combat COVID-19 [42]. These data may also be supported by the correlation between agreeableness and a fear of COVID-19.

A significant finding supported by studies in the literature is the correlation between fear of COVID-19 and depression [43–45]. Indeed, many research paths have supported the study's results. Indeed, a fear of COVID-19 has been positively correlated with mental health consequences such as depression, stress, and anxiety symptoms, indicating that the higher the FCV-19S score, the higher the level of mental health issues such as depression [46]. Çıkrıkçı et al. [47] have shown that the fear of illness and infection can lead to depression, anxiety, and stress in some people. In a similar vein, Huang and Zhao [48] have observed that many individuals experienced moderate-to-severe levels of depression, anxiety, and stress during the initial phase of the COVID-19 pandemic. Yet, another study described the positive relationship between anxiety, stress, depression, intolerance to uncertainty, FCV-19S, and positivity, finding mediators. This research indicated a statistically significant positive correlation between FCV-19S and depression, intolerance to uncertainty, anxiety, and stress [49].

Equally significant is the difference between the mean scores of men and women regarding the scores reported on the BDI; women displayed higher scores, indicating, according to the scoring provided by the psychometric tool, the presence of a mild mood disorder. This finding is also supported by already published studies which emphasize how depression is the condition most widespread among infertile women [50], compared to men who report lower scores [51,52].

There are many studies in the literature regarding degrees of depression because depression is a widespread condition and it is often related to infertility [50,53]. At present, depression is the most frequently diagnosed psychiatric condition worldwide [54,55]. Moreover, even after treatments with assisted reproduction techniques, couples sometimes fail to overcome the feelings of mourning and loss associated with infertility [56]. Additionally, it is important to highlight that infertility also contributes to the risk of depression. According to Nik Hazlina et al. [57], women experiencing infertility are 1.4 times more likely to suffer from depression. This indicates that infertility elevates the risk of depression. Therefore, this finding should be considered a guiding factor for clinical and research interventions.

Of greater significance is the average score reported by women on the BDI (>10), which highlights the presence of a mild mood disorder, suggesting clinical indications regarding the intervention to be made with these women. Indeed, even regarding couples undergoing their first attempt of ART, health professionals should bear in mind these clinically significant data and particularly consider the emotional aspect of the infertility condition, often omitted in the gynecology department [58,59].

Moreover, the mediation analysis revealed how neuroticism predicted a fear of COVID-19, as well as having a significant effect on depression. Neuroticism is a personality trait which was originally defined to include anxiety, emotional instability, worry, tension, and self-pity. This negative affectivity can be accompanied by a pervasive perception that the world is a dangerous and threatening place, along with beliefs about one's inability to manage or cope with difficult events [60]. In agreement with previous studies [24,61,62], the results confirmed Taylor's [63] prediction that individuals with a high level of neuroticism are vulnerable to significant discomfort during pandemics because they are sensitive to stress and infection threats. Thus, having a personality with high levels of neuroticism can predict a real fear of COVID-19.

The role of neuroticism as a predictor of depression is also supported by the literature in this field [64,65]. Such studies suggest, for example, a relationship mediated by the environment between neuroticism and depression. This personality factor interacts with stressful life events, triggering new episodes of depression at young and more advanced ages [66,67]. Similarly, the pandemic can be understood in this sense as a definitively stressful life event, which, in addition to predicting the depression variable, permits the results obtained from the mediation model within the considerations already made by studies in the literature. A note of caution is that although these direct and indirect relationships in the mediation model are significant (with some aligning with the existing literature), the fact that the total effect of the mediation model is not significant suggests the need to consider other variables not examined in this study in order to explain the relationship between neuroticism and depression, with a fear of COVID-19 as a mediator.

## 5. Conclusions

The study has highlighted how the well-being of infertile couples can be significantly compromised by certain personality traits and the potential presence of depression, especially during global emergencies such as the COVID-19 pandemic. Some correlations, such as the relationship between neuroticism and a fear of COVID-19, are supported by the current literature. Other innovative findings have also been highlighted in this study; for example, the correlation between agreeableness and a fear of COVID-19 diverge from the current literature in the field.

The presence of mild mood disorders in the average scores of infertile women underscores the importance of addressing the well-being of these patients from their initial consultation regarding ART services. This suggests a shift in clinical practice which should focus not only on addressing infertility itself but also on empowering infertile women psychologically by leveraging their resources. In addition, and as highlighted by the mediation model, certain personality traits, such as neuroticism, are effective predictors of the fear of COVID-19 and the presence of depressive symptoms. Similarly, the authors of this study noted that perceiving an intense fear of COVID-19 predicted significant depression. However, while these individual relationships are significant, the total impact of the model cannot be said to be significant, indicating that the mediation model is not fully explained by the variables examined. This suggests that the study may have required the elaboration of additional variables.

The consequences of this study may have an impact on various fields, including clinical practice, future research, and the understanding of psychological dynamics in healthcare emergencies. The finding that neuroticism is a strong predictor of depression and a fear of COVID-19 highlights the importance of assessing personality traits in the psychological evaluations of patients. Mental health professionals may find it efficacious to implement more targeted screenings and personalized interventions in addressing symptoms of depression and anxiety, especially in emergency contexts such as pandemics. The presence of mild mood disorders among women suggests the need for additional psychological support, even during the initial consultation with assisted reproduction services. Specialists in the field might consider integrating psychological interventions into treatment protocols to improve the overall well-being of patients.

Finally, the insignificance of the overall effect of the mediation model suggests that other variables might influence the relationship between neuroticism, a fear of COVID-19, and depression. Future research could explore additional confounding or mediating factors, such as social support, resilience, or past trauma experiences. Since the mediation model did not demonstrate a significant effect on the mental health of patients, longitudinal studies tracking participants over time could provide further insights into how these relationships evolve and impact on mental health.

In light of the considerations presented in this paper, infertility in couples can be said to be a heterogeneous condition, with great variability. Studying the personalities of men and women who access ART services, and the potential impact of depression, are undoubtedly variables of primary importance when dealing with infertility. This is particularly relevant if studies can promptly increase the quantity and quality of evidence-based clinical interventions. Of the limitations of this study, the lack of a variable with which to measure anxiety should certainly be highlighted; such an inclusion may have clarified the relationship between neuroticism and depression.

**Author Contributions:** Conceptualization, S.B., C.P., M.A., A.P., G.C. and G.G.; methodology, S.B., G.G. and A.V.; software, G.G.; validation, Y.K., A.L. and S.B.; formal analysis, G.G. and S.B.; investigation, S.B., Y.K., A.P., A.L., A.V. and G.G.; resources, G.G. and S.B.; data curation, G.G. and S.B.; writing—original draft preparation, S.B.; writing—review and editing, A.P., M.A., C.P. and G.G.; visualization, S.B. and G.C.; supervision, G.G.; project administration, C.P. and M.A. All authors have read and agreed to the published version of the manuscript.

**Funding:** This research received no external funding.

**Institutional Review Board Statement:** The study was conducted in accordance with the Declaration of Helsinki and it was approved by the Palermo 2 Ethical Committee (registry number 60AOR2020 dated 12 March 2020).

**Informed Consent Statement:** Informed consent was obtained from all subjects involved in the study. Written informed consent was obtained from the patients to publish this paper.

**Data Availability Statement:** The data presented in this study are available on request from the corresponding author.

**Conflicts of Interest:** The authors declare no conflicts of interest.

## References

1. Ionio, C.; Mascheroni, E.; Colombo, C.; Lista, G. Prenatal attachment in twin pregnancy. In *Multiple Pregnancy-New Challenges*; IntechOpen: Rijeka, Croatia, 2018.
2. Activities of the Italian National ART Registry. 2021. Available online: https://www.iss.it/rpma-dati-registro (accessed on 10 June 2024).
3. Zegers-Hochschild, F.; Adamson, G.D.; Dyer, S.; Racowsky, C.; de Mouzon, J.; Sokol, R.; Rienzi, L.; Sunde, A.; Schmidt, L.; Cooke, I.D.; et al. The international glossary on infertility and fertility care. *Fertil. Steril.* **2017**, *108*, 393–406. [CrossRef] [PubMed]
4. Borght, M.V.; Wyns, C. Fertility and infertility: Definition and epidemiology. *Clin. Biochem.* **2018**, *62*, 2–10. [CrossRef]
5. Hayden, R.P.; Flannigan, R.; Schlegel, P.N. The role of lifestyle in male infertility: Diet, physical activity, and body habitus. *Curr. Urol. Rep.* **2018**, *19*, 56. [CrossRef]
6. Italian Ministry of Health. Piano Nazionale per la Fertilità. Available online: https://www.salute.gov.it/imgs/C_17_pubblicazioni_2367_allegato.pdf (accessed on 10 June 2024).

7. Babore, A.; Stuppia, L.; Trumello, C.; Candelori, C.; Antonucci, I. Male factor infertility and lack of openness about infertility as risk factors for depressive symptoms in males undergoing assisted reproductive technology treatment in Italy. *Fertil. Steril.* **2017**, *107*, 1041–1047. [CrossRef]
8. Matthiesen SM, S.; Frederiksen, Y.; Ingerslev, H.J.; Zachariae, R. Stress, distress, and outcome of assisted reproductive technology (ART): A meta-analysis. *Hum. Reprod.* **2011**, *26*, 2763–2776. [CrossRef] [PubMed]
9. Volgsten, H.; Ekselius, L.; Poromaa, I.S.; Svanberg, A.S. Personality traits associated with depressive and anxiety disorders in infertile women and men undergoing in vitro fertilization treatment. *Acta Obs. Gyn. Scan* **2010**, *89*, 27–34. [CrossRef]
10. Chiaffarino, F.; Baldini, M.P.; Scarduelli, C.; Bommarito, F.; Ambrosio, S.; D'Orsi, C.; Torretta, R.; Bonizzoni, M.; Ragni, G. Prevalence and incidence of depressive and anxious symptoms in couples undergoing assisted reproductive treatment in an Italian infertility department. *EJOG* **2011**, *158*, 235–241. [CrossRef] [PubMed]
11. Zarbo, C.; Brugnera, A.; Compare, A.; Candeloro, I.; Secomandi, R.; Betto, E.; Fusi, F.; Marabini, R.; Malandrino, C.; Carnelli, M.; et al. Perfectionistic traits and importance given to parenthood are associated with infertility-related quality of life in a sample of infertile women with and without endometriosis. *SRH* **2018**, *17*, 86–90. [CrossRef] [PubMed]
12. Costa, P.T.; McCrae, R.R. The revised neo personality inventory (neo-pi-r). *SAGE Handb. Personal. Theory Assess.* **2008**, *2*, 179–198.
13. Dragan, W.Ł.; Bates, J.E.; Lansford, J.E.; Dodge, K.A.; Pettit, G.S. Individual and Environmental Predictors of Age of First Intercourse and Number of Children by Age 27. *Front. Psychol.* **2020**, *11*, 1639. [CrossRef]
14. Jokela, M. Characteristics of the first child predict the parents' probability of having another child. *Dev. Psychol.* **2010**, *46*, 915–926. [CrossRef] [PubMed]
15. Saeed Abbasi, I.; Rattan, N.; Kousar, T.; Khalifa Elsayed, F. Neuroticism and close relationships: How negative affect is linked with relationship disaffection in couples. *Am. J. Fam. Ther.* **2018**, *46*, 139–152. [CrossRef]
16. Kreuzer, M.; Gollwitzer, M. Neuroticism and satisfaction in romantic relationships: A systematic investigation of intra-and interpersonal processes with a longitudinal approach. *EJP* **2022**, *36*, 149–179. [CrossRef]
17. Pinquart, M.; Stotzka, C.; Silbereisen, R.K. Personality and ambivalence in decisions about becoming parents. *Soc. Behav. Pers.* **2008**, *36*, 87–95. [CrossRef]
18. Giorli, A.; Ferretti, F.; Biagini, C.; Salerni, L.; Bindi, I.; Dasgupta, S.; Pozza, A.; Gualtieri, G.; Gusinu, R.; Coluccia, A.; et al. A literature systematic review with meta-analysis of symptoms prevalence in COVID-19: The relevance of olfactory symptoms in infection not requiring hospitalization. *Curr. Treat. Option Ne* **2020**, *22*, 36. [CrossRef] [PubMed]
19. ESHRE—European Society for Human Reproduction and Embryology. Coronavirus COVID-19: ESHRE Statement on Pregnancy and Conception. Available online: https://www.eshre.eu/Europe/Position-statements/COVID19 (accessed on 19 March 2020).
20. IFFS. IFFS Statements on COVID-19 and Reproduction. Available online: https://www.iffsreproduction.org/iffs-COVID-19-task-force-statements/ (accessed on 19 March 2020).
21. Souza, M.; Nakagawa, H.; Taitson, P.F.; Cordts, E.B.; Antunes, R.A. Management of ART and COVID-19: Infertility in times of pandemic. What now? *JBRA Assist. Reprod.* **2020**, *24*, 231–232. [CrossRef]
22. Kohút, M.; Kohútová, V.; Halama, P. Big Five predictors of pandemic-related behavior and emotions in the first and second COVID-19 pandemic wave in Slovakia. *Personal. Individ. Differ.* **2021**, *180*, 110934. [CrossRef] [PubMed]
23. Cusinato, M.; Iannattone, S.; Spoto, A.; Poli, M.; Moretti, C.; Gatta, M.; Miscioscia, M. Stress, resilience, and well-being in Italian children and their parents during the COVID-19 pandemic. *Int. J. Environ. Res. Public Health* **2020**, *17*, 8297. [CrossRef]
24. Caci, B.; Miceli, S.; Scrima, F.; Cardaci, M. Neuroticism and Fear of COVID-19. The Interplay between Boredom, Fantasy Engagement, and Perceived Control Over Time. *Front. Psychol.* **2020**, *11*, 574393. [CrossRef] [PubMed]
25. Polizzi, C.; Giordano, G.; Burgio, S.; Lavanco, G.; Alesi, M. Maternal Competence, Maternal Burnout and Personality Traits in Italian Mothers after the First COVID-19 Lockdown. *Int. J. Environ. Res. Public Health* **2022**, *19*, 9791. [CrossRef]
26. Pozza, A.; Marazziti, D.; Mucci, F.; Angelo, N.; Prestia, D.; Dèttore, D. Sexual response in obsessive-compulsive disorder: The role of obsessive beliefs. *CNS Spectr.* **2020**, *26*, 528–537. [CrossRef]
27. Vaughan, D.A.; Shah, J.S.; Penzias, A.S.; Domar, A.D.; Toth, T.L. Infertility remains a top stressor despite the COVID-19 pandemic. *Reprod. Biomed. Online* **2020**, *41*, 425–427. [CrossRef] [PubMed]
28. Turocy, J.M.; Robles, A.; Hercz, D.; D'Alton, M.; Forman, E.J.; Williams, Z. The emotional impact of the SRM Guidelines on fertility patients during the COVID-19 pandemic. *Fertil. Steril.* **2020**, *114*, e63. [CrossRef]
29. Caci, B.; Cardaci, M.; Tabacchi, M.E.; Scrima, F. Personality variables as predictors of Facebook usage. *Psychol. Rep.* **2014**, *114*, 528–539. [CrossRef] [PubMed]
30. Beck, A.T.; Steer, R.A.; Brown, G. Beck Depression Inventory–II (BDI-II) [Database Record]. *APA PsycTest* **1996**. [CrossRef]
31. Ahorsu, D.K.; Lin, C.; Imani, V.; Saffari, M.; Griffiths, M.D.; Pakpour, A.H. The Fear of COVID-19 Scale: Development and initial validation. *Int. J. Ment. Health Addict.* **2020**, *20*, 1537–1545. [CrossRef] [PubMed]
32. MacKinnon, D.P.; Fairchild, A.J.; Fritz, M.S. Mediation analysis. *Annu. Rev. Psychol.* **2007**, *58*, 593–614. [CrossRef] [PubMed]
33. Hayes, A.F. An index and test of linear moderated mediation. *Multivar. Behav. Res.* **2015**, *50*, 1–22. [CrossRef]
34. Wilt, J.; Oehlberg, K.; Revelle, W. Anxiety in personality. *Personal. Individ. Differ.* **2011**, *50*, 987–993. [CrossRef]
35. Mezquita, L.; Bravo, A.J.; Morizot, J.; Pilatti, A.; Pearson, M.R.; Ibáñez, M.I.; Cross-Cultural Addictions Study Team. Cross-cultural examination of the Big Five Personality Trait Short Questionnaire: Measurement invariance testing and associations with mental health. *PLoS ONE* **2019**, *14*, e0226223. [CrossRef]

36. Wang, Y.; Zhang, B. Impact of Personality Trait and Professional Identity on Work-Related Depression, Anxiety and Irritation among Chinese Nurses. *Southeast Asian J. Trop. Med. Public Health* **2017**, *48*, 447–454. [PubMed]
37. Montag, C.; Sindermann, C.; Rozgonjuk, D.; Yang, S.; Elhai, J.D.; Yang, H. Investigating Links between Fear of COVID-19, Neuroticism, Social Networks Use Disorder, and Smartphone Use Disorder Tendencies. *Front. Psychol.* **2021**, *12*, 682837. [CrossRef] [PubMed]
38. Odachi, R.; Takahashi, S.; Sugawara, D.; Tabata, M.; Kajiwara, T.; Hironishi, M.; Buyo, M. The Big Five personality traits and the fear of COVID-19 in predicting depression and anxiety among Japanese nurses caring for COVID-19 patients: A cross-sectional study in Wakayama prefecture. *PLoS ONE* **2022**, *17*, e0276803. [CrossRef] [PubMed]
39. Nazari, N.; Safitri, S.; Usak, M.; Arabmarkadeh, A.; Griffiths, M.D. Psychometric Validation of the Indonesian Version of the Fear of COVID-19 Scale: Personality Traits Predict the Fear of COVID-19. *Int. J. Ment. Health Addict.* **2023**, *21*, 1348–1364. [CrossRef] [PubMed]
40. Al-Omiri, M.K.; Alzoubi, I.A.; Al Nazeh, A.A.; Alomiri, A.K.; Maswady, M.N.; Lynch, E. COVID-19 and Personality: A Cross-Sectional Multicenter Study of the Relationship between Personality Factors and COVID-19-Related Impacts, Concerns, and Behaviors. *Front. Psychiatry* **2021**, *12*, 608730. [CrossRef] [PubMed]
41. Fink, M.; Bäuerle, A.; Schmidt, K.; Rheindorf, N.; Musche, V.; Dinse, H.; Moradian, S.; Weismüller, B.; Schweda, A.; Teufel, M.; et al. COVID-19-fear affects current safety behavior mediated by neuroticism—Results of a large cross-sectional study in Germany. *Front. Psychol.* **2021**, *12*, 671768. [CrossRef] [PubMed]
42. Asselmann, E.; Borghans, L.; Montizaan, R.; Seegers, P. The role of personality in the thoughts, feelings, and behaviors of students in Germany during the first weeks of the COVID-19 pandemic. *PLoS ONE* **2020**, *15*, e0242904. [CrossRef] [PubMed]
43. Erbiçer, E.S.; Metin, A.; Çetinkaya, A.; Şen, S. The relationship between fear of COVID-19 and depression, anxiety, and stress. In *European Psychologist*; Hogrefe Publishing: Göttingen, Germany, 2022.
44. Tsang, S.; Avery, A.R.; Duncan, G.E. Fear and depression linked to COVID-19 exposure A study of adult twins during the COVID-19 pandemic. *Psychiatry Res.* **2021**, *296*, 113699. [CrossRef]
45. Kausar, N.; Ishaq, A.; Qurban, H.; Rashid, H.A. Fear of COVID-19 and depression: Mediating role of anxiety and stress among university students. *JBM* **2021**, *8*, 9. [CrossRef]
46. Fitzpatrick, K.M.; Harris, C.; Drawve, G. Fear of COVID-19 and the mental health consequences in America. *Psychol. Trauma* **2020**, *12* (Suppl. S1), S17. [CrossRef]
47. Çıkrıkçı, Ö.; Çıkrıkçı, N.; Griffiths, M. Fear of COVID-19, stress and depression: A meta-analytic test of the mediating role of anxiety. *Psychol Psychother.* **2022**, *95*, 853–874. [CrossRef] [PubMed]
48. Huang, Y.; Zhao, N. Generalized anxiety disorder, depressive symptoms and sleep quality during COVID-19 outbreak in China: A web-based cross-sectional survey. *Psychiatry Res.* **2020**, *288*, 112954. [CrossRef] [PubMed]
49. Bakioğlu, F.; Korkmaz, O.; Ercan, H. Fear of COVID-19 and positivity: Mediating role of intolerance of uncertainty, depression, anxiety, and stress. *Int. J. Ment. Health Addict.* **2021**, *19*, 2369–2382. [CrossRef]
50. Burgio, S.; Polizzi, C.; Buzzaccarini, G.; Laganà, A.S.; Gullo, G.; Perricone, G.; Perino, A.; Cucinella, G.; Alesi, M. Psychological variables in medically assisted reproduction: A systematic review. *Przegląd Menopauzalny* **2022**, *21*, 47–63. [CrossRef] [PubMed]
51. Galhardo, A.; Pinto-Gouveia, J.; Cunha, M.; Matos, M. The impact of shame and self-judgment on psychopathology in infertile patients. *Hum. Reprod.* **2011**, *26*, 2408–2414. [CrossRef]
52. Wichman, C.L.; Ehlers, S.L.; Wichman, S.E.; Weaver, A.L.; Coddington, C. Comparison of multiple psychological distress measures between men and women preparing for in vitro fertilization. *Fertil Steril* **2011**, *95*, 717–721. [CrossRef]
53. Van Vleet, T.; Stark-Inbar, A.; Merzenich, M.M.; Jordan, J.T.; Wallace, D.L.; Lee, M.B.; Dawes, H.E.; Chang, E.F.; Nahum, M. Biases in processing of mood-congruent facial expressions in depression. *Psychiatry Res.* **2019**, *275*, 143–148. [CrossRef]
54. Downs, J.; Blackmore, A.M.; Epstein, A.; Skoss, R.; Langdon, K.; Jacoby, P.; Whitehouse, A.J.O.; Leonard, H.; Rowe, P.W.; Glasson, E.J.; et al. The prevalence of mental health disorders and symptoms in children and adolescents with cerebral palsy: A systematic review and meta-analysis. *Dev. Med. Child. Neurol.* **2018**, *60*, 30–38. [CrossRef]
55. Leung, D.K.Y.; Chan, W.C.; Spector, A.; Wong, G.H.Y. Prevalence of depression, anxiety, and apathy symptoms across dementia stages: A systematic review and meta-analysis. *Int. J. Geriatr. Psychiatry* **2021**, *36*, 1330–1344. [CrossRef] [PubMed]
56. Darwiche, J.; Milek, A.; Antonietti, J.P.; Vial, Y. Partner support during the prenatal testing period after assisted conception. *Women Bith* **2019**, *32*, e264–e271. [CrossRef]
57. Nik Hazlina, N.H.; Norhayati, M.N.; Shaiful Bahari, I.; Nik Muhammad Arif, N.A. Worldwide prevalence, risk factors and psychological impact of infertility among women: A systematic review and meta-analysis. *BMJ Open* **2022**, *12*, e057132. [CrossRef] [PubMed]
58. Yasini, M.; Khalili, M.A.; Hashemian, Z. The level of anxiety and depression among Iranian infertile couples undergoing in vitro fertilization or intra cytoplasmic sperm injection cycles. *Res. J. Med. Sci.* **2005**, *10*, 358–362.
59. Salk, R.H.; Hyde, J.S.; Abramson, L.Y. Gender differences in depression in representative national samples: Meta-analyses of diagnoses and symptoms. *Psychol. Bull.* **2017**, *143*, 783–822. [CrossRef] [PubMed]
60. Barlow, D.H.; Ellard, K.K.; Sauer-Zavala, S.; Bullis, J.R.; Carl, J.R. The origins of neuroticism. *Perspect. Psychol. Sci.* **2014**, *9*, 481–496. [CrossRef] [PubMed]
61. Lee, S.A.; Crunk, E.A. Fear and psychopathology during the COVID-19 crisis: Neuroticism, hypochondriasis, reassurance-seeking, and coronaphobia as fear factors. *OMEGA-J. Death Dying* **2022**, *85*, 483–496. [CrossRef] [PubMed]

62. Liu, S.; Lithopoulos, A.; Zhang, C.Q.; Garcia-Barrera, M.A.; Rhodes, R.E. Personality and perceived stress during COVID-19 pandemic: Testing the mediating role of perceived threat and efficacy. *Personal. Individ. Differ.* **2021**, *168*, 110351. [CrossRef] [PubMed]
63. Taylor, S. The psychology of pandemics. *Annu. Rev. Clin. Psychol.* **2022**, *18*, 581–609. [CrossRef] [PubMed]
64. Weber, K.; Giannakopoulos, P.; Herrmann, F.R.; Bartolomei, J.; Digiorgio, S.; Ortiz Chicherio, N.; Delaloye, C.; Ghisletta, P.; Lecerf, T.; De Ribaupierre, A.; et al. Stressful life events and neuroticism as predictors of late-life versus early-life depression. *Psychogeriatrics* **2013**, *13*, 221–228. [CrossRef]
65. Kikhavani, S.; Taghinejad, H. Personality Factor as a Predictor of Depression Score among Depressed and CHD Patients. *JCDR* **2015**, *9*, VC04–VC07. [CrossRef] [PubMed]
66. Assari, S. Neuroticism Predicts Subsequent Risk of Major Depression for Whites but Not Blacks. *Behav. Sci.* **2017**, *7*, 64. [CrossRef]
67. Liu, R.T.; Alloy, L.B. Stress generation in depression: A systematic review of the empirical literature and recommendations for future study. *Clin. Psychol. Rev.* **2010**, *30*, 582–593. [CrossRef] [PubMed]

Journal of
*Clinical Medicine*

MDPI

*Article*

# Maternal and Fetal Outcomes of COVID-19 According to the Trimester of Diagnosis: A Cross-Sectional Prospective Study in a Tertiary University Hospital

**Naser Al-Husban [1,*], Rahaf Mohammad Di'bas [2], Sara Salem Karadsheh [2], Lara Ali Alananzeh [2], Iman Aolymat [3], Asma Kilani [4], Ala'eddien Obeidat [4], Alhareth Eid Alhusban [4] and Hedaieh Al-Husban [5]**

1 Department of Obstetrics and Gynecology, School of Medicine, The University of Jordan, P.O. Box 2194, Amman 11941, Jordan
2 Jordan University Hospital, Amman 11942, Jordan; rahafdibas47@yahoo.com (R.M.D.); karadshehsarah@gmail.com (S.S.K.); ananzeh_l@yahoo.com (L.A.A.)
3 Department of Anatomy, Physiology and Biochemistry, Faculty of Medicine, The Hashemite University, P.O. Box 330127, Zarqa 13133, Jordan; imank@hu.edu.jo
4 School of Medicine, The University of Jordan, Amman 11942, Jordan; asma_kilani@yahoo.com (A.K.); alaaobeidat2001@gmail.com (A.O.); alh0211493@ju.edu.jo (A.E.A.)
5 Ibn AlHaitham Hospital, Amman 11942, Jordan; husban99@yahoo.com
* Correspondence: n.alhusban@ju.edu.jo

**Abstract: Objectives:** Pregnant women are considered a high-risk group because they may be particularly susceptible to COVID-19. Our study tried to relate fetomaternal outcomes and trimester-specific infection. **Methods:** A prospective study on 224 pregnant women with confirmed antenatal infections at a tertiary hospital. Data from the antenatal clinic records, admission files, labor ward and neonatal notes, lab results, respiratory consultations, and ICU admission were analyzed using Jamovi 2.2.5, with $p < 0.05$ indicating significance. **Results:** A total of 224 patients were included—10, 32, and 182 patients were diagnosed in the first, second, and third trimesters, respectively. Neonatal NICU admissions were significantly higher among those with infections in the third trimester compared to those in the first trimester ($p = 0.008$). Significant differences in Apgar scores at 1 and 5 min emerged between the second and third trimesters ($p = 0.014$ and $p = 0.037$, respectively). However, no significant differences were observed in Apgar scores between the first and second trimesters ($p = 0.341$, $p = 0.108$) or the first and third trimesters ($p = 0.545$, $p = 0.755$). Complications of pregnancy, including maternal mortality and various conditions (respiratory, obstetrical, sepsis, DIC), neonatal outcomes, ICU admission, and cesarean section indications, showed no significant differences related to the trimester of infection ($p$-values: 0.989, 0.892). Study limitations include sample size impacting generalization, higher COVID-19 cases in the third trimester than other trimesters, and potential historical data availability and accuracy issues. **Conclusions:** In the third trimester, COVID-19 caused more neonatal ICU admissions than the first trimester, with lower Apgar scores at 1 and 5 min compared to the second trimester, indicating an increasing susceptibility and vulnerability to COVID-19 infection with an increasing pregnancy age. Other fetal and maternal outcomes showed no significant differences in infection timing.

**Keywords:** COVID-19; fetomaternal; outcome; pregnancy; trimester

## 1. Introduction

The coronavirus disease 2019 (COVID-19) is caused by a single-stranded RNA-enveloped virus, which causes a wide range of symptoms with an incubation period varying from 2 to 12 days.

It began in Wuhan, China, in December 2019, and since then, the number of confirmed cases and associated mortality and morbidity have increased rapidly. By 12 March 2020, the World Health Organization (WHO) classified the outbreak as a pandemic [1]. This pandemic negatively affected many people, including pregnant women and their fetuses, increasing the maternal death rates from 5.17 per 100,000 pregnancies in the year prior to the pandemic to 8.69 fatalities per 100,000 during the pandemic [2]. There were also nationwide lockdowns, disruption of healthcare services, and fear of attending healthcare facilities that affected the well-being of pregnant people and their babies, thus increasing maternal mental health issues and rates of stillbirth and preterm birth, especially in low- and middle-income countries [3,4].

### 1.1. *Physiological and Immunological Vulnerabilities of Pregnant Women to COVID-19*

Pregnant women are considered a high-risk group because they may be particularly susceptible to COVID-19 due to the physiologic changes of pregnancy involving the cardiorespiratory system in which the enlarged uterus raises abdominal pressure and lifts the diaphragm. Also, hormonal changes increase the subcostal angle and outward expansion of the rib cage while decreasing chest wall compliance, leading to "physiologic dyspnea" in many pregnant women and decreasing functional residual capacity, resulting in compensatory respiratory alkalemia. This change can shift the oxygen dissociation curve to the right, which is beneficial in transferring oxygen to the fetus but may hinder respiratory function in pregnant women with pulmonary complications resulting in altered response to COVID-19 infection in pregnancy, with the third trimester being the riskiest because the heavily pregnant uterus compresses the lungs more than in early pregnancy [2,5].

Another system is the immune system; pregnancy is an immunologically vulnerable period because of the dilutional anemia that happens in 38% of pregnant women, leading to reduced blood oxygen content, prioritizing vital organs like the heart and brain over immune organs, potentially compromising immune function. Also, hormonal changes, particularly human chronic gonadotropin and progesterone, modulate immune responses and fetal tolerance. These factors result in placing pregnant women at risk for more severe illness and complications from infections [5].

### 1.2. *Impact of COVID-19-Induced Cytokine Storm on Fetomaternal Outcomes*

It has been reported that COVID-19, especially in severe cases, can lead to a cytokine storm. Additionally, pregnant women in their first and third trimesters of pregnancy are in a pro-inflammatory state due to the complex interaction between the immune system and sex hormones. Therefore, the cytokine storm induced by SARS-CoV-2 in these periods may exacerbate the severity of the inflammatory state, potentially resulting in adverse obstetric outcomes [5].

Even without a placental infection, raised inflammatory cytokines levels were seen in the neonates' cord blood. It is still not obvious if these cytokines were fetal or maternal in origin. Immune cells in cord blood were shown in research to exhibit higher cytokine production in SARS-CoV-2-infected pregnancies [6].

### 1.3. *COVID-19 Impact on the Placenta*

Placental infection by COVID-19 appears to be uncommon. Even without placental infection, CoVID-2-related inflammation and coagulation still occur and manifest most commonly as thrombosis and fibrin deposition in the intervillous spaces [6]. COVID-19 increases the risk of thromboembolic complications in the general population, and while pregnancy is, by itself, a hypercoagulable state with increased thrombin production and an increase in intravascular inflammation, COVID-19 increases the risk of preeclampsia, preterm birth, and other adverse pregnancy outcomes as an additive or synergistic risk factor for thrombosis during pregnancy, leading to uteroplacental malperfusion. To avoid these events, the RCOG recommended that all pregnant women admitted with confirmed COVID-19 should receive prophylactic low-molecular-weight heparin (LMWH) [7,8].

### 1.4. The Increased Risk of Complications Associated with COVID-19 during Pregnancy

Taking all of this into consideration, it is understandable why pregnant individuals were found to be at a heightened risk of more severe symptoms than people who were not pregnant. One study showed that the risk of adult respiratory distress syndrome and acute renal failure was between 1.66 and 2.22 times higher in mothers with COVID-19 infections during pregnancy compared to those without [9], and also were more likely to be admitted to an intensive care unit (4%), require invasive ventilation [10], need a C-section (45.4 versus 32.4 percent), deliver preterm (26.9 versus 14.1 percent), die around the time of birth, and experience postpartum hemorrhage [11]. Other recent studies concluded that severe COVID-19 is strongly associated with preeclampsia, gestational diabetes, preterm birth, and low birth weight [12].

### 1.5. Vertical Transmission and Breastfeeding Considerations in COVID-19

Fortunately, the rate of vertical transmission of the virus to the fetus transplacentally reported in women with COVID-19 proved to be a minority, and most of the cases of neonatal SARS-CoV-2 are due to postnatal infection [13,14]. This could be because the virus is known to have a very low level of viremia, and the level of virus receptor expression in the placenta that facilitates viral entry is very low [12].

In addition, breastmilk transmission was unlikely [3]. In contrast, when breastfeeding, secretory IgA antibodies and other immunologically active substances in breast milk are passed to the suckling infant, supporting their immature adaptive immune system. Therefore, breastfeeding by infected mothers was encouraged [12].

### 1.6. COVID-19 Vaccination in Pregnancy: Safety, Efficacy, and Fetal Outcomes

In pregnancy, COVID-19 vaccine adverse events have not been shown to be different from those of the general population. In addition, no adverse outcomes were reported for obstetric, fetal, or neonatal patients [12]. On the contrary, they found that severe complications, such as critical care admission, stillbirths, and early neonatal deaths, were more common in those who were unvaccinated compared with those who were vaccinated [15] and that there is 89% vaccine effectiveness against COVID-19 hospitalizations when given during pregnancy [2]. As for the effect of vaccination on fetal outcomes, it was found that the risk of infant hospitalization for COVID-19 up to 4–6 months of age could be reduced by 30–70% by vaccinating pregnant women [12].

## 2. Methods and Population

### 2.1. Study Population

Pregnant women who have had a confirmed COVID-19 infection by nasopharyngeal swab(s) at a University Hospital in the period February 2020–August 2022. These women were infected in different trimesters of pregnancy.

### 2.2. Follow-up

They were followed from the time of infection until 6 weeks postpartum. They were assessed regarding hospitalization due to the infection and/or its complications, sepsis, death, respiratory complications, disseminated intravascular coagulation (DIC), ICU admission, antenatal clinic visits, miscarriages, preterm deliveries, development of pre-eclampsia, induction of labor, mode of delivery, indications for cesarean sections (CS), complications of delivery, intrauterine growth restriction (IUGR), stillbirths, neonatal intensive care unit (NICU) admission and its outcome, and breastfeeding practices in these women.

### 2.3. Data Collection and Sources

The obstetric outcomes were obtained from the antenatal clinic and admission notes, labor ward data, postnatal clinic notes, or admissions. The respiratory variables were obtained from respiratory consultations and interventions, anesthesia notes and the intensive care unit admissions notes. The fetal variables were obtained from the nursery and neonatal intensive care unit notes and neonatologists' notes.

### 2.4. Inclusion and Exclusion Criteria

The inclusion criteria included all those who had a confirmed infection and completed data.

The exclusion criteria included women with multiple pregnancies, those with suspected but not confirmed infections, those with chronic underlying medical disorders, and those with missing data.

### 2.5. Ethical Considerations and Registration

Ethics approval for this study was obtained from the institutional review board (IRB) at Jordan University Hospital (Decision number 307/2020, dated 29 December 2020). The study involved a prospective review of obstetric, medical, and respiratory clinical data and notes collected over a specified period. As the data did not include any personal, individual, or identifying information, written informed consent was not required. Throughout the study, all information was anonymized, and strict measures were implemented to ensure participant confidentiality. No identifying data will be shared.

The study was registered in clinicaltrials.gov with a ClinicalTrials.gov Identifier: NCT04869202.

This study has been reported in line with the STROCSS criteria [16].

### 2.6. Statistical Analysis

Data were entered into and analyzed using Jamovi 2.2.5. $p \leq 0.05$ was considered significant. Data was assessed for normality using Kolmogorov–Smirnov test.

Descriptive analysis was applied to calculate the frequencies and percentages for categorical variables and the means (standard deviations) and medians (interquartile ranges) for continuous variables according to the normality of distribution.

The Chi-squared (2) test was used to test for association between categorical variables.

The Mann–Whitney test was used to find if there are significant differences in gestational age at delivery, birth weight, and Apgar scores between first and second, first and third, and second and third trimesters.

The Kruskal–Wallis test was used to examine the differences in Apgar scores and birth weight and gestational age (GA) at delivery in relation to the trimester in which the patient became infected.

### 2.7. Definitions

Preeclampsia is characterized by new-onset hypertension after 20 weeks of gestation, defined by a systolic blood pressure of 140 mm Hg or more or diastolic blood pressure of 90 mm Hg or more on two occasions at least 4 h apart or more severe values (diastolic $\geq$ 110 mm Hg or systolic $\geq$ 160 mm Hg) [15].

Fetal death, according to the United States Center for Health Statistics, is the delivery of a fetus showing no signs of life, regardless of pregnancy duration. Stillbirth is defined as fetal death at or beyond 20 weeks gestation or with a birth weight of 350 g or more, aiming to standardize definitions [17].

Early pregnancy loss is now described using terms like "miscarriage" or "intrauterine pregnancy loss" for pregnancies lost before 20 weeks gestation, reflecting a shift toward clearer and less stigmatized terminology in medical practice [18,19].

The aim of this study is to assess the fetomaternal outcomes of pregnancies complicated by COVID-19 infection according to trimester at diagnosis in a tertiary university hospital.

## 3. Results

### 3.1. The Study Population Demographics

The study's significant contribution lies in its utilization of a distinct dataset sourced specifically from Jordan. This unique dataset offers valuable insights that are contextually relevant to Jordan, thereby enhancing the significance and applicability of the study findings within this regional setting.

Among the participants, a total of 224 patients who had confirmed COVID-19 during pregnancy were included. Most patients (182) were diagnosed in the third trimester.

A detailed description of the study population is shown in Tables 1 and 2.

**Table 1.** An overview of the means (standard deviations) and medians (interquartile ranges) according to the normality of distribution and probability values for several variables in relation to trimester at the time of diagnosis.

| | First Trimester | Second Trimester | Third Trimester | *p*-Value |
|---|---|---|---|---|
| Age | 32.4 (SD 5.19) | 32.1 (SD 5.14) | 31 (IQR 27.75–35) | 0.51 |
| GA at delivery | 38.1 (SD 1.10) | 38 (IQR 36.25–40) | 38 (IQR 36–39) | 0.829 |
| Birth weight | 3.11 (SD 0.48) | 2.85 (IQR 2.56–3.1) | 3 (IQR 2.7–3.26) | 0.304 |
| Apgar (min 1) | 8 (IQR 8–8) | 8 (IQR 8–8) | 8 (IQR 8–8) | 0.017 |
| Apgar (min 5) | 9 (IQR 9–9) | 9 (IQR 9–9) | 9 (IQR 9–9) | 0.037 |

*p*-value; probability value.

**Table 2.** An overview of the frequencies, percentages, and probability values for several variables in relation to the gestational period at diagnosis.

| | N | % | First (N = 10) | Second (N = 32) | Third (N = 182) | *p*-Value |
|---|---|---|---|---|---|---|
| Parity | 224 | | | | | |
| Nulliparity | 1 | 0.4% | 0/10 | 0/32 | 1/182 | |
| Multiparity | 152 | 67.9% | 5/10 | 16/32 | 131/182 | |
| Grand multiparity | 71 | 31.7% | 5/10 | 16/32 | 50/182 | |
| Complications | 39 | | | | | $p = 0.989$ |
| Death | 2 | 5.1% | 0/1 | 0/7 | 2/31 | $p = 0.762$ |
| Sepsis | 2 | 5.1% | 0/1 | 0/7 | 2/31 | $p = 0.762$ |
| Respiratory | 7 | 17.9% | 0/1 | 0/7 | 7/31 | $p = 0.333$ |
| Obstetric | 16 | 41% | 0/1 | 3/7 | 13/31 | $p = 0.699$ |
| Neonatal | 18 | 46.2% | 1/1 | 5/7 | 12/31 | $p = 0.161$ |
| DIC | 3 | 7.7% | 0/1 | 0/7 | 3/31 | $p = 0.657$ |
| ICU | 5 | 12.8% | 0/1 | 0/7 | 5/31 | $p = 0.477$ |
| NICU admission | 224 | | | | | $p = 0.008$ |
| Dead | 4 | 1.8% | 0/10 | 3/32 | 1/182 | |
| Admitted to the NICU | 58 | 25.9% | 1/10 | 7/32 | 50/182 | |
| Not admitted to the NICU | 162 | 72.3% | 9/10 | 22/32 | 131/182 | |
| Indications of NICU admission | 58 | | | | | $p = 0.387$ |
| Non-COVID-related | 34 | 58.6% | 0/1 | 5/7 | 29/50 | |
| COVID-related | 24 | 41.4% | 1/1 | 2/7 | 21/50 | |
| Mode of delivery | 224 | | | | | $p = 0.391$ |
| Normal vaginal delivery | 112 | 50% | 6/10 | 19/32 | 87/182 | |
| Cesarean section | 112 | 50% | 4/10 | 13/32 | 95/182 | |
| Indications of Caesarean section | 112 | | | | | $p = 0.892$ |
| IUGR | 5 | 4.5% | 0/4 | 0/13 | 5/95 | $p = 0.626$ |
| Oligohydramnios | 1 | 0.9% | 0/4 | 0/13 | 1/95 | $p = 0.914$ |
| Maternal respiratory condition | 3 | 2.7% | 0/4 | 0/13 | 3/95 | $p = 0.759$ |
| Fetal distress | 14 | 12.5% | ¼ | 3/13 | 10/95 | $p = 0.326$ |
| Elective | 89 | 79.5% | ¾ | 10/13 | 76/95 | $p = 0.943$ |
| Breastfeeding | 224 | | | | | $p = 0.604$ |
| Yes | 175 | 78.1% | 9/10 | 24/32 | 142/182 | |
| No | 49 | 21.9% | 1/10 | 8/32 | 40/182 | |

*N* is the number of non-missing values. *p*-value—probability value.

### 3.2. Complications of Pregnancy

There was no significant difference in complications of pregnancy, including maternal mortality, respiratory conditions (pneumonia, hypoxia, respiratory failure, pulmonary hypertension), obstetrical conditions (severe preeclampsia, oligohydramnios, gestational hypertension, uncontrolled gestational diabetes, and placenta accreta), sepsis, DIC and ICU admission in relation to the trimester in which the patient became infected ($p = 0.989$) (Table 2). Perhaps the overall fetomaternal complications in our study were low because we excluded patients with comorbidities such as hypertension, diabetes mellitus, lupus, nephropathy, antiphospholipid antibody syndrome, and others.

### 3.3. *Indications for CS*

There was no significant difference in indications for CS, including elective, fetal distress, IUGR, maternal respiratory conditions, and oligohydramnios, in relation to the trimester in which the patient became infected ($p = 0.892$) (Table 2). A total of 86% of CS was done under spinal anesthesia.

### 3.4. *Neonatal Outcome*

There was a significant difference in the neonatal admission to the NICU ($p = 0.008$) in relation to the gestational period at diagnosis. The indications for these admissions were divided into COVID-related and non-COVID-related categories.

### 3.5. *Apgar Score*

There were significant differences in Apgar scores at 1 and 5 min after birth in relation to the trimester at which the patient contracted COVID-19 infection, with *p*-values of 0.017 and 0.037, respectively.

The percentages of infants with low Apgar scores ($\leq 5$) at 1 and 5 min varied by trimester: In the first trimester, 10% (1/10) had low Apgar scores at 1 min, and 0% (0/10) at 5 min. In the second trimester, 12.5% (4/32) had low Apgar scores at 1 min and 6.3% (2/32) at 5 min. In the third trimester, 2.2% (4/182) had low Apgar scores at 1 min and 0.5% (1/182) at 5 min.

There was a significant difference in Apgar 1 and 5 between the second and third trimesters ($p = 0.014$ and $p = 0.037$, respectively). However, there were no significant differences in Apgar 1 and 5 between the first and second trimesters ($p = 0.509$, $p = 0.321$) or the first and third trimesters ($p = 0.480$, $p = 0.683$) (Table 3).

**Table 3.** The probability values of comparing the trimesters in which the patient contracted COVID.

| | | ***p*-Value** | | | |
|---|---|---|---|---|---|
| **Trimester at Time of Diagnosis** | | **Birth Weight** | **Gestational Age at Delivery** | **Apgar (1 min)** | **Apgar (5 min)** |
| First | Second | 0.183 | 0.695 | 0.509 | 0.321 |
| First | Third | 0.276 | 0.539 | 0.48 | 0.683 |
| Second | Third | 0.299 | 0.877 | 0.014 | 0.037 |

*p*-value—probability value.

### 3.6. *GA at Delivery and Birth Weight*

There were no significant differences in GA at delivery or birth weight in relation to the trimester in which the patient became infected with COVID-19; *p*-values are 0.829 and 0.304, respectively. The Mann–Whitney test revealed no significant differences in birth weight and GA at delivery between the first, second, and third trimesters, as shown in (Table 3).

## 4. Discussion

Many data and recommendations have changed regarding guidelines, virus profile and administration of patients and pregnant women with COVID-19. All patients in our study received one or another form of treatment ranging from nothing to decongestants and antipyretics to the extreme situation of antiviral, steroids and ventilatory support.

As there were very little data considering the effects of COVID-19 infection in relation to the trimester of infection and a robust collection of maternal data by trimester of exposure, including the periconception period, was required to determine these effects, we conducted such a study.

### 4.1. Complications of Pregnancy and Maternal Outcomes

Infection during the third trimester poses a higher risk for ICU admission, critical illness, mechanical ventilation, and death [20,21]. A recent study observed higher maternal and fetal complications in women diagnosed in the third trimester with higher maternal mortality rates and a greater frequency of pregnancy-induced hypertension compared to other trimesters [22]. On the other hand, a study of 114 infected women discovered that higher GA was protective against severe illness [23]. Our findings align with this study, revealing that advanced gestational infection does not carry more adverse maternal outcomes than early infection. Hypertension amplifies the risk of death in the third trimester [24]. However, we excluded mothers with co-existing medical disorders such as hypertension from our study to ensure consistency in the study population and rule out contributing factors to adverse fetomaternal outcomes.

A study showed that women with active infections by the time of delivery had a significantly higher rate of hospital admission for COVID-19 and ICU admission than the recovered group [25]. We did not specifically study those cases with an active, symptomatic intrapartum infection.

UK data showed that early pregnant women with COVID-19 represented a minority of hospitalized pregnant women [21]. Maternal outcomes were favorable when infection occurred in the first trimester, and women who experienced spontaneous abortion in the first trimester had similar antibody prevalence to those with ongoing pregnancies [26]. The minimal respiratory changes during this phase may explain this. However, first-trimester infection could still lead to complications due to SARS-CoV-2 invasion of the placental villi in subsequent weeks of gestation [27]. A study found that there was a higher proportion of placentas from patients with COVID-19 in earlier gestations with evidence of placental infection-associated features [6].

It was found in small case reports of COVID-19-infected pregnant women that no miscarriages occurred in the first trimester of pregnancy and, in fact, they all were second or third-trimester miscarriages [28]. Meanwhile, in asymptomatic pregnant women, the COVID-19 environment did not appear to influence rates of first-trimester miscarriage [29]. On the other hand, research suggested that miscarriage was more commonly seen in patients who became ill in the first trimester compared to the second trimester [20].

One study revealed a significant association between miscarriage and trimester at diagnosis of infection but no significant association between stillbirth, pre-eclampsia, or trimester at diagnosis [30]. Our study had the same result concerning stillbirth and pre-eclampsia: we found no significant association between complications of pregnancy that included maternal mortality, obstetrical conditions involving pre-eclampsia, ICU admission, intrauterine fetal demise, and trimester at diagnosis ($p = 0.989$) (Table 2).

### 4.2. GA at Delivery and NICU Admission

Fetal loss during the first 24 weeks of gestation was due to several systematic inflammatory events, including the placenta with subsequent premature labor, rupture of membranes, or placental insufficiency [31,32].

Among infants born to mothers who tested positive 0–14 days before delivery, more were admitted to the NICU than those born to mothers who tested positive more than 14 days before delivery and were also born earlier [33]. We did not examine the impact of infection timing in the third trimester on fetomaternal outcomes. Prematurity may be due to maternal complications, intrauterine infection, the perceived need for early antiviral treatment in the disease course [34], or it may be iatrogenic [35].

Our study found no significant association between GA at diagnosis and GA at delivery, as well as NICU admission, which is consistent with previous research [30]. However, we did find a significant association between the trimester at diagnosis and NICU admission ($p = 0.008$), which is an interesting finding. That could be explained by the fact that most of the neonatal complications in COVID-19-positive mothers were due to prematurity and not COVID-19 infection. A multicenter study showed that if mothers were admitted for COVID-19 infection, their newborns had a higher risk of premature delivery [36]. Women with COVID-19 infection in their third trimester had the highest frequencies of preterm labor and are at higher risk of adverse outcomes [20,22], which increases the likelihood of NICU admission. All these facts together could explain the results of our study, which found an association between NICU admission and trimester at diagnosis.

There was a lack of information on the vertical transmission potential, resulting in understandable anxiety among women and obstetricians, which in turn was reflected in the high rates of preterm birth [21], which was similarly explained in our study. The evidence inferred that vertical transmission of SARS-CoV-2 was rare [37]. In our study, the number of neonates born to COVID-19-infected mothers was zero, and similarly, no cases of vertical or horizontal transmission were found in another study [36]. The chance that congenital anomalies were caused by COVID-19 was low [37].

A decline in the number of NICU admissions and neonatal resuscitations during the pandemic was seen, which might have been explained by travel bans and strict measures of infection prevention and control [38]. In our study, the indications for admission were 41.4% COVID-related and 58.6% non-COVID-related.

### 4.3. Apgar Score

Our study found that neonates whose mothers were diagnosed with infections in the second trimester had significantly different Apgar scores at 1 and 5 min compared to those diagnosed in the third trimester. However, there were no significant differences in Apgar scores between the first and second or first and third trimesters. In a recent study, it was observed that women with COVID-19 infection in the third trimester had the lowest Apgar scores and highest in patients with COVID-19 infection in the first trimester [22]. We could not draw clear conclusions about the risk of low Apgar scores due to insufficient evidence. It is possible that pregnant women experience a transition to a pro-inflammatory state in the third trimester and an anti-inflammatory state in the second trimester. Given the association of COVID-19 with cytokine storms, pregnant women infected during the third trimester might exhibit reduced Apgar scores due to the heightened inflammatory response, potentially impacting fetal health [5]. Contrary to expectations, there were no significant differences in Apgar scores between the first and third trimesters, possibly due to the small number of pregnant women diagnosed in the first trimester ($n = 10$) compared to the third trimester ($n = 182$). Larger studies are needed to establish the true association.

### 4.4. Birth Weight

The pathological placental features, including multiple villous infarcts, could result in subsequent miscarriage or IUGR [32]. Placental hypoperfusion was associated with occlusive fibrin deposition and non-occlusive thrombi [21,30]. The small for gestational age (SGA) risk was found to be comparable across all trimesters [39]. Another study revealed that there was no significant difference in birthweight, birthweight percentile, or rates of SGA infants (5.95% in the active-infection group, which was low when compared to 8.75% in the recovered group) [25]. Similarly, there was no significant association between IUGR and trimester at diagnosis [30]. These findings were consistent with our study, as we did not find a significant association between birth weight and trimester at diagnosis ($p = 0.304$).

### 4.5. Mode of Delivery

During the initial stages of the pandemic in China, 90% of infected women were delivered by CS [36], which might indicate that obstetricians lack enough knowledge about the effects of COVID-19 on pregnancy or that cesarean was necessary because of worsening maternal symptoms [35]. Those who required hospitalization had a high cesarean section rate. Following current obstetric guidelines over time, indications for CS were gradually reduced to scenarios with maternal or fetal compromise [36]. The rate of CS in our study was 50%, with elective indications being the highest and oligohydramnios being the least. Similar to our findings, there was no significant association between the mode of delivery and the trimester of infection diagnosis [25].

### 4.6. Breastfeeding

WHO and CDC recommended the wearing of a facemask and continued breastfeeding by infected mothers. While one study reported finding the virus in breastmilk one week after delivery, two small studies found no molecular evidence of the virus in breastmilk [26].

Providing support to breastfeeding mothers was very important, as this infection was a major cause of anxiety [35]. Fortunately, the rate of mothers breastfeeding in our study was 78.1%. This might be partly due to the strong societal and cultural ties and partly to the early widespread vaccination, which caused relatively mild infection in most cases and decreased anxiety in pregnant women.

### 4.7. Limitations

There are some potential limitations to our study. It is a single-centered study. The sample size of the study may be limited, potentially reducing the generalization of the findings to a broader population. The number of pregnant women who became infected with COVID-19 in the third trimester is much higher than in the second and first trimesters. Lastly, there may be limitations in terms of the availability and accuracy of historical data. This could introduce errors in the documentation of events and outcomes.

It is important to differentiate this kind of infection from other infections like ZIKA VIRUS, considering the relatively recent discovery of this congenital infectious syndrome. Further studies and updated long-term follow-up are needed [40]. In Jordan, termination of pregnancy is totally prohibited and illegal unless the pregnancy is threatening the mother's life. In our hospital, there were no pregnancy terminations due to COVID infection, and there was no evidence of vertical transmission [41]. In our hospital, we did not study the different variants of the virus. The delta variant was found to be associated with more adverse fetomaternal outcomes than other variants [42]. Around the same period of time of our study, it was found that there were moderate scores in COVID-19 vaccine hesitancy among Jordanian pregnant women despite the current international recommendations for its safety for women and their fetuses or neonates [43]. Moreover, it was found that about a third of pregnant women were still hesitant about the vaccine, probably because of the conflicting information [44].

## 5. Conclusions

In the third trimester, COVID-19 caused more neonatal ICU admissions than in the first trimester, with lower Apgar scores at 1 and 5 min compared to the second trimester, indicating an increasing susceptibility and vulnerability to COVID-19 infection with an increasing pregnancy age. Other fetal and maternal outcomes showed no significant differences in infection timing.

**Author Contributions:** Methodology, N.A.-H.; Software, A.E.A. and H.A.-H.; Validation, N.A.-H., I.A. and A.K.; Formal analysis, N.A.-H., R.M.D., S.S.K. and L.A.A.; Investigation, I.A., A.K., A.O. and H.A.-H.; Resources, A.O. and A.E.A.; Data curation, R.M.D., S.S.K. and L.A.A.; Writing—original draft, N.A.-H.; Supervision, N.A.-H. All authors have read and agreed to the published version of the manuscript.

**Funding:** This research received no external funding.

**Institutional Review Board Statement:** Ethics approval was obtained by the institutional review board (IRB) at Jordan University Hospital (decision number 307/2020, dated 29 December 2020). ClinicalTrials.gov Identifier: NCT04869202. https://clinicaltrials.gov/ct2/show/NCT04869202 (accessed on 18 June 2023).

**Informed Consent Statement:** Patient consent was waived by the IRB due to non-identifying and total maintenance of confidentiality all through the study period until submission.

**Data Availability Statement:** All data are available from the corresponding author on reasonable request.

**Conflicts of Interest:** The authors declare no conflicts of interest.

## References

1. Allotey, J.; Stallings, E.; Bonet, M.; Yap, M.; Chatterjee, S.; Kew, T.; Debenham, L.; Llavall, A.C.; Dixit, A.; Zhou, D.; et al. Clinical manifestations, risk factors, and maternal and perinatal outcomes of coronavirus disease 2019 in pregnancy: Living systematic review and meta-analysis. *BMJ* **2020**, *370*, m3320. [CrossRef] [PubMed] [PubMed Central]
2. Marshall, M. Does covid-19 affect pregnancies? *New Sci.* **2023**, *258*, 14–15. [CrossRef]
3. Kotlar, B.; Gerson, E.M.; Petrillo, S.; Langer, A.; Tiemeier, H. The impact of the COVID-19 pandemic on maternal and perinatal health: A scoping review. *Reprod. Health* **2021**, *18*, 1–39. [CrossRef] [PubMed]
4. Chmielewska, B.; Barratt, I.; Townsend, R.; Kalafat, E.; van der Meulen, J.; Gurol-Urganci, I.; O'Brien, P.; Morris, E.; Draycott, T.; Thangaratinam, S.; et al. Effects of the COVID-19 pandemic on maternal and perinatal outcomes: A systematic review and meta-analysis. *Lancet Glob. Health* **2021**, *9*, e759–e772. [CrossRef]
5. Chen, M.; Zeng, J.; Liu, X.; Sun, G.; Gao, Y.; Liao, J.; Yu, J.; Luo, X.; Qi, H. Changes in physiology and immune system during pregnancy and coronavirus infection: A review. *Eur. J. Obstet. Gynecol. Reprod. Biol.* **2020**, *255*, 124–128. [CrossRef]
6. Corbetta-Rastelli, C.M.; Altendahl, M.; Gasper, C.; Goldstein, J.D.; Afshar, Y.; Gaw, S.L. Analysis of placental pathology after COVID-19 by timing and severity of infection. *Am. J. Obstet. Gynecol. MFM* **2023**, *5*, 100981. [CrossRef]
7. Regan, A.K.; A Arah, O.; Fell, D.B.; Sullivan, S.G. Risk of Severe Maternal Morbidity Associated With Severe Acute Respiratory Syndrome Coronavirus 2 Infection During Pregnancy. *Open Forum Infect. Dis.* **2023**, *10*, ofad613. [CrossRef]
8. Jamil, R.; Shah, N.; Butt, S.; Shah, T.; Kazi, S.; Perveen, F.; Hossain, N. Clinical characteristics, obstetric and perinatal outcome of Covid-19 infection in pregnant women. *J. Pak. Med Assoc.* **2022**, *72*, 1391–1395. [CrossRef]
9. Metz, T.D.; Clifton, R.G.; Hughes, B.L.; Sandoval, G.J.; Grobman, W.A.; Saade, G.R.; Manuck, T.A.; Longo, M.; Sowles, A.; Clark, K.; et al. Association of SARS-CoV-2 Infection With Serious Maternal Morbidity and Mortality From Obstetric Complications. *JAMA* **2022**, *327*, 748–759. [CrossRef] [PubMed]
10. Wei, S.Q.; Bilodeau-Bertrand, M.; Liu, S.; Auger, N. The impact of COVID-19 on pregnancy outcomes: A systematic review and meta-analysis. *Can. Med Assoc. J.* **2021**, *193*, E540–E548. [CrossRef]
11. Al-Rawaf, S.A.; Mousa, E.T.; Kareem, N.M. Correlation between Pregnancy Outcome and Placental Pathology in COVID-19 Pregnant Women. *Infect. Dis. Obstet. Gynecol.* **2022**, *2022*, 1–5. [CrossRef]
12. Chambers, C.; Krogstad, P.; Bertrand, K.; Contreras, D.; Tobin, N.H.; Bode, L.; Aldrovandi, G. Evaluation for SARS-CoV-2 in Breast Milk From 18 Infected Women. *JAMA* **2020**, *324*, 1347–1348. [CrossRef]
13. Edlow, A.G.; Li, J.Z.; Collier, A.-R.Y.; Atyeo, C.; James, K.E.; Boatin, A.A.; Gray, K.J.; Bordt, E.A.; Shook, L.L.; Yonker, L.M.; et al. Assessment of Maternal and Neonatal SARS-CoV-2 Viral Load, Transplacental Antibody Transfer, and Placental Pathology in Pregnancies During the COVID-19 Pandemic. *JAMA Netw. Open* **2020**, *3*, e2030455. [CrossRef]
14. Ouyang, Y.; Bagalkot, T.; Fitzgerald, W.; Sadovsky, E.; Chu, T.; Martínez-Marchal, A.; Brieño-Enríquez, M.; Su, E.J.; Margolis, L.; Sorkin, A.; et al. Term Human Placental Trophoblasts Express SARS-CoV-2 Entry Factors ACE2, TMPRSS2, and Furin. *mSphere* **2021**, *6*. [CrossRef]
15. Karrar, S.A.; Martingano, D.J.; Hong, P.L. (Last Update: 2024, February 25). Preeclampsia. StatPearls—NCBI Bookshelf. Available online: https://www.ncbi.nlm.nih.gov/books/NBK570611/ (accessed on 19 August 2024).
16. Mathew, G.; Agha, R.; for the STROCSS Group. STROCSS 2021: Strengthening the Reporting of cohort, cross-sectional and case-control studies in Surgery. *Int. J. Surg.* **2021**, *96*, 106165. [CrossRef]
17. Maslovich, M.M.; Burke, L.M. (Last Update: 2022, October 31). Intrauterine Fetal Demise. StatPearls—NCBI Bookshelf. Available online: https://www.ncbi.nlm.nih.gov/books/NBK557533/ (accessed on 19 August 2024).
18. Dugas, C.; Slane, V.H. (Last Update: 2022, June 27). Miscarriage (Archived). StatPearls—NCBI Bookshelf. Available online: https://www.ncbi.nlm.nih.gov/books/NBK532992/ (accessed on 19 August 2024).
19. Alves, C.; Jenkins, S.M.; Rapp, A. (Last Update: 2023, October 12). Early Pregnancy Loss (Spontaneous Abortion). StatPearls—NCBI Bookshelf. Available online: https://www.ncbi.nlm.nih.gov/books/NBK560521/ (accessed on 19 August 2024).
20. Boushra, M.N.; Koyfman, A.; Long, B. COVID-19 in pregnancy and the puerperium: A review for emergency physicians. *Am. J. Emerg. Med.* **2020**, *40*, 193–198. [CrossRef]
21. Turan, O.; Hakim, A.; Dashraath, P.; Jeslyn, W.J.L.; Wright, A.; Abdul-Kadir, R. Clinical characteristics, prognostic factors, and maternal and neonatal outcomes of SARS-CoV-2 infection among hospitalized pregnant women: A systematic review. *Int. J. Gynecol. Obstet.* **2021**, *151*, 7–16. [CrossRef]

22. Siahafshari, K.; Movahedi, M.; Hajhashemi, M.; Khorvash, F.; Saeidi, M.; Allameh, Z. Evaluation of maternal and fetal outcomes in pregnant women with COVID-19 based on different trimesters. *Adv. Biomed. Res.* **2023**, *12*, 165. [CrossRef]
23. Tutiya, C.; Mello, F.; Chaccur, G.; Almeida, C.; Galvão, E.; de Souza, A.C.B.; Kondo, M.M.; Torloni, M.R.; Siaulys, M. Risk factors for severe and critical Covid-19 in pregnant women in a single center in Brazil. *J. Matern. Neonatal Med.* **2021**, *35*, 5389–5392. [CrossRef]
24. Basu, J.K.; Chauke, L.; Magoro, T. Maternal mortality from COVID 19 among South African pregnant women. *J. Matern. Neonatal Med.* **2021**, *35*, 5932–5934. [CrossRef]
25. Zlatkin, R.; Dollinger, S.; Jacoby, C.; Shmueli, A.; Barbash-Hazan, S.; Chen, R.; Wiznitzer, A.; Hadar, E. Obstetric and perinatal outcomes in parturients with active SARS-CoV-2 infection during labor and delivery: A retrospective cohort study. *BMC Pregnancy Childbirth* **2022**, *22*, 511. [CrossRef]
26. Cosma, S.; Carosso, A.R.; Cusato, J.; Borella, F.; Carosso, M.; Bovetti, M.; Filippini, C.; D'avolio, A.; Ghisetti, V.; Di Perri, G.; et al. Coronavirus disease 2019 and first-trimester spontaneous abortion: A case-control study of 225 pregnant patients. *Am. J. Obstet. Gynecol.* **2020**, *224*, 391.e1–391.e7. [CrossRef]
27. Algarroba, G.N.; Rekawek, P.; Vahanian, S.A.; Khullar, P.; Palaia, T.; Peltier, M.R.; Chavez, M.R.; Vintzileos, A.M. Visualization of severe acute respiratory syndrome coronavirus 2 invading the human placenta using electron microscopy. *Am. J. Obstet. Gynecol.* **2020**, *223*, 275–278. [CrossRef]
28. Papapanou, M.; Papaioannou, M.; Petta, A.; Routsi, E.; Farmaki, M.; Vlahos, N.; Siristatidis, C. Maternal and Neonatal Characteristics and Outcomes of COVID-19 in Pregnancy: An Overview of Systematic Reviews. *Int. J. Environ. Res. Public Health* **2021**, *18*, 596. [CrossRef]
29. Rotshenker-Olshinka, K.; Volodarsky-Perel, A.; Steiner, N.; Rubenfeld, E.; Dahan, M.H. COVID-19 pandemic effect on early pregnancy: Are miscarriage rates altered, in asymptomatic women? *Arch. Gynecol. Obstet.* **2020**, *303*, 839–845. [CrossRef]
30. Sunder, A.; Varghese, B.; Darwish, B.; Shaikho, N.; Rashid, M. Impacts and effects of COVID-19 infection in pregnancy. *SciVee* **2022**, *43*, 67–74. [CrossRef]
31. Wastnedge, E.A.N.; Reynolds, R.M.; van Boeckel, S.R.; Stock, S.J.; Denison, F.C.; Maybin, J.A.; Critchley, H.O.D. Pregnancy and COVID-19. *Physiol. Rev.* **2021**, *101*, 303–318. [CrossRef]
32. Kazemi, S.N.; Hajikhani, B.; Didar, H.; Hosseini, S.S.; Haddadi, S.; Khalili, F.; Mirsaeidi, M.; Nasiri, M.J. COVID-19 and cause of pregnancy loss during the pandemic: A systematic review. *PLoS ONE* **2021**, *16*, e0255994. [CrossRef]
33. Flaherman, V.J.; Afshar, Y.; Boscardin, W.J.; Keller, R.L.; Mardy, A.H.; Prahl, M.K.; Phillips, C.T.; Asiodu, I.V.; Berghella, V.; Chambers, B.D.; et al. Infant Outcomes Following Maternal Infection With Severe Acute Respiratory Syndrome Coronavirus 2 (SARS-CoV-2): First Report From the Pregnancy Coronavirus Outcomes Registry (PRIORITY) Study. *Clin. Infect. Dis.* **2020**, *73*, e2810–e2813. [CrossRef]
34. Liu, D.; Li, L.; Wu, X.; Zheng, D.; Wang, J.; Yang, L.; Zheng, C. Pregnancy and Perinatal Outcomes of Women With Coronavirus Disease (COVID-19) Pneumonia: A Preliminary Analysis. *Am. J. Roentgenol.* **2020**, *215*, 127–132. [CrossRef]
35. Elsaddig, M.; Khalil, A. Effects of the COVID pandemic on pregnancy outcomes. *Best Pr. Res. Clin. Obstet. Gynaecol.* **2021**, *73*, 125–136. [CrossRef]
36. Gabriel, M.A.M.; Vergeli, M.R.; Carbonero, S.C.; Sole, L.; Molina, T.C.; Calle, I.R.; Pérez, I.C.; Fernández, B.; Buratti, A.F.; Morillo, A.F.-C.; et al. Maternal, Perinatal and Neonatal Outcomes With COVID-19: A Multicenter Study of 242 Pregnancies and Their 248 Infant Newborns During Their First Month of Life. *Pediatr. Infect. Dis. J.* **2020**, *39*, e393–e397. [CrossRef]
37. Khalil, A.; Kalafat, E.; Benlioglu, C.; O'Brien, P.; Morris, E.; Draycott, T.; Thangaratinam, S.; Le Doare, K.; Heath, P.; Ladhani, S.; et al. SARS-CoV-2 infection in pregnancy: A systematic review and meta-analysis of clinical features and pregnancy outcomes. *eClinicalMedicine* **2020**, *25*, 100446. [CrossRef]
38. Maeda, Y.; Nakamura, M.; Ninomiya, H.; Ogawa, K.; Sago, H.; Miyawaki, A. Trends in intensive neonatal care during the COVID-19 outbreak in Japan. *Arch. Dis. Child. - Fetal Neonatal Ed.* **2020**, *106*, 327–329. [CrossRef] [PubMed]
39. Fallach, N.; Segal, Y.; Agassy, J.; Perez, G.; Peretz, A.; Chodick, G.; Gazit, S.; Patalon, T.; Ben Tov, A.; Goldshtein, I. Pregnancy outcomes after SARS-CoV-2 infection by trimester: A large, population-based cohort study. *PLoS ONE* **2022**, *17*, e0270893. [CrossRef] [PubMed]
40. Gullo, G.; Scaglione, M.; Cucinella, G.; Riva, A.; Coldebella, D.; Cavaliere, A.F.; Signore, F.; Buzzaccarini, G.; Spagnol, G.; Laganà, A.S.; et al. Congenital Zika Syndrome: Genetic Avenues for Diagnosis and Therapy, Possible Management and Long-Term Outcomes. *J. Clin. Med.* **2022**, *11*, 1351. [CrossRef]
41. Maranto, M.; Zaami, S.; Restivo, V.; Termini, D.; Gangemi, A.; Tumminello, M.; Culmone, S.; Billone, V.; Cucinella, G.; Gullo, G. Symptomatic COVID-19 in Pregnancy: Hospital Cohort Data between May 2020 and April 2021, Risk Factors and Medicolegal Implications. *Diagnostics* **2023**, *13*, 1009. [CrossRef]
42. Incognito, G.G.; Distefano, R.E.C.; Campo, G.; Gulino, F.A.; Gulisano, C.; Gullotta, C.; Gullo, G.; Cucinella, G.; Tuscano, A.; Bruno, M.T.; et al. Comparison of Maternal and Neonatal Outcomes between SARS-CoV-2 Variants: A Retrospective, Monocentric Study. *J. Clin. Med.* **2023**, *12*, 6329. [CrossRef]

43. Masa'deh, R.; Momani, A.; Rayan, A.; Hamaideh, S.H.; Masadeh, O.M.; Al-Yateem, N. COVID-19 vaccine hesitancy among women planning for pregnancy, pregnant or breastfeeding mothers in Jordan: A cross-sectional study. *PLoS ONE* **2023**, *18*, e0286289. [CrossRef]
44. Maranto, M.; Gullo, G.; Bruno, A.; Minutolo, G.; Cucinella, G.; Maiorana, A.; Casuccio, A.; Restivo, V. Factors Associated with Anti-SARS-CoV-2 Vaccine Acceptance among Pregnant Women: Data from Outpatient Women Experiencing High-Risk Pregnancy. *Vaccines* **2023**, *11*, 454. [CrossRef]

Journal of
*Clinical Medicine*

MDPI

*Article*

# Shedding Light on the COVID-19 Pandemic: Placental Expression of Cell Biomarkers in Negative, Vaccinated, and Positive Pregnant Women

**Constantin Condac [1,2,†], Ludmila Lozneanu [3,†], Daniela Roxana Matasariu [4,5,*], Alexandra Ursache [4,*], Iuliana Elena Bujor [4], Maria Elena Niță [5], Vasile Lucian Boiculese [6] and Victoria Bîrluțiu [2]**

1 Department of Anesthesia and Intensive Care, "Cuza Vodă" Hospital, 700038 Iasi, Romania; costicondac@gmail.com
2 Department of Infectious Diseases, University of Medicine and Pharmacy "Lucian Blaga", 550169 Sibiu, Romania; victoria.birlutiu@ulbsibiu.ro
3 Department of Morpho-Functional Sciences I—Histology, University of Medicine and Pharmacy "Gr. T. Popa", 700115 Iasi, Romania; ludmila.lozneanu@umfiasi.ro
4 Department of Obstetrics and Gynecology, University of Medicine and Pharmacy "Gr. T. Popa", 700115 Iasi, Romania; iuliana-elena.bujor@d.umfiasi.ro
5 Department of Obstetrics and Gynecology, "Cuza Vodă" Hospital, 700038 Iasi, Romania; elemarni28@gmail.com
6 Biostatistics, Department of Preventive Medicine and Interdisciplinarity, University of Medicine and Pharmacy "Gr. T. Popa", 700115 Iasi, Romania; lboiculese@gmail.com
* Correspondence: daniela.matasariu@umfiasi.ro (D.R.M.); alexandra.ursache@umfiasi.ro (A.U.)
† These authors contributed equally to this work.

**Abstract: Background**: We investigated the expression of inflammation, placental development, and function markers, including cluster of differentiation 44 (CD44), osteopontin (OPN), and cyclooxygenase-2 (COX-2), to shed light on the controversy regarding the impact of the COVID-19 epidemic on fetal development and pregnancy outcomes. **Methods**: We immunohistochemically analyzed placental tissue from 170 patients (65 COVID-positive and unvaccinated women; 35 Pfeizer-vaccinated and COVID-negative women; and 70 COVID-negative and unvaccinated women, without any other associated pathology) for particularities in the expression of these three molecules. **Results**: CD44 expression was highest in COVID-negative and unvaccinated women, moderate in COVID-positive cases, and lowest in vaccinated and COVID-negative women. OPN expression was highest in COVID-negative and Pfeizer-vaccinated cases, moderate in COVID-negative and unvaccinated cases, and lowest in COVID-positive cases. COX-2 expression was increased in COVID-negative and unvaccinated women, modestly elevated in COVID-positive and unvaccinated cases, and lowest in vaccinated cases. **Conclusions**: These findings reflected an alteration in the placental structure and consequent function due to altered expression of the three studied molecules.

**Keywords:** COVID-19; placenta; immunohistochemistry; diagnosis; SARS-CoV-2; Pfizer vaccine; CD44; osteopontin; COX2

## 1. Introduction

The impact of coronavirus disease (COVID) infection on pregnant women and their infants is of particular interest to obstetricians, pediatricians, and patients [1]. In past epidemics of emerging infections, the pathological analysis of placentas has proven to be a highly informative technique for understanding the mechanism of transmission to the fetus [2].

This infection manifests with a wide range of organ damage, resulting in a diverse constellation of clinical conditions [3]. Human cell viral access is mediated by angiotensin-converting enzyme 2 (ACE-2), receptors for which are abundant on the placental syncytiotrophoblast, underlying a potential connection between the infection and altered placental function [4,5]. Although the pathophysiology is not yet completely understood, there is evidence that the timeframe in which infection appears might play a crucial role in maternal and fetal outcomes. Less mature placentas seem to be more vulnerable to certain types of viral-mediated damage than mature placentas, due to the systemic inflammatory response and hypercoagulation [6].

Cluster of differentiation 44 (CD44) is a widespread, well-known molecule that plays a key role in many cell processes (regulation of vascular permeability, inflammatory response, signaling pathways, cell activation, cell adhesion, cell migration, and cell-to-cell and cell-to-matrix interaction). Hyaluronic acid (HA) is the intermediary for cell-to-cell and cell-to-matrix CD44 interactions [7–9]. This molecule can exhibit other ligands as well, and is capable of interactions with osteopontin, collagen, and matrix metalloproteinases. The CD44 molecule seems to be involved in the stabilization and orientation of the HA grid, both of which are essential in maintaining the placental integrity in normal pregnancy [8,9].

Osteopontin (OPN) is another important CD44 counterpart. It is a major non-collagenous bone matrix protein that is involved in both normal and pathological calcification processes, and also in angiogenesis via CD44 and integrin interactions [10,11]. In the placenta tissue, this effector molecule is expressed by the cytotrophoblasts of chorionic villi, augmenting both ion and nutrient transport [12]. Although osteopontin expression is only present in immature tissue, it becomes visible in a series of processes such as wound healing and pathological calcification (atherosclerosis, breast cancer, and renal stones) [10].

As a part of the cyclooxygenase (COX) family, cyclooxygenase-2 (COX-2) is the base enzyme responsible for the synthesis of prostaglandins from arachidonic acid. Its involvement in angiogenesis, by promoting the proliferation of vascular endothelial cells, inhibiting inflammation, and cell apoptosis, has been acknowledged. It has been demonstrated that abnormal COX-2 levels are associated with ovulation failure, infertility, and implantation disorders [13]. It is an important marker for decidualization, and is highly expressed around the embryo invasion site [14].

The study of CD44, OPN, and COX-2 expression in placental tissue might provide valuable insights into the effects of COVID infection and vaccination during pregnancy. Each marker plays a distinct role in cellular processes and immune responses, making them crucial for understanding placental pathology under different conditions. Our goal was to evaluate CD44, OPN, and COX-2 expression in three groups of pregnant women (healthy and unvaccinated, COVID-positive and unvaccinated, and COVID-vaccinated and COVID-negative) to assess possible physiopathological pathways for the alterations in placental architecture consecutive to inflammatory responses, which may be influenced by viral infections or vaccine-induced immune modulation.

## 2. Materials and Methods

### 2.1. Patients and Tissue Samples

The study period was from January 2021 to January 2023. All of the patients provided written informed consent. The study was by the Ethics Committee of the University of Medicine and Pharmacy "Lucian Blaga", Sibiu (1442/19.03.2024) and of the Obstetrics and Gynecology Hospital "Cuza-Voda" in Iasi, Romania (10426/24.08.2021 and 19/04.08.2023).

Specimens were collected from women who gave birth at term without complications, associated disease, or chronic treatment (toxoplasma, rubella, cytomegalovirus, herpes with no acute infection detected; hepatitis B and C, HIV, and syphilis-negative women). Formalin-fixed, paraffin-embedded tissue samples were collected from pregnant women who gave birth at the Obstetrics and Gynecology Hospital "Cuza-Voda" in Iasi.

The pregnant women were divided into three groups: COVID-positive and unvaccinated women, COVID-negative and vaccinated women, and COVID-negative and unvaccinated women. The COVID-positive and unvaccinated group included asymptomatic women, with the disease detected anytime during pregnancy but at least 14 days before birth. The diagnosis of COVID positivity was established using Polymerase Chain Reaction (PCR) testing. The second group included Pfeizer-vaccinated women, with the first or second dose administered at least 14 days before birth, who never tested positive for COVID during the pandemic, and with a negative rapid COVID test confirmed every three weeks during pregnancy. The control group included COVID-negative and unvaccinated women who gave birth at term without any complications or associated pathology (all the women included in the third group had not tested positive during the pandemic until inclusion in our study, and had negative rapid COVID tests every three weeks during pregnancy).

Exclusion Criteria

Women with obstetrical and/or other medical complications were excluded from our analysis. Patients with COVID infection at the time of giving birth; malignancy; depression; genetic syndromes; infectious or autoimmune diseases; pre-existing or gestational diabetes; hypertension and its complications, such as preeclampsia; premature rupture of membranes; oligohydramnios; intrauterine growth restriction, defined as ultrasound estimated fetal weight less than the 10th percentile for gestational age; chorioamnionitis; and smoking were excluded.

### 2.2. *Immunohistochemistry*

We collected four tissue samples from each placenta, one for each of the four quadrants. Hematoxylin and eosin (H&E) sections were examined, and immunohistochemistry (IHC) was evaluated by two pathologists. IHC staining was performed on formalin-fixed, paraffin-embedded tissues for immunohistochemistry utilizing monoclonal antibodies against cluster of differentiation 44 (CD44), osteopontin (OPN), and cyclooxygenase-2 (COX-2). Four-micrometer-thick serial sections were prepared in citrate buffer (pH 6) after deparaffinization in xylene and rehydration in ethanol series. Endogenous peroxidase activity was inhibited with 0.3% $H_2O_2$ for 20 min at room temperature. IHC was used to determine the expressions of CD44, OPN, and anti-COX2 using specific Abcam Company dilutions for CD44 of 1:250 (catalog no. ab157107, Abcam, Cambridge, UK), OPN of 1:200 (catalog no. ab8448, Abcam, Cambridge, UK), and anti-COX-2 of 1:100 (catalog no. ab15191, Abcam, Cambridge, UK), and were incubated overnight at 4 °C. The sections were washed, exposed to the secondary antibody for 45 min at 37 °C, and cleaned with phosphate-buffered saline (PBS). Hematoxylin was used as a counterstain in the standard avidin–biotin–peroxidase technique, using a liquid DAB (diaminobenzidine) substrate and chromogen system. Human jejunum served as a positive control for CD44, OPN, and anti-COX-2.

All the placental samples were examined for CD44, OPN, and anti-COX-2 presence. Positive cells (brown or yellowish-brown color in the nucleus) in the epithelial and stromal compartments were considered CD44, OPN, and anti-COX-2 positive, regardless of staining intensity or the number of positive cells.

### 2.3. *Statistical Analysis*

The data were imported into Microsoft Excel and analyzed in SPSS 24 (IBM Corp. Released 2016. IBM SPSS Statistics for Windows, Version 24.0. IBM Corp., Armonk, NY, USA). The descriptive statistics included sample size (N absolute and N% relative frequencies), mean, standard deviation, and the 95% confidence interval for the mean, quartiles, minimum, and maximum. Statistical hypothesis tests included nonparametric tests like Kruskal–Wallis for three-sample and post hoc tests for two-sample comparisons with Bonferroni–Dunn corrections. These were applied to the analysis of continuous numerical variables. The Chi-square or Fisher exact tests were used for categorical variables. Pearson's correlation coefficient was used to evaluate the correlation between biomarkers. A standard significance level of 0.05 was used.

## 3. Results

After applying the inclusion and the exclusion criteria, 170 pregnant women were included in the study: 65 unvaccinated COVID-positive women in group 1, 35 vaccinated and COVID-negative women in group 2, and 70 unvaccinated COVID-negative women in group 3. All of the COVID-positive study patients were asymptomatic. The ages of our patients ranged from 18 to 39 years (Figure 1).

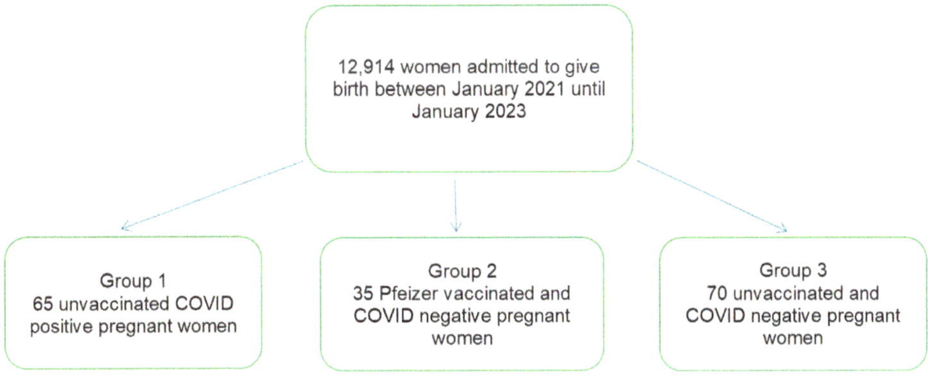


**Figure 1.** Flow chart of our included cases.

All of the study patients were asymptomatic. None required supplemental oxygen administration or admission to the intensive care unit. Laboratory testing, such as complete blood count, inflammatory markers, and biochemical profile, was performed. Neonatal outcomes, including birthweight, APGAR scores, and neonatal intensive care unit (NICU) admissions, were similar between the three groups (Table 1).

**Table 1.** Clinical and demographic characteristics of the pregnant women.

| Clinical and Demographic Characteristics of the Women | | No. | Mean | St. Dev. | Percentile 25 | Median | Percentile 75 | Min | Max | Kruskal–Wallis *p*-Value |
|---|---|---|---|---|---|---|---|---|---|---|
| Maternal age (years) | Negative and unvaccinated | 70 | 28 | 4 | 27 | 29 | 31 | 19 | 34 | <0.001 |
| | Positive | 65 | 31 | 5 | 28 | 33 | 34 | 18 | 39 | |
| | Pfizer vaccinated | 35 | 30 | 5 | 27 | 30 | 33 | 18 | 39 | |
| Gestational age at delivery (weeks) | Negative and unvaccinated | 70 | 40 | 1 | 38 | 40 | 41 | 37 | 41 | <0.001 |
| | Positive | 65 | 38 | 3 | 37 | 38 | 39 | 28 | 40 | |
| | Pfizer vaccinated | 35 | 38 | 3 | 37 | 39 | 40 | 29 | 41 | |
| Fetal weight (grams) | Negative and unvaccinated | 70 | 3507 | 354 | 3260 | 3495 | 3670 | 2800 | 4490 | 0.01 |
| | Positive | 65 | 3237 | 536 | 2920 | 3300 | 3600 | 1980 | 4540 | |
| | Pfizer vaccinated | 35 | 3291 | 522 | 2920 | 3390 | 3650 | 1990 | 4570 | |
| Apgar score at 1 min (point) | Negative and unvaccinated | 70 | 9 | 1 | 8 | 9 | 9 | 8 | 9 | 0.67 |
| | Positive | 65 | 8 | 1 | 8 | 9 | 9 | 4 | 9 | |
| | Pfizer vaccinated | 35 | 8 | 1 | 8 | 9 | 9 | 4 | 10 | |
| Hemoglobin antepartum (milligrams/deciliter) | Negative and unvaccinated | 70 | 12.3 | 1.1 | 11.8 | 12.1 | 13.6 | 10.0 | 13.7 | 0.76 |
| | Positive | 65 | 12.2 | 0.8 | 11.9 | 12.3 | 12.5 | 9.7 | 13.4 | |
| | Pfizer vaccinated | 35 | 12.3 | 0.9 | 11.9 | 12.3 | 13.0 | 9.8 | 14.3 | |
| Hematocrit antepartum (%) | Negative and unvaccinated | 70 | 36.3 | 3.4 | 35.0 | 37.0 | 38.9 | 28.1 | 40.0 | 0.578 |
| | Positive | 65 | 36.4 | 2.6 | 35.3 | 36.0 | 38.0 | 29.3 | 41.0 | |
| | Pfizer vaccinated | 35 | 36.8 | 2.9 | 35.3 | 36.9 | 38.8 | 28.1 | 42.1 | |

**Table 1.** *Cont.*

| Clinical and Demographic Characteristics of the Women | | No. | Mean | St. Dev. | Percentile 25 | Median | Percentile 75 | Min | Max | Kruskal–Wallis *p*-Value |
|---|---|---|---|---|---|---|---|---|---|---|
| Hemoglobin postpartum (milligrams/deciliter) | Negative and unvaccinated | 70 | 10.9 | 0.8 | 10.4 | 10.9 | 11.4 | 9.0 | 13.0 | 0.61 |
| | Positive | 65 | 11.0 | 0.9 | 10.4 | 11.0 | 11.6 | 8.9 | 12.8 | |
| | Pfizer vaccinated | 35 | 11.1 | 0.8 | 10.5 | 11.0 | 11.6 | 9.7 | 12.9 | |
| Hematocrite postpartum (%) | Negative and unvaccinated | 70 | 31.8 | 2.9 | 29.0 | 31.1 | 34.3 | 27.8 | 37.0 | 0.52 |
| | Positive | 65 | 32.3 | 2.8 | 30.4 | 32.3 | 33.6 | 27.7 | 38.5 | |
| | Pfizer vaccinated | 35 | 32.4 | 2.8 | 29.9 | 32.5 | 34.3 | 27.5 | 37.5 | |
| Leucocyte value ($10^3$/L) | Negative and unvaccinated | 70 | 12,293 | 2272 | 10,350 | 11,485 | 14,600 | 9900 | 16,500 | <0.001 |
| | Positive | 65 | 10,186 | 2590 | 8280 | 10,120 | 12,100 | 5390 | 16,400 | |
| | Pfizer vaccinated | 35 | 10,936 | 2922 | 8320 | 10,350 | 12,280 | 5390 | 16,500 | |
| Platelet value ($10^6$/L) | Negative and unvaccinated | 70 | 220,500 | 78,240 | 149,000 | 217,500 | 278,000 | 122,000 | 355,000 | 0.76 |
| | Positive | 65 | 218,523 | 63,791 | 156,000 | 211,000 | 260,000 | 132,000 | 355,000 | |
| | Pfizer vaccinated | 35 | 227,543 | 71,222 | 156,000 | 218,000 | 278,000 | 135,000 | 360,000 | |
| CRP (C-reactive protein) value (milligrams/deciliter) | Negative and unvaccinated | 70 | 3.12 | 1.52 | 2.00 | 2.75 | 4.10 | 0.90 | 10.00 | 0.89 |
| | Positive | 65 | 3.09 | 1.30 | 1.90 | 3.00 | 4.80 | 1.07 | 4.90 | |
| | Pfizer vaccinated | 35 | 3.18 | 1.20 | 2.30 | 2.80 | 4.10 | 1.00 | 4.90 | |

When examining the H&E sections, pathological changes were noted. In COVID-positive and vaccinated women, we observed signs of inflammation, such as villitis or intervillositis, increased fibrin deposition, and possibly microthrombi. These changes indicated an immune response or vascular involvement associated with COVID. Conversely, in non-COVID and unvaccinated women, the placenta showed typical histological features without these specific inflammatory or vascular alterations (Figure 2A–C).

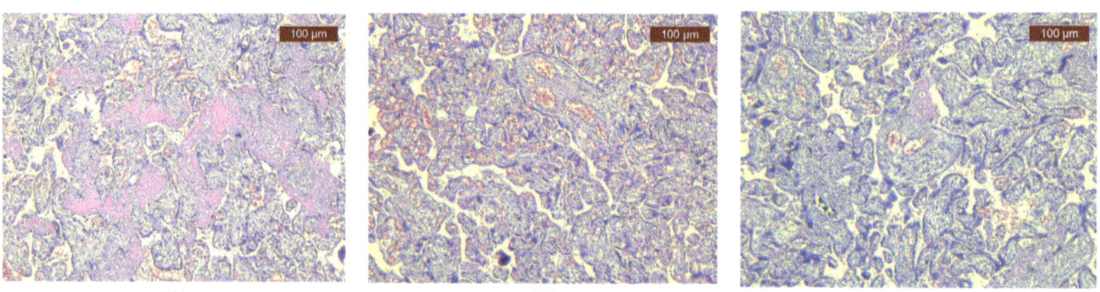


(A) (B) (C)

**Figure 2.** Representative histopathological changes in the placenta (HE). (**A**) COVID-19-positive pregnant women: small, well-vascularized chorionic villi. Syncytial knots and intervillous fibrin (HEx10). (**B**) COVID-19-vaccinated pregnant women: chorionic villi, congestion, and fibrosis (HEx20). (**C**) COVID-19-negative and unvaccinated pregnant women: different size of chorionic villi, congestion, and area of fibrosis (HEx10).

Strikingly, our analysis identified a more intensive CD44 expression on the surface of placental connective tissue stroma within healthy unvaccinated placental tissue (Figure 3C, Table 2). In placental tissues from COVID-positive pregnant women, we observed a more subtle decrease in CD44 expression (Figure 3B, Table 2). Comparatively, CD44 expression was the lowest in COVID-vaccinated placental tissues (Figure 3B, Table 2).

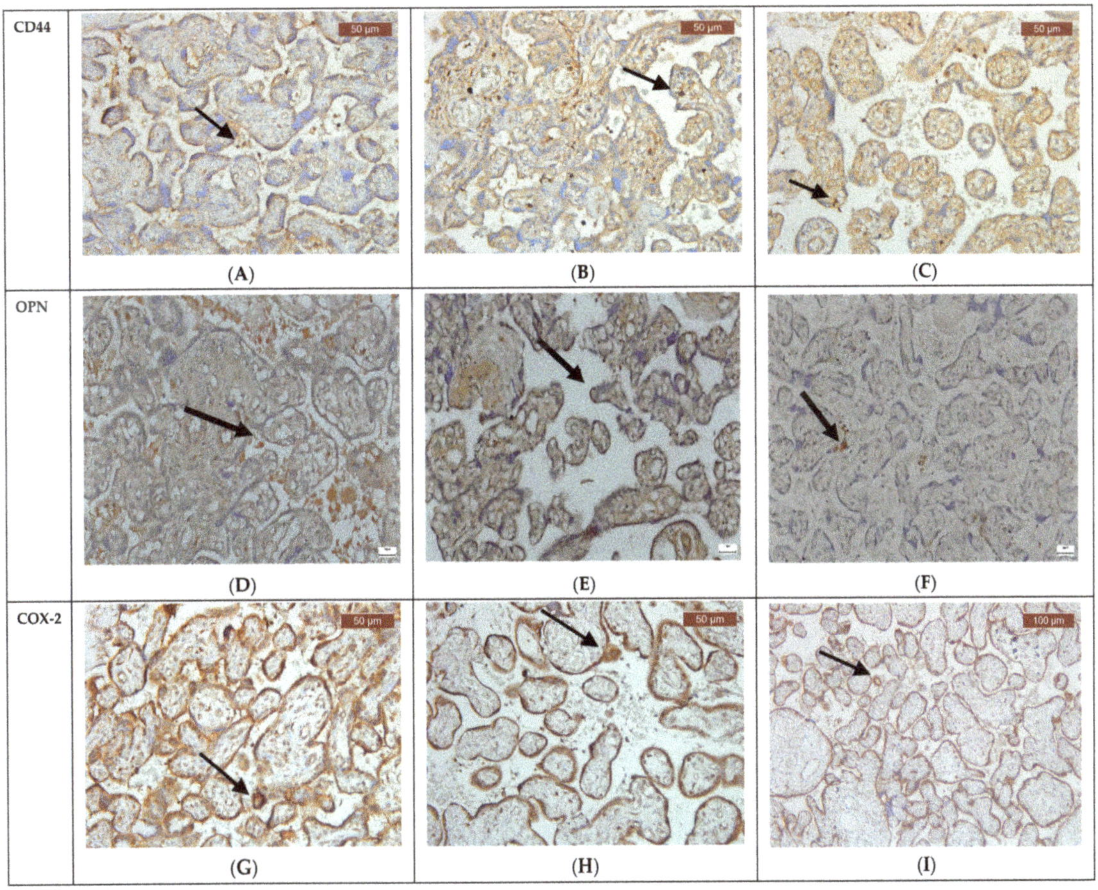


**Figure 3.** Representative immunohistochemical analysis of CD44, OPN, and anti-COX-2 in trophoblastic mononuclear cells. The arrows indicate positive staining. (**A**) COVID-19-positive pregnant women (×20). (**B**) COVID-19-vaccinated pregnant women (×20). (**C**) COVID-19-negative and unvaccinated pregnant women (×20). (**D**) COVID-19-positive pregnant women (×20). (**E**) COVID-19-vaccinated pregnant women (×20). (**F**) COVID-19-negative and unvaccinated pregnant women (×20). (**G**) COVID-19-posietive pregnant women (×20). (**H**) COVID-19-vaccinated pregnant women (×20). (**I**) COVID-19-negative and unvaccinated pregnant women (×20).

**Table 2.** CD44, OPN, and anti-COX-2 placental expression in our three groups of pregnant women.

| | | | CD44 (Cluster of Differentiation 44) | | p-Value | OPN (Osteopontin) | | p-Value | COX-2 (Cyclooxygenase-2) | | p-Value | |
|---|---|---|---|---|---|---|---|---|---|---|---|---|
| | | | Negative | Positive | | Negative | Positive | | Negative | Positive | | Total |
| Group | COVID-positive | Count | 23 | 42 | <0.001 * Positive vs. vaccinated | 53 | 12 | <0.001 * Positive vs. vaccinated | 4 | 61 | 0.295 F Positive vs. vaccinated | 65 |
| | | % within lot | 35.4% | 64.6% | | 81.5% | 18.5% | | 6.2% | 93.8% | | 100.0% |
| | Pfeizer vaccinated | Count | 0 | 35 | 0.004 F Vaccinated vs. negative | 11 | 24 | <0.001 * Vaccinated vs. negative | 0 | 35 | All positive Vaccinated vs. negative | 35 |
| | | % within lot | 0.0% | 100.0% | | 31.4% | 68.6% | | 0.0% | 100.0% | | 100.0% |
| | Negative and unvaccinated | Count | 14 | 56 | 0.045 * Positive vs. negative | 56 | 14 | 0.82 * Positive vs. negative | 0 | 70 | 0.051 F Positive vs. negative | 70 |
| | | % within lot | 20.0% | 80.0% | | 80.0% | 20.0% | | 0.0% | 100.0% | | 100.0% |
| Total | | Count | 37 | 133 | | 120 | 50 | | 4 | 166 | | 170 |
| | | % within lot | 21.8% | 78.2% | | 70.6% | 29.4% | | 2.4% | 97.6% | | 100.0% |

F—Fisher's exact test. *—Chi-square test.

Furthermore, our analysis demonstrated an upregulation of OPN expression in the placental tissues of COVID-vaccinated women, evident in both the epithelial and stromal compartments (Figure 3E, Table 2). COVID-negative and unvaccinated women showed a slight upregulation of OPN expression in placental tissues (Figure 3F, Table 2). In contrast, the OPN expression in COVID-positive placentas was the lowest (Figure 3D, Table 2). Surprisingly, both healthy and COVID-positive cases registered similar percentages of OPN within the stromal and epithelial compartments of the trophoblast, suggesting a relatively stable, non-inflammatory state. However, as reflected in the table above, a significant proportion of the cases were OPN-negative, particularly among the COVID-positive and healthy unvaccinated groups. The most notable difference was observed in the vaccinated group, where the number of OPN-positive cases was double that of the OPN-negative cases (Table 2).

In COVID-negative and unvaccinated placentas, we detected an increased expression of anti-COX-2 in trophoblasts, decidua cells, and infiltrating immune cells. Following COVID infection, anti-COX-2 expression was modestly elevated compared to its low expression levels in vaccinated placentas, with no negative cases of anti-COX-2 in healthy and vaccinated pregnant women (Figure 3G–I, Table 2).

The correlations between the biomarkers were relatively low, indicating a weak linear relationship: 0.121 correlation between CD44 and OPN; 0.200 correlation between CD44 and COX-2; and 0.100 correlation between OPN and COX-2. The Cohen's power analysis computed 87 participants per group to detect a medium effect size with a significance level of 0.05 and a power of 0.8. We used a simplified logistic regression model using only the main effects the groups and CD44, due to limited data that made it difficult to estimate the effects with accuracy. The results indicated that women from the vaccinated group were significantly more likely to have a positive OPN expression compared to those from the COVID-positive group, with no significant differences in OPN positivity between the control group and the COVID-negative group, and without any significant impact of CD44 positivity on the likelihood of OPN being positive. Fisher's exact test results for each biomarker across our group comparisons reinforced our results, indicating that COVID vaccination is associated with a higher expression of CD44 and OPN, while COX-2 expression remains unaffected (Figure 4).

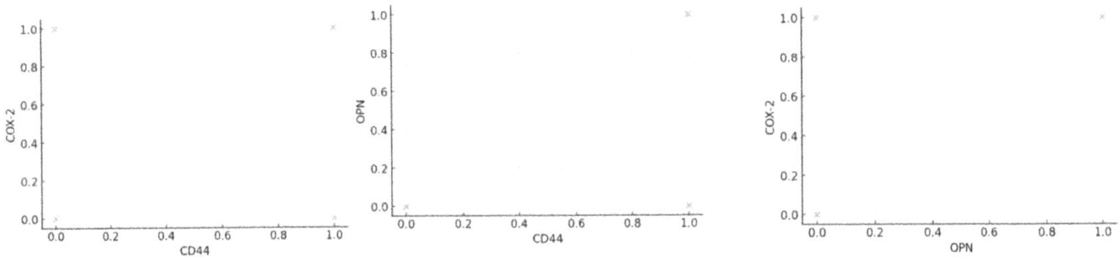


**Figure 4.** Scatterplots representing the correlations between our three biomarkers.

## 4. Discussion

A wide range of placental histopathologic abnormalities secondary to COVID infection during pregnancy have been reported in the literature, with central findings represented by vascular malperfusion and villitis. The fact that these placental alterations are present regardless of the symptomatic or asymptomatic status of the pregnant women suggests a direct viral causative effect. The presence of virions in the placental villis further supports this. A severe systemic inflammatory response and hypercoagulable state, with widespread microthrombi, induced by COVID infection, are certainties [1,4,6,15]. Garg et al., Debelenko et al., and Chen et al. described decidual arteriopathy, with utero-placental insufficiency and consecutive hypoxia, accompanied by fibrinoid necrosis, increased syncytial knots, and inflammatory villitis processes [5,16,17]. Information about placental injury in COVID-asymptomatic women is scarce, so we investigated whether this viral infection has a significant impact on cluster of differentiation 44 (CD44), osteopontin (OPN), and cyclooxygenase-2 (COX-2) placental inflammatory markers. We investigated the expression of these three key molecules in a placental study to clarify some of the ongoing debates surrounding previous epidemics.

Often, secondary tissue hypoxia, together with widespread anemia in pregnancy in our region, significantly decrease the oxygen transport capacity [18]. Although significant therapeutic efforts are devoted to preventing and correcting anemia in pregnancy, a high proportion of low hemoglobin levels in our entire cohort of pregnant women, regardless of their infectious or vaccinated status, was still observed. Up-to-date evidence suggests that COVID vaccination has a low impact on the placenta, without significant differences compared to healthy subjects [19].

Routine blood analysis is also impacted by this disease. The most encountered alteration in COVID infection is lymphopenia with elevated neutrophil count levels [20]. Although frequently described in the literature, our study did not detect such changes. This might have been due to the asymptomatic state of our patients, the small number of cases, or unknown region particularities.

Despite the fact that the literature has often described a multitude of unfavorable neonatal outcomes, our study only identified two: a lower birth weight and a lower gestational age at birth [3,20]. This was also reflected in the study by Maranto et al., 2023, which noted a higher prematurity rate in COVID-positive women, especially in symptomatic cases, with higher rates of delivery through cesarean sections in these cases [21], as in our research. Icognito et al. conducted a study that revealed variations in maternal–fetal severity of outcomes based on the COVID infection subtype. The findings highlighted the significant impact of early subtypes, like Delta, in contrast to later subtypes, such as Alpha and Omicron, with milder maternal–fetal impacts [22]. Maranto et al. underlined the importance of COVID vaccination in this reluctant but very vulnerable obstetric population, with the purpose of enhancing maternal–fetal outcomes [23]. Another aspect of interest to researchers is the fact that cesarean section is associated in some studies with an increased rate of neonatal secondary infection [24]. This was not observed in our results. Despite the fact that all of our neonates were accommodated with their mothers, and all of them were exclusively breastfed, none became infected. However, despite positive short-term fetal outcomes, we cannot exclude the possibility of long-term consequences arising from this disease [25].

The interaction between CD44 and HA is important in angiogenesis, particularly in the differentiation of endothelial cells, but also in their proliferation and migration [8,26]. This seems to play a central role, especially in the first trimester of pregnancy, with CD44 having a high degree of expression in almost every placental structure (decidua, syncytial knots and bridges, fibroblast and muscle cells, and mucosal connective tissue) [8,27]. Our results reflected an increased CD44 expression in COVID-negative unvaccinated pregnancy placentas, suggesting that in these cases placentation evolves in a natural physiological manner. The alterations in placental architecture and angiogenesis, consequent to COVID infection and vaccination, are reflected by a more discrete presence of CD44 in the epithelial and stromal compartments.

Another interesting aspect is the fact that placental first trimester macrophages, the Hofbauer cells, with less accurate detected functions, secrete a number of placental angiogenesis and remodeling molecules, such as OPN. OPN seems to be involved in implantation and placentation, favoring the angiogenesis process [11,28]. Our results showed that the majority of our pregnant women, regardless of group, had a negative expression of OPN in their placentas. The rates of positive cases were similar between COVID-positive and COVID-negative cases. This might have been secondary to our case enrolment process, as we did not separately analyze cases with COVID in each trimester of pregnancy, and perhaps more pronounced OPN positivity results from an early viral infection, with altered placentation and Hofbauer cell function. However, COVID vaccinations administered during earlier gestation led to subtle alterations in the proportion of OPN-positive cells, with the number of positive cells nearly double the negative cells.

Increased COX-2 expression in tissues is related to an inflammatory response. This molecule has a markedly low expression in normal tissue but dramatically increases in some conditions, related to an inflammatory state [29–33]. COX-2 is a central player in the human decidualization process, as a modulator of mitogenesis, differentiation, and angiogenesis [33,34]. A deficit is linked to unfavorable pregnancy outcomes [30–32,35]. Our findings clearly underlined high COX-2 positivity in normal unaffected unvaccinated pregnancies compared to COVID-positive or vaccinated cases. The downregulation of COX-2 in vaccinated cases, although subtler, might have been secondary to reduced inflammation and immunomodulation due to the vaccine.

Zika infection shares many similarities with COVID but more seriously affects fetal development due to its high tropism in trophoblastic cells, causing inflammation and metabolic impairment with mitochondrial dysfunction. COVID infection has modestly negative pregnancy outcomes, with severity varying depending on the viral subtype and mother's symptoms [18,36]. Despite this, research is still needed to fully understand the disease and better prepare for possible future pandemics. The significant differences between the groups in the CD44 and OPN status suggested that vaccination may enhance certain immune pathways, potentially offering greater protection or a more vigilant immune state compared to natural infection or the unvaccinated state. This has implications for understanding the long-term benefits of vaccination in terms of immune system activation.

Our study had limitations due to the limited number of cases and the lack of a separate pregnancy trimester analysis. However, data from the literature remain scarce and we believe that our results are meaningful. Further research is essential to fully elucidate the implications of the expression of these markers and to confirm these findings.

## 5. Conclusions

The findings in this work reflected an alteration in the placental structure and consequent function due to altered expression of the three studied molecules. We detected high levels of CD44 and COX-2 expression in normal uninfected and unvaccinated pregnancies as a result of the normal process of placentation, with downregulation of these molecules in COVID-infected women and more subtle changes in vaccinated individuals. The OPN levels remained similar, potentially due to late pregnancy COVID infection with less affected placentation. This underlines the need for closer obstetric monitoring due to a high risk of unfavorable maternal and fetal outcomes.

**Author Contributions:** Conceptualization, C.C. and D.R.M.; methodology, C.C. and V.B.; software, V.L.B. and A.U.; validation, L.L. and D.R.M.; formal analysis, L.L. and I.E.B.; investigation, D.R.M.; resources, C.C. and L.L.; data curation, A.U.; writing—original draft preparation, C.C. and M.E.N.; writing—review and editing, D.R.M. and A.U.; visualization, L.L.; supervision, V.B.; project administration, C.C. All authors have read and agreed to the published version of the manuscript.

**Funding:** This research received no external funding.

**Institutional Review Board Statement:** The study was conducted in accordance with the Declaration of Helsinki, and approved by the Ethics Committee of the UNIVERSITY OF MEDICINE AND PHARMACY "Lucian Blaga", Sibiu (1442/19 March 2024) and of the Obstetrics and Gynecology Hospital "Cuza-Voda" in Iasi, Romania (10426/24 August 2021 and 19/4 August 2023).

**Informed Consent Statement:** Written informed consent has been obtained from the patients to publish this paper.

**Data Availability Statement:** The data used to support the findings of this study are available upon request to the corresponding author.

**Acknowledgments:** The authors would like to acknowledge the contribution of Department of Obstetrics and Gynecology, Women's Hospital, Universities of Medicine and Pharmacy "Gr. T. Popa" Sibiu, Romania for supporting this study. We are also greatly indebted to all participants for donating their tissue/placenta.

**Conflicts of Interest:** The authors declare no conflicts of interest.

## References

1. Shanes, E.D.; Mithal, L.B.; Otero, S.; Azad, H.A.; Miller, E.S.; Goldstein, J.A. Placental Pathology in COVID-19. *Am. J. Clin. Pathol.* **2020**, *154*, 23–32. [CrossRef] [PubMed]
2. Schwartz, D.A.; Bugatti, M.; Santoro, A.; Facchetti, F. Molecular Pathology Demonstration of SARS-CoV-2 in Cytotrophoblast from Placental Tissue with Chronic Histiocytic Intervillositis, Trophoblast Necrosis and COVID-19. *J. Dev. Biol.* **2021**, *9*, 33. [CrossRef] [PubMed]
3. Bertero, L.; Borella, F.; Botta, G.; Carosso, A.; Cosma, S.; Bovetti, M.; Carosso, M.; Abbona, G.; Collemi, G.; Papotti, M.; et al. Placenta histopathology in SARS-CoV-2 infection: Analysis of a consecutive series and comparison with control cohorts. *Virchows Arch.* **2021**, *479*, 715–728. [CrossRef] [PubMed]
4. Di Girolamo, R.; Khalil, A.; Alameddine, S.; D'Angelo, E.; Galliani, C.; Matarrelli, B.; Buca, D.; Liberati, M.; Rizzo, G.; D'Antonio, F. Placental histopathology after SARS-CoV-2 infection in pregnancy: A systematic review and meta-analysis. *Am. J. Obstet. Gynecol. MFM* **2021**, *3*, 100468. [CrossRef] [PubMed]
5. Garg, R.; Agarwal, R.; Yadav, D.; Singh, S.; Kumar, H.; Bhardwaj, R. Histopathological Changes in Placenta of Severe Acute Respiratory Syndrome Coronavirus 2 (SARS-CoV-2) Infection and Maternal and Perinatal Outcome in COVID-19. *J. Obstet. Gynaecol. India* **2023**, *73*, 44–50. [CrossRef] [PubMed]
6. Patberg, E.T.; Adams, T.; Rekawek, P.; Vahanian, S.A.; Akerman, M.; Hernandez, A.; Rapkiewicz, A.V.; Ragolia, L.; Sicuranza, G.; Chavez, M.R.; et al. Coronavirus disease 2019 infection and placental histopathology in women delivering at term. *Am. J. Obstet. Gynecol.* **2021**, *224*, 382.e1–382.e18, Erratum in: *Am. J. Obstet. Gynecol.* **2023**, *228*, 128. https://doi.org/10.1016/j.ajog.2021.04.255. [CrossRef]
7. Vikesaa, J.; Hansen, T.V.; Jønson, L.; Borup, R.; Wewer, U.M.; Christiansen, J.; Nielsen, F.C. RNA-binding IMPs promote cell adhesion and invadopodia formation. *EMBO J.* **2006**, *25*, 1456–1468. [CrossRef]
8. Obut, M.; Oğlak, S.C. Expression of CD44 and IL-10 in normotensive and preeclamptic placental tissue. *Ginekol. Pol.* **2020**, *91*, 334–341. [CrossRef]
9. Thapa, R.; Wilson, G.D. The Importance of CD44 as a Stem Cell Biomarker and Therapeutic Target in Cancer. *Stem Cells Int.* **2016**, *2016*, 2087204. [CrossRef]
10. Higashibata, Y.; Sakuma, T.; Kawahata, H.; Fujihara, S.; Moriyama, K.; Okada, A.; Yasui, T.; Kohri, K.; Kitamura, Y.; Nomura, S. Identification of promoter regions involved in cell- and developmental stage-specific osteopontin expression in bone, kidney, placenta, and mammary gland: An analysis of transgenic mice. *J. Bone Miner. Res.* **2004**, *19*, 78–88. [CrossRef]
11. Thomas, J.R.; Appios, A.; Zhao, X.; Dutkiewicz, R.; Donde, M.; Lee, C.Y.C.; Naidu, P.; Lee, C.; Cerveira, J.; Liu, B.; et al. Phenotypic and functional characterization of first-trimester human placental macrophages, Hofbauer cells. *J. Exp. Med.* **2021**, *218*, e20200891. [CrossRef] [PubMed]

12. Wu, G.; Li, X.; Seo, H.; McLendon, B.A.; Kramer, A.C.; Bazer, F.W.; Johnson, G.A. Osteopontin (OPN)/Secreted Phosphoprotein 1 (SPP1) Binds Integrins to Activate Transport of Ions across the Porcine Placenta. *Front. Biosci.* **2022**, *27*, 117. [CrossRef] [PubMed]
13. Szczuko, M.; Kikut, J.; Komorniak, N.; Bilicki, J.; Celewicz, Z.; Ziętek, M. The Role of Arachidonic and Linoleic Acid Derivatives in Pathological Pregnancies and the Human Reproduction Process. *Int. J. Mol. Sci.* **2020**, *21*, 9628. [CrossRef] [PubMed]
14. Hwang, Y.J.; Sung, G.J.; Marquardt, R.; Young, S.L.; Lessey, B.A.; Kim, T.H.; Cheon, Y.P.; Jeong, J.W. SIRT1 plays an important role in implantation and decidualization during mouse early pregnancy. *Biol. Reprod.* **2022**, *106*, 1072–1082. [CrossRef] [PubMed]
15. Helmi, Z.; Al-Badri, H. Association of placental histopathological findings with COVID-19 and its predictive factors. *Rev. Bras. Ginecol. Obstet.* **2024**, *46*, e-rbgo3. [CrossRef]
16. Debelenko, L.; Katsyv, I.; Chong, A.M.; Peruyero, L.; Szabolcs, M.; Uhlemann, A.C. Trophoblast damage with acute and chronic intervillositis: Disruption of the placental barrier by severe acute respiratory syndrome coronavirus 2. *Hum. Pathol.* **2021**, *109*, 69–79. [CrossRef]
17. Chen, J.; Du, L.; Wang, F.; Shao, X.; Wang, X.; Yu, W.; Bi, S.; Chen, D.; Pan, X.; Zeng, S.; et al. Cellular and molecular atlas of the placenta from a COVID-19 pregnant woman infected at midgestation highlights the defective impacts on foetal health. *Cell Prolif.* **2022**, *55*, e13204. [CrossRef]
18. Surekha, M.V.; Suneetha, N.; Balakrishna, N.; Putcha, U.K.; Satyanarayana, K.; Geddam, J.J.B.; Sreenu, P.; Tulja, B.; Mamidi, R.S.; Rutter, G.A.; et al. Impact of COVID-19 during pregnancy on placental pathology, maternal and neonatal outcome—A cross-sectional study on anemic term pregnant women from a tertiary care hospital in southern India. *Front. Endocrinol.* **2023**, *14*, 1092104. [CrossRef]
19. Tartaglia, S.; Di Ilio, C.; Romanzi, F.; Moresi, S.; Nardi, E.; Bevilacqua, E.; Arena, V.; Lanzone, A. Effects of SARS-CoV-2 mRNA vaccine on placental histopathology: Comparison of a population of uncomplicated COVID-19 positive pregnant women. *Placenta* **2024**, *149*, 64–71. [CrossRef]
20. Valdespino-Vázquez, M.Y.; Helguera-Repetto, C.A.; León-Juárez, M.; Villavicencio-Carrisoza, O.; Flores-Pliego, A.; Moreno-Verduzco, E.R.; Díaz-Pérez, D.L.; Villegas-Mota, I.; Carrasco-Ramírez, E.; López-Martínez, I.E.; et al. Fetal and placental infection with SARS-CoV-2 in early pregnancy. *J. Med. Virol.* **2021**, *93*, 4480–4487. [CrossRef]
21. Maranto, M.; Zaami, S.; Restivo, V.; Termini, D.; Gangemi, A.; Tumminello, M.; Culmone, S.; Billone, V.; Cucinella, G.; Gullo, G. Symptomatic COVID-19 in Pregnancy: Hospital Cohort Data between May 2020 and April 2021, Risk Factors and Medicolegal Implications. *Diagnostics* **2023**, *13*, 1009. [CrossRef] [PubMed]
22. Incognito, G.G.; Distefano, R.E.C.; Campo, G.; Gulino, F.A.; Gulisano, C.; Gullotta, C.; Gullo, G.; Cucinella, G.; Tuscano, A.; Bruno, M.T.; et al. Comparison of Maternal and Neonatal Outcomes between SARS-CoV-2 Variants: A Retrospective, Monocentric Study. *J. Clin. Med.* **2023**, *12*, 6329. [CrossRef] [PubMed] [PubMed Central]
23. Maranto, M.; Gullo, G.; Bruno, A.; Minutolo, G.; Cucinella, G.; Maiorana, A.; Casuccio, A.; Restivo, V. Factors Associated with Anti-SARS-CoV-2 Vaccine Acceptance among Pregnant Women: Data from Outpatient Women Experiencing High-Risk Pregnancy. *Vaccines* **2023**, *11*, 454. [CrossRef] [PubMed] [PubMed Central]
24. Kreis, N.N.; Ritter, A.; Louwen, F.; Yuan, J. A Message from the Human Placenta: Structural and Immunomodulatory Defense against SARS-CoV-2. *Cells* **2020**, *9*, 1777. [CrossRef]
25. Sarno, L.; Locci, M.; Fulgione, C.; Perillo, F.; Dell'Isola, A.; Mantelli, D.; Sibillo, C.; Saccone, G.; Maruotti, G.M.; Terracciano, D.; et al. Characteristics of Placental Histopathology in Women with Uncomplicated Pregnancies Affected by SARS-CoV-2 Infection at the Time of Delivery: A Single-Center Experience. *Biomedicines* **2022**, *10*, 3003. [CrossRef]
26. Balsak, D.; Togrul, C.; Ekinci, C.; Cavus, Y.; Tahaoglu, A.E.; Deveci, E.; Gül, T.; Karaman, E.; Ekinci, A.; Sakar, N. Severe pre-eclampsia complicated by HELLP syndrome alterations in the structure of the umbilical cord (morphometric and immunohistochemical study). *Biotechnol. Biotechnol. Equip.* **2015**, *29*, 345–350. [CrossRef]
27. Zhu, R.; Wang, S.C.; Sun, C.; Tao, Y.; Piao, H.L.; Wang, X.Q.; Du, M.R.; Li, D.-J. Hyaluronan-CD44 interaction promotes growth of decidual stromal cells in human first-trimester pregnancy. *PLoS ONE* **2013**, *8*, e74812. [CrossRef]
28. Li, M.C.; Fang, Q.; He, Z.M.; Gao, Y.; Zhou, Y. Placental expression of osteopontin(OPN) in monochorionic twins with discordant growth. *Placenta* **2013**, *34*, 288–290. [CrossRef]
29. Song, Y.B.; Sun, M.Y. Correlation analysis between COX-2 gene polymorphism and eclampsia. *Eur. Rev. Med. Pharmacol. Sci.* **2019**, *23*, 6404–6410. [CrossRef]
30. Pannunzio, A.; Coluccia, M. Cyclooxygenase-1 (COX-1) and COX-1 Inhibitors in Cancer: A Review of Oncology and Medicinal Chemistry Literature. *Pharmaceuticals* **2018**, *11*, 101. [CrossRef]
31. Gately, S. The Contributions of Cyclooxygenase-2 to Tumor Angiogenesis. *Cancer Metastasis* **2000**, *19*, 19–27. [CrossRef] [PubMed]
32. Mancini, A.D.; Di Battista, J.A. The cardinal role of the phospholipase $A_2$/cyclooxygenase-2/prostaglandin E synthase/prostaglandin $E_2$ (PCPP) axis in inflammostasis. *Inflamm. Res.* **2011**, *60*, 1083–1092. [CrossRef] [PubMed]
33. Tang, H.; Pan, L.; Tang, L.; Liu, J. Alpha-enolase 1 knockdown facilitates the proliferation and invasion of villous trophoblasts by upregulating COX-2. *Mol. Genet. Genom. Med.* **2023**, *11*, e2220. [CrossRef] [PubMed]
34. Zhang, D.; Chang, X.; Bai, J.; Chen, Z.J.; Li, W.P.; Zhang, C. The Study of Cyclooxygenase 2 in Human Decidua of Preeclampsia. *Biol. Reprod.* **2016**, *95*, 56. [CrossRef] [PubMed]

35. Shah, B.H.; Catt, K.J. Roles of LPA3 and COX-2 in implantation. *Trends Endocrinol. Metab.* **2005**, *16*, 397–399. [CrossRef]
36. Gullo, G.; Scaglione, M.; Cucinella, G.; Riva, A.; Coldebella, D.; Cavaliere, A.F.; Signore, F.; Buzzaccarini, G.; Spagnol, G.; Laganà, A.S.; et al. Congenital Zika Syndrome: Genetic Avenues for Diagnosis and Therapy, Possible Management and Long-Term Outcomes. *J. Clin. Med.* **2022**, *11*, 1351. [CrossRef]

Journal of
*Clinical Medicine*

MDPI

*Article*

# Vitamin D Receptor—Interplay in COVID-19-Negative, -Infected, and -Vaccinated Women during Pregnancy

**Constantin Condac [1,2,†], Ludmila Lozneanu [3,†], Daniela Roxana Matasariu [4,5,*], Alexandra Ursache [4,*], Iuliana Elena Bujor [4], Maria Elena Niță [5], Vasile Lucian Boiculese [6], Mihai Sava [7], Paula Țăroi [8] and Victoria Bîrluțiu [2]**

1 Department of Anesthesia and Intensive Care, "Cuza Vodă" Hospital, 700038 Iasi, Romania; costicondac@gmail.com
2 Department of Infectious Diseases, University of Medicine and Pharmacy "Lucian Blaga", 550169 Sibiu, Romania; victoria.birlutiu@ulbsibiu.ro
3 Department of Morpho-Functional Sciences I—Histology, University of Medicine and Pharmacy "Gr. T. Popa", 700115 Iasi, Romania; ludmila.lozneanu@umfiasi.ro
4 Department of Obstetrics and Gynecology, University of Medicine and Pharmacy "Gr. T. Popa", 700115 Iasi, Romania; iuliana-elena.bujor@d.umfiasi.ro
5 Department of Obstetrics and Gynecology, "Cuza Vodă" Hospital, 700038 Iasi, Romania; elemarni28@gmail.com
6 Biostatistics, Department of Preventive Medicine and Interdisciplinarity, University of Medicine and Pharmacy "Gr. T. Popa", 700115 Iasi, Romania; lboiculese@gmail.com
7 Department of Anesthesia and Intensive Care, University of Medicine and Pharmacy "Lucian Blaga", 550169 Sibiu, Romania; mihai.sava@ulbsibiu.ro
8 Department of Obstetrics and Gynecology, University of Medicine and Pharmacy "Lucian Blaga", 550169 Sibiu, Romania; paula.nita@ulbsibiu.ro
* Correspondence: daniela.matasariu@umfiasi.ro (D.R.M.); alexandra.ursache@umfiasi.ro (A.U.)
† These authors contributed equally to this work.

**Abstract: Background:** The trophoblast is a significant source of vitamin D synthesis during pregnancy, with the literature suggesting its role in fetal growth. We aim to underline a possible mechanism that would explain negative fetal outcomes in COVID-19-positive mothers by examining the relationship between altered placental structure and function and throphoblast cells' vitamin D receptor levels. **Methods:** The study included 170 placental samples collected from women who gave birth at term without complications, divided into three groups: COVID-19-positive and unvaccinated, COVID-19-negative and vaccinated, and COVID-19-negative and unvaccinated, with exclusion criteria for any other medical complications. Immunohistochemistry (IHC) was performed to detect vitamin D receptor (VDR) expression, and immediate fetal outcomes (weight and Apgar score) were assessed. **Results:** We found lower gestational age at birth, lower birth weight, and reduced placental VDR (vitamin D receptor) levels in COVID-19-positive women compared to COVID-19-vaccinated and COVID-19-negative women. **Conclusions:** The presence of the vitamin D receptor in the placenta is related to fetal and placental growth. Its deficiency may contribute to negative fetal outcomes in COVID-19-positive cases.

**Keywords:** placenta; SARS-CoV-2; COVID-19; vitamin D receptor; immunohistochemistry; diagnosis; Pfizer vaccine

## 1. Introduction

Coronavirus disease 2019 (COVID-19) is an acute respiratory illness caused by SARS-CoV-2 infection [1,2]. COVID-19 infection can negatively impact various organs and tissues, leading to diverse clinical manifestations [3]. Beyond respiratory symptoms, it can impact gastrointestinal function; cause preeclampsia in pregnant women; affect liver function; impair renal, cardiac, and male fertility function; and cause neurological, immune, and endocrine system dysfunction [4–6]. The virus accesses human cells via the angiotensin-converting enzyme 2 (ACE-2), which is abundantly present on the placental syncytiotrophoblast, suggesting a possible connection between infection and impaired placental function [7,8].

The impact of COVID-19 on pregnant women and infants is of particular interest to obstetricians, pediatricians, and patients [9]. Pregnancy increases the vulnerability to severe forms of COVID-19 due to physiological changes, particularly in the cardiovascular and immune systems. However, its impact on maternal and fetal outcomes remains a topic of debate. There is evidence linking COVID-19 in pregnancy to complications such as hypertensive disorders, preterm birth, fetal growth pathology, gestational diabetes, increased neonatal intensive care admission, and stillbirth. Discrepancies in the literature are further pronounced when considering the effects of different viral strains and the outcomes for asymptomatic or mildly symptomatic pregnant women. There is also persistent controversy about the vertical transmission of COVID-19 infection, either mediated by angiotensin-converting enzyme 2, or through hypoxemia-injured placenta [10,11]. The pathological analysis of placenta during past epidemics has been informative regarding the resulting negative outcomes and the mechanisms of disease transmission to the fetus. Extensive research has been conducted to explain the physiological and pathological mechanisms of COVID-19, to limit its spread and consequences [12–14].

Vitamin D plays multiple roles in the human organism, including the development of the reproductive axis, homeostasis, bone formation, and the modulation of both innate and adaptive immune systems. It supports placental development and function by regulating calcium transport, which is essential for pregnancy maintenance, and preventing a maternal immune response against the embryo, playing a pivotal role in fetal growth and development [15–17]. The literature is abundant in studies that relate low vitamin D serum levels to the severity of the COVID-19 infection, underlining vitamin D's well-known role in modulating the immune response, depending on the expression of its receptor [17–20]. From the first trimester of pregnancy, the placental levels of vitamin D receptor (VDR) increase significantly, underlining vitamin D's importance in fetal development and placental physiology, with some authors suggesting that it shows antimicrobial and anti-inflammatory activity [21].

The available literature contains limited data on vitamin D levels in COVID-19-positive pregnant women [20,22], with only one study by Moreno-Fernandez et al. evaluating placental vitamin D levels [23], which prompted our study to try to clarify the connection between COVID-19 infection and adverse obstetrical outcomes. We aimed to underline a possible mechanism that would explain negative fetal outcomes in COVID-19-positive mothers by examining the relationship between altered placental structure and function and trophoblast cells' vitamin D receptor levels.

## 2. Materials and Methods

### 2.1. Patients and Tissue Samples

The study period was from January 2021 to January 2023. All of the patients provided written informed consent. The study was approved by the ethics committees of the University of Medicine and Pharmacy "Lucian Blaga", Sibiu (1442/19 March 2024) and the Obstetrics and Gynecology Hospital "Cuza-Voda" in Iasi, Romania (No. 10426/24 August 2021 and No. 19/4 August 2023).

Specimens were collected from women who gave birth at term without complications, associated disease, or chronic treatment (for toxoplasma; rubella; cytomegalovirus; herpes with no acute infection detected; hepatitis B or C; HIV; or syphilis).

The pregnant women were divided into three groups: COVID-19-positive and unvaccinated women; COVID-19-negative and vaccinated women; and COVID-19-negative and unvaccinated women. Group 1, comprising the COVID-19-positive and unvaccinated women, included asymptomatic patients, with the disease detected at any time during pregnancy but at least 14 days before birth. The diagnosis of COVID-19 positivity was confirmed using Polymerase Chain Reaction (PCR) testing. The second group included Pfizer-vaccinated women, with the first or second dose administered at least 14 days before birth, who never tested positive for COVID-19 during the pandemic and achieved negative results for all their rapid COVID-19 tests, which were taken every three weeks during pregnancy. The control group included COVID-19-negative and unvaccinated women who gave birth at term without any complications or associated pathology (all the women included in the third group never tested positive during the pandemic until inclusion in our study, and had returned negative rapid COVID-19 tests every three weeks during pregnancy).

Exclusion Criteria

Women with obstetrical and/or other medical complications were excluded from our analysis. Patients with COVID-19 infection at the time of giving birth; malignancy; depression; genetic syndromes; infectious or autoimmune diseases; pre-existing or gestational diabetes; hypertension and its complications, such as preeclampsia; premature rupture of membranes; oligohydramnios; intrauterine growth restriction, defined as ultrasound-estimated fetal weight less than the 10th percentile for gestational age; or chorioamnionitis and those who smoked were excluded.

### 2.2. *Immunohistochemistry*

We collected four tissue samples from each placenta, one for each of the four quadrants. Hematoxylin and eosin (H&E) sections were examined, and immunohistochemistry (IHC) was evaluated by two pathologists. IHC staining was performed on formalin-fixed, paraffin-embedded tissues for immunohistochemistry utilizing monoclonal antibodies against VDR. Four-micrometer-thick serial sections were prepared in citrate buffer (pH 6) after deparaffinization in xylene and rehydration in ethanol series. Endogenous peroxidase activity was inhibited with 0.3% $H_2O_2$ for 20 min at room temperature. IHC was used to determine the expression of vitamin D receptor (VDR) that was diluted at 1:3000 (catalog no ab3508 Abcam, Cambridge, UK) and incubated overnight at 4 °C. The sections were washed, exposed to the secondary antibody for 45 min at 37 °C, and cleaned with phosphate-buffered saline (PBS). Hematoxylin was used as a counterstain in the standard avidin-biotin-peroxidase technique, using a liquid DAB (diaminobenzidine) substrate and chromogen system. Human jejunum tissue was used as a positive control.

One hundred and seventy placental samples were examined for VDR presence. Positive cells (with a brown or yellowish-brown color in the nucleus) in epithelial and stromal compartments were considered VDR-positive, regardless of the intensity of staining or the number of positive cells.

### 2.3. *Statistical Analysis*

Data were imported into Microsoft Excel and analyzed in SPSS 24 (IBM Corp. Released 2016. IBM SPSS Statistics for Windows, Version 24.0. Armonk, NY, USA: IBM Corp.). Descriptive statistics included sample size (N), mean, standard deviation, standard error, 95% confidence interval, minimum, maximum, and absolute and relative frequencies. Non-parametric statistical hypothesis tests, such as the Kruskal–Wallis test for 3 samples and post hoc tests using Bonferroni–Dunn corrections for 2-sample comparisons, were applied. These have been applied to the analysis of continuous numerical variables. Chi-square or Fisher exact tests were applied for categorical variables. A significance level of 0.05 was considered statistically significant.

Since we had small sample volumes, we performed a statistical power analysis using the G*power 3.1.9.7 application. Post hoc power analysis was conducted based on the sample sizes, the effect, and the type I error rate of $\alpha = 0.05$. We simulated different scenarios for real continuous variable hypotheses tests using the Kruskal–Wellis test, and also for frequency comparisons with chi-square distribution. The power 1-$\beta$ ranges between 0.09 and 0.93.

## 3. Results

After applying the inclusion and the exclusion criteria, 170 pregnant women were included in the study: 65 unvaccinated COVID-19-positive women in group 1, 35 vaccinated and COVID-19-negative women in group 2, and 70 unvaccinated COVID-19-negative women in group 3. All of the COVID-19-positive patients in the study were asymptomatic. The ages of our patients ranged from 18 to 39 years.

All of the study patients were asymptomatic. None required supplemental oxygen administration or admission to the intensive care unit. Laboratory testing, involving complete blood counts, inflammatory markers, and biochemical profiles, was performed. Neonatal outcomes, including birth weights, APGAR scores, and neonatal intensive care unit (NICU) admissions, were similar between the three groups (Table 1).

**Table 1.** Distribution of included cases.

| Group | Frequency | Percent | Valid Percent | Cumulative Percent |
|---|---|---|---|---|
| COVID-19-positive pregnant women | 65 | 38.2 | 38.2 | 38.2 |
| COVID-19-vaccinated pregnant women | 35 | 20.6 | 20.6 | 58.8 |
| COVID-19-negative and unvaccinated pregnant women | 70 | 41.2 | 41.2 | 100 |
| Total | 170 | 100 | 100 | |

The unvaccinated pregnant women had a mean age that was 3 years lower than that of the vaccinated women. When we analyzed our groups based on their urban or rural provenance, we detected that in the COVID-19-positive group, 73% of the included cases had urban residency, as did almost 69% from the vaccinated group, while in the COVID-19-negative unvaccinated group, the distribution by residency was equal.

A significant positive correlation was observed between birth gestational age and birth weight. The mean gestational delivery age in our three groups showed significant differences: COVID-19-positive and COVID-19-vaccinated pregnant women had a lower birth gestational age compared to the COVID-19-negative unvaccinated group (Table 2). Another statistically significant difference between the three groups became evident when analyzing the birth weights of the newborns, with children from the COVID-19-negative and unvaccinated group having a higher birth weight compared to those born to vaccinated or COVID-19-positive pregnant women. However, when we analyzed the immediate after-birth statuses of the newborns as reflected by the Apgar scores, we found no significant difference between the three groups (Table 2).

**Table 2.** Clinical and demographic characteristics of included women.

| Clinical and Demographic Characteristics of Women | | No | Mean | St. Dev. | Percentile 25 | Median | Percentile 75 | Min | Max | Kruskal–Wallis $p$-Value |
|---|---|---|---|---|---|---|---|---|---|---|
| Maternal age (years) | Negative and unvaccinated | 70 | 28 | 4 | 27 | 29 | 31 | 19 | 34 | <0.001 |
| | Positive | 65 | 31 | 5 | 28 | 33 | 34 | 18 | 39 | |
| | Pfizer-vaccinated | 35 | 30 | 5 | 27 | 30 | 33 | 18 | 39 | |
| Gestational age at delivery (weeks) | Negative and unvaccinated | 70 | 40 | 1 | 38 | 40 | 41 | 37 | 41 | <0.001 |
| | Positive | 65 | 38 | 3 | 37 | 38 | 39 | 28 | 40 | |
| | Pfizer-vaccinated | 35 | 38 | 3 | 37 | 39 | 40 | 29 | 41 | |
| Fetal weight (grams) | Negative and unvaccinated | 70 | 3507 | 354 | 3260 | 3495 | 3670 | 2800 | 4490 | 0.01 |
| | Positive | 65 | 3237 | 536 | 2920 | 3300 | 3600 | 1980 | 4540 | |
| | Pfizer-vaccinated | 35 | 3291 | 522 | 2920 | 3390 | 3650 | 1990 | 4570 | |
| Apgar score at 1 min (point) | Negative and unvaccinated | 70 | 9 | 1 | 8 | 9 | 9 | 8 | 9 | 0.67 |
| | Positive | 65 | 8 | 1 | 8 | 9 | 9 | 4 | 9 | |
| | Pfizer-vaccinated | 35 | 8 | 1 | 8 | 9 | 9 | 4 | 10 | |

**Table 2.** *Cont.*

| Clinical and Demographic Characteristics of Women | | No | Mean | St. Dev. | Percentile 25 | Median | Percentile 75 | Min | Max | Kruskal–Wallis *p*-Value |
|---|---|---|---|---|---|---|---|---|---|---|
| Hemoglobin antepartum (milligrams/deciliter) | Negative and unvaccinated | 70 | 12.3 | 1.1 | 11.8 | 12.1 | 13.6 | 10.0 | 13.7 | 0.76 |
| | Positive | 65 | 12.2 | 0.8 | 11.9 | 12.3 | 12.5 | 9.7 | 13.4 | |
| | Pfizer-vaccinated | 35 | 12.3 | 0.9 | 11.9 | 12.3 | 13.0 | 9.8 | 14.3 | |
| Hematocrit antepartum (%) | Negative and unvaccinated | 70 | 36.3 | 3.4 | 35.0 | 37.0 | 38.9 | 28.1 | 40.0 | 0.578 |
| | Positive | 65 | 36.4 | 2.6 | 35.3 | 36.0 | 38.0 | 29.3 | 41.0 | |
| | Pfizer-vaccinated | 35 | 36.8 | 2.9 | 35.3 | 36.9 | 38.8 | 28.1 | 42.1 | |
| Hemoglobin postpar-tum(milligrams/deciliter) | Negative and unvaccinated | 70 | 10.9 | 0.8 | 10.4 | 10.9 | 11.4 | 9.0 | 13.0 | 0.61 |
| | Positive | 65 | 11.0 | 0.9 | 10.4 | 11.0 | 11.6 | 8.9 | 12.8 | |
| | Pfizer-vaccinated | 35 | 11.1 | 0.8 | 10.5 | 11.0 | 11.6 | 9.7 | 12.9 | |
| Hematocrite postpartum (%) | Negative and unvaccinated | 70 | 31.8 | 2.9 | 29.0 | 31.1 | 34.3 | 27.8 | 37.0 | 0.52 |
| | Positive | 65 | 32.3 | 2.8 | 30.4 | 32.3 | 33.6 | 27.7 | 38.5 | |
| | Pfizer-vaccinated | 35 | 32.4 | 2.8 | 29.9 | 32.5 | 34.3 | 27.5 | 37.5 | |
| Leucocyte value ($10^3$/liter) | Negative and unvaccinated | 70 | 12,293 | 2272 | 10,350 | 11,485 | 14,600 | 9900 | 16,500 | <0.001 |
| | Positive | 65 | 10,186 | 2590 | 8280 | 10,120 | 12,100 | 5390 | 16,400 | |
| | Pfizer-vaccinated | 35 | 10,936 | 2922 | 8320 | 10,350 | 12,280 | 5390 | 16,500 | |
| Platelet value ($10^6$/liter) | Negative and unvaccinated | 70 | 220,500 | 78,240 | 149,000 | 217,500 | 278,000 | 122,000 | 355,000 | 0.76 |
| | Positive | 65 | 218,523 | 63,791 | 156,000 | 211,000 | 260,000 | 132,000 | 355,000 | |
| | Pfizer-vaccinated | 35 | 227,543 | 71,222 | 156,000 | 218,000 | 278,000 | 135,000 | 36,0000 | |
| CRP (C-reactive protein) value (milligrams/deciliter) | Negative and unvaccinated | 70 | 3.12 | 1.52 | 2.00 | 2.75 | 4.10 | 0.90 | 10.00 | 0.89 |
| | Positive | 65 | 3.09 | 1.30 | 1.90 | 3.00 | 4.80 | 1.07 | 4.90 | |
| | Pfizer-vaccinated | 35 | 3.18 | 1.20 | 2.30 | 2.80 | 4.10 | 1.00 | 4.90 | |

The serum infection/inflammation markers showed no statistical difference in CRP values among the pregnant participants. However, pregnant women who were neither infected with the virus nor vaccinated had significantly higher leucocyte values (Table 2).

When examining H&E sections, pathological changes were depicted. In COVID-19-positive and vaccinated women, we observed signs of inflammation, such as villitis or intervillositis, increased fibrin deposition, and possibly microthrombi. These changes indicate an immune response or vascular involvement associated with the virus. Conversely, in non-infected and unvaccinated women, the placenta showed typical histological features without these specific inflammatory or vascular alterations (Figure 1A–C).

IHC analysis revealed differences in VDR expression among the three groups, with a statistically significantly higher number of VDR-negative cases in tissue samples originating from the placenta of COVID-19-vaccinated women ($p < 0.001$). The number of VDR-positive cases was higher in non-vaccinated COVID-19-negative pregnant women compared to COVID-19-positive and vaccinated ones (Figure 2A–C and Table 3).

**Table 3.** VDR status in our three groups of pregnant women.

| Group | | VDR | | Total | *p*-Value |
|---|---|---|---|---|---|
| | | Negative | Positive | | |
| COVID-19-positive pregnant women | Count | 29 | 36 | 65 | 0.044 |
| | % within group | 44.6% | 55.4% | 100.0% | COVID-positive vs. COVID-vaccinated |

**Table 3.** *Cont.*

| Group | | VDR | | Total | p-Value |
|---|---|---|---|---|---|
| | | Negative | Positive | | |
| Pfizer-vaccinated pregnant women | Count | 23 | 12 | 35 | <0.001 |
| | % within group | 65.7% | 34.3% | 100.0% | COVID-vaccinated vs. control |
| COVID-19-negative and unvaccinated pregnant women | Count | 14 | 56 | 70 | 0.002 |
| | % within group | 20.0% | 80.0% | 100.0% | COVID-positive vs. control |
| Total | Count | 66 | 104 | 170 | |
| | % within group | 38.8% | 61.2% | 100.0% | |

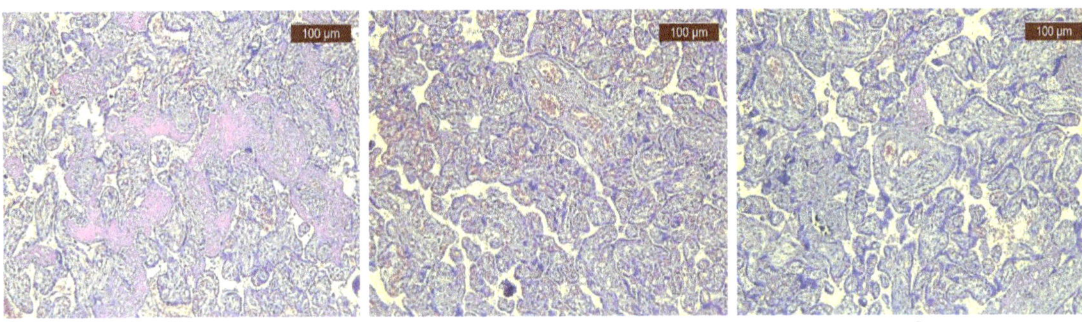


(A) (B) (C)

**Figure 1.** Representative histopathological changes in placenta (H&E). (**A**) COVID-19-positive pregnant women: small, well-vascularized chorionic villi. Syncytial knots and intervillous fibrin (HE × 10). (**B**) COVID-19-vaccinated pregnant women: chorionic villi, congestion, and fibrosis (HE × 20). (**C**) COVID-19-negative and unvaccinated pregnant women: different sizes of chorionic villi, congestion, and area of fibrosis (HE × 10).

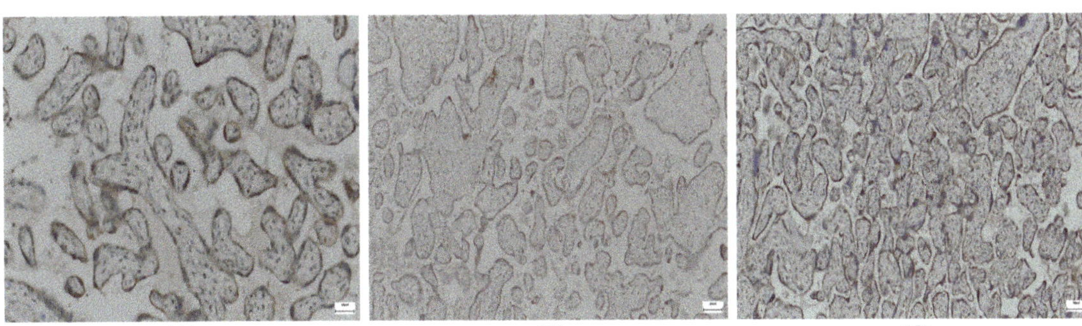

(A) (B) (C)

**Figure 2.** Representative images—immunohistochemical visualization of VDR in mononuclear cells of trophoblasts. (**A**) COVID-19-positive pregnant women (×20). (**B**) COVID-19-vaccinated pregnant women (×20). (**C**) COVID-19-negative and unvaccinated pregnant women (×10).

## 4. Discussion

The COVID-19 pandemic had a profound socio-economic impact, resulting in significant alterations to daily behavior and routine. It emphasized depression, underlining the importance of assessing personality traits in patients for more effective health management. The healthcare system was particularly strained, with increasing reports of heightened patient admissions and hospitalizations, largely due to reduced outpatient services in both gynecology and obstetrics departments. In gynecology, the most common presenting complaint was lower abdominal pain, alongside oncological emergencies. In addition to the psychological stress associated with gynecological conditions, women were further burdened by concerns over potential contagion. Similarly, obstetrics departments saw a rise in emergency cases, accompanied by a decline in non-urgent cases, likely driven by fears of infection [23–25].

A classification system for maternal, fetal, and neonatal COVID-19 infections was proposed by Shah et al. [26]. According to this classification, virus detection by PCR or electron microscopy using fetal or placental tissue, as well as the definitive or probable maternal status, defines a confirmed congenital infection [26,27]. The placenta often has a protective role, inhibiting the transmission of infectious agents from the mother to the fetus [1]. Diverse maternal conditions, including morphological changes, can influence the placenta's function. For example, tissue hypoxia, a common adverse effect of COVID-19 that is caused by a hypercoagulable state, together with anemia (an independent risk factor), can lower the physiological capacity for oxygen transport when faced with increased demand, such as in placental tissue [28]. Although there were no statistically significant differences in hemoglobin and hematocrit levels among our three groups, the overall incidence of anemia remains high in our region's pregnant population. Therefore, we may assume that anemia, as an independent risk factor, uniformly impacts all three included groups.

The immunocompromised state of pregnancy makes patients more susceptible to viral respiratory infections, due to the attenuated immune response of the placenta. Hypoxia, inflammatory activation, increased thrombotic events—secondary to COVID-19—due to turbulent and slow blood flow, progressive rises in fibrin degradation products, and decreased fibrinolysis may lead to adverse pregnancy outcomes due to pathological insult of the placenta, whether acute or chronic (such as miscarriage, oligohydramnios, fetal growth restriction, silent placental abruption, postpartum hemorrhage, unexplained stillbirth, lower Apgar score, congenital viral syndrome, birth defect, preeclampsia, preterm birth, cesarean section) [8,14,29–33]. These placental changes can be highly unpredictable and subtle, varying with the severity of the disease and with the viral subtype, with early variants of COVID-19 registering a more significant negative impact on maternal and fetal outcomes compared to later viral subtypes, such as Omicron, making early detection and intervention extremely challenging [32]. Therefore, vigilant antenatal and intrapartum monitoring is essential in such cases [29,32], especially because many pregnant women remain reluctant to undergo vaccination [34].

Our analysis did not reveal any alterations in newborn status besides a lower birth weight in COVID-19-positive and vaccinated mothers, similar to results described in the literature [31,32]. Lymphopenia with a higher neutrophil count has been associated with COVID-19 infection in pregnant women compared to non-pregnant ones [35]. Our study results reflected quite the opposite, with similar CRP levels among our three groups and higher leucocyte values in the COVID-19-negative and unvaccinated groups. The source of this inconsistency might be the low number of cases included in our research, due to stringent inclusion and exclusion criteria, or perhaps due to some regional particularities.

The neonatal outcomes described were Apgar score, fetal birth weight, the need for neonatal intensive care admission, and fetal demise. Immediately after birth, the Apgar scores of and the three days spent in hospital by the newborns from our included cases did not reveal any negative impact of the infection or vaccination on the newborns. No fetal demise was detected, and there was no need for intensive care admission in our cases. Despite the lack of negative impact on our newborns, the infection and multi-organ fetal inflammation (including lung and kidney) produced by COVID-19 infection during early pregnancy, described in the literature, should alert clinicians involved in the assessment and management of pregnant women to possible fetal consequences and adverse perinatal outcomes [27,36]. Even with a normal short-term outcome, long-term sequelae, such as consequences for the neurodevelopment of newborns, cannot be excluded [30,33].

Compared to placentas from non-infected unvaccinated pregnant women, there were no significant differences in macroscopic and microscopic placental appearance, including placental weight, abnormal cord insertion, and maternal or fetal vascular malperfusion. However, because the majority of our analyzed placentas were not infected and the majority of neonates were negative for coronavirus infection, our findings largely came from examining healthy placentas from uninfected fetuses, similar to those obtained by Schwartz et al. [12]. Many authors have reported no definitive vertical transmission of COVID-19, but the findings in the literature are inconsistent [1,3,37–39]. Additionally, limited positive cases have been reported (mostly case reports or small case series) in the late pregnancy stage with possible postpartum infections, with a rate of transmission ranging from 0% to 9% [30]. Given the extensive literature supporting the benefits of vitamin D supplementation in COVID-19-positive patients, particularly pregnant women, and the well-documented adverse maternal and fetal outcomes associated with low vitamin D serum levels, we sought to evaluate vitamin D status in such cases [40–42]. Assessing serum vitamin D levels in a standardized manner poses serious challenges, as numerous studies report conflicting results due to variations in quantification methods and the wide range of factors influencing vitamin D levels [19,42]. To avoid these limitations, we focused on detecting VDR expression in placental tissue, which may prove to be a more accurate assessment of the impact of COVID-19 infection and vaccination on the levels of vitamin D, an essential molecule with a critical role in placentation and fetal well-being [40–43]. Since both vitamin D and VDR levels fluctuate throughout pregnancy [19,40–43], we specifically selected placentas only from women in their third trimester of pregnancy for our IHC analysis.

To the best of our knowledge, apart from a single study by Moreno-Fernandez et al., which evaluated placental vitamin D levels [22], this is the first study to assess VDR expression in placental tissue from COVID-19-positive, COVID-19-negative but Pfizer-vaccinated, and COVID-19-negative and unvaccinated pregnant women. By focusing on VDR rather than serum vitamin D, our study offers a novel approach to understanding how COVID-19 infection and vaccination influence vitamin D pathways during pregnancy, with potential implications for maternal and fetal health. Our results further support the well-established fact that vitamin D supplementation is required in COVID-19-positive cases that exhibit a depletion of this essential compound. Also, the fact that both COVID-19-positive and Pfizer-vaccinated pregnant women revealed lower levels of placental VDR supports this observation even further. Vitamin D supplementation increases VDR expression [28,40]. Thus, vitamin D supplementation might prove to be useful both during COVID-19 infection and also after vaccination, with a potential to improve maternal and fetal outcomes.

The trophoblast is a significant source of vitamin D synthesis in pregnancy, with the literature proving its role in fetal growth [40,41,43]. Vitamin D is involved in a wide range of placental processes, being responsible for immune modulation and impacting hormonal secretion at this level. Its receptor's presence is also related to immune reactions, as well as fetal and placental growth [40,41,43]. Therefore, our two main findings seem to be related, with the lack of VDR expression impacting fetal growth, although in a non-statistically significant manner. It is important to differentiate the effects of COVID-19 from causes of maternal and fetal malperfusion, such as preexisting pregnancy-induced hypertension and disseminated intravascular coagulation during pregnancy [8], twin pregnancy, smoking, and preeclampsia [19,43]. That is one of the main reasons for our small number of cases—we used very strict inclusion and exclusion criteria to ensure the accuracy of this study's results.

According to Joshi et al., the placental abnormalities in their study were not related to the symptoms or severity of COVID-19, with no correlation between maternal and fetal disease characteristics [29]. Even with a normal fetal and maternal outcome, most of the placentas (82.6%) presented signs of maternal vascular malperfusion, with features of fetal vascular malperfusion in almost half of the cases [29]. This aspect underlines once more the importance of studying the placenta's structure and function in viral infections for a better understanding of their exact impact. Despite the fact that COVID-19 infection shares similarities with Zika infection, without the same catastrophic fetal malformation effect, its frequent silent and subtle alteration of the maternal–fetal unit might not be minor at all. It is important to mention that we did not find any maternal symptoms or clinical details that could predict abnormal placental findings in pregnancy complicated by COVID-19 infection [44]. The duration of COVID-19 infection is approximately 20 days, ranging from 5 to 60 days, so the virus may reach and affect the placenta before delivery. This means that the virus can be cleared and no longer be detectable in a placental specimen obtained at childbirth [45]. On the other hand, infection in the late stage of gestation may indicate no evidence of vertical trans-placental COVID-19 transmission, without significant impact on the perinatal outcomes of newborns, in both mild and severe cases [1]. Another important aspect to consider is that these studies included a heterogeneous population for the timing of infection. A small series has reported that in cases of adverse outcomes, a specific placentitis—characterized by trophoblast degeneration, intervillositis, and massive perivillous fibrinoid deposits—has been identified, with similar findings observed in our cases [30].

The limitations of the above-mentioned studies include limited sample sizes and the fact that the asymptomatic forms of COVID-19 included cases with no mild, moderate, or severe disease-affected patients. Also, our group sizes were unequal, with the imbalance resulting in possible bias and impaired generalizability of the results. Our study only focused on short-term fetal outcomes, with limited understanding of the long-term impact of COVID-19 infection on children born from COVID-19-infected asymptomatic mothers. As this is a single-center study, our findings may not be fully representative of other populations from other regions, highlighting the need for further research using a larger cohort to better understand the exact pathophysiological mechanisms behind impaired fetal growth and adverse pregnancy outcomes. Such insights could improve pregnancy management in future epidemics. Another limitation is that we did not analyze or subdivide our COVID-19-infected group based on their gestational age at the time of infection. We plan to expand our research in this area to determine whether specific outcomes and VDR expression are influenced by the timing of the infection during pregnancy, or by disease severity. Also, we want to try to correlate vitamin D serum levels with placental VDR expression and pregnancy outcomes in COVID-19-positive, vaccinated, and control groups, to obtain more insights into the implications of vitamin D in pregnancy, in the context of COVID-19 infection. We also evaluated additional placental markers related to immune response, structure, and function in another study we performed on vaccinated COVID-19-positive and unvaccinated COVID-19-negative women, to explore potential pathways and provide explanations for the increased maternal and fetal morbidity observed during the pandemic.

## 5. Conclusions

Although we detected lower birth weights in COVID-19-positive and COVID-19-vaccinated pregnant women compared to the control group, the difference was not statistically significant. However, we uncovered a higher expression of VDR in placental tissue from unvaccinated COVID-19-negative cases compared to the other two groups in our study. These two findings seem to be connected, serving as a starting point for future pregnancy management during epidemics. The presence of the vitamin D receptor in the placenta is related to fetal and placental growth. Its deficiency may contribute to negative maternal and fetal outcomes in COVID-19-positive cases, suggesting that vitamin D supplementation could help mitigate the negative effects of viral infection.

**Author Contributions:** Conceptualization, C.C. and D.R.M.; methodology, C.C. and V.B.; software, V.L.B. and A.U.; validation, L.L., D.R.M. and A.U.; formal analysis, L.L. and I.E.B.; investigation, P.T. and D.R.M.; resources, C.C. and L.L.; data curation, A.U. and M.S.; writing—original draft preparation, C.C. and M.E.N.; writing—review and editing, D.R.M. and A.U.; visualization, L.L. and M.S.; supervision, V.B.; project administration, C.C. All authors have read and agreed to the published version of the manuscript.

**Funding:** This research received no external funding.

**Institutional Review Board Statement:** This study was conducted in accordance with the Declaration of Helsinki, and approved by the ethics committees of the UNIVERSITY OF MEDICINE AND PHARMACY "Lucian Blaga", Sibiu (1442/19 March 2024) and the Obstetrics and Gynecology Hospital "Cuza-Voda" in Iasi, Romania (10426/24 August 2021 and 19/4 August 2023).

**Informed Consent Statement:** Written informed consent has been obtained from the patients to publish this paper.

**Data Availability Statement:** The data used to support the findings of this study are available upon request to the corresponding author.

**Acknowledgments:** The authors would like to acknowledge the contribution of the Department of Obstetrics and Gynecology at the Women's Hospital of the University of Medicine and Pharmacy "Gr. T. Popa" Sibiu, Romania, for supporting this study. We are also greatly indebted to all participants for donating their tissue/placenta.

**Conflicts of Interest:** The authors declare no conflicts of interest.

## References

1. Giordano, G.; Petrolini, C.; Corradini, E.; Campanini, N.; Esposito, S.; Perrone, S. COVID-19 in pregnancy: Placental pathological patterns and effect on perinatal outcome in five cases. *Diagn. Pathol.* **2021**, *16*, 88. [CrossRef] [PubMed]
2. He, M.; Skaria, P.; Kreutz, K.; Chen, L.; Hagemann, I.S.; Carter, E.B.; Mysorekar, I.U.; Nelson, D.M.; Pfeifer, J.; Dehner, L.P. Histopathology of Third Trimester Placenta from SARS-CoV-2-Positive Women. *Fetal Pediatr. Pathol.* **2022**, *41*, 403–412. [CrossRef] [PubMed]
3. Bertero, L.; Borella, F.; Botta, G.; Carosso, A.; Cosma, S.; Bovetti, M.; Carosso, M.; Abbona, G.; Collemi, G.; Papotti, M.; et al. Placenta histopathology in SARS-CoV-2 infection: Analysis of a consecutive series and comparison with control cohorts. *Virchows Arch.* **2021**, *479*, 715–728. [CrossRef] [PubMed]
4. El-Kassas, M.; Alboraie, M.; Elbadry, M.; El Sheemy, R.; Abdellah, M.; Afify, S.; Madkour, A.; Zaghloul, M.; Awad, A.; Wifi, M.N.; et al. Non-pulmonary involvement in COVID-19: A systemic disease rather than a pure respiratory infection. *World J. Clin. Cases* **2023**, *11*, 493–505. [CrossRef]
5. Tossetta, G.; Fantone, S.; Delli Muti, N.; Balercia, G.; Ciavattini, A.; Giannubilo, S.R.; Marzioni, D. Preeclampsia and severe acute respiratory syndrome coronavirus 2 infection: A systematic review. *J. Hypertens.* **2022**, *40*, 1629–1638. [CrossRef]
6. Delli Muti, N.; Finocchi, F.; Tossetta, G.; Salvio, G.; Cutini, M.; Marzioni, D.; Balercia, G. Could SARS-CoV-2 infection affect male fertility and sexuality? *APMIS* **2022**, *130*, 243–252. [CrossRef]
7. Di Girolamo, R.; Khalil, A.; Alameddine, S.; D'Angelo, E.; Galliani, C.; Matarrelli, B.; Buca, D.; Liberati, M.; Rizzo, G.; D'Antonio, F. Placental histopathology after SARS-CoV-2 infection in pregnancy: A systematic review and meta-analysis. *Am. J. Obstet. Gynecol. MFM* **2021**, *3*, 100468. [CrossRef]
8. Garg, R.; Agarwal, R.; Yadav, D.; Singh, S.; Kumar, H.; Bhardwaj, R. Histopathological Changes in Placenta of Severe Acute Respiratory Syndrome Coronavirus 2 (SARS-Cov-2) Infection and Maternal and Perinatal Outcome in COVID-19. *J. Obstet. Gynaecol. India* **2023**, *73*, 44–50. [CrossRef]
9. Shanes, E.D.; Mithal, L.B.; Otero, S.; Azad, H.A.; Miller, E.S.; Goldstein, J.A. Placental Pathology in COVID-19. *Am. J. Clin. Pathol.* **2020**, *154*, 23–32. [CrossRef]
10. Libretti, A.; Troìa, L.; Cappello, A.M.; Casarotti, C.; D'Amato, A.T.; Dallarda, G.; Ghio, M.; Nicosia, A.; Ricci, D.; Savasta, F.; et al. Pregnancy and neonatal outcomes of SARS-CoV-2 infection discovered at the time of delivery: A tertiary center experience in North Italy. *J. Perinat. Med.* **2023**, *52*, 215–221. [CrossRef]
11. Juan, J.; Gil, M.M.; Rong, Z.; Zhang, Y.; Yang, H.; Poon, L.C. Effect of coronavirus disease 2019 (COVID-19) on maternal, perinatal and neonatal outcome: Systematic review. *Ultrasound Obstet. Gynecol.* **2020**, *56*, 15–27. [CrossRef] [PubMed]
12. Schwartz, D.A.; Bugatti, M.; Santoro, A.; Facchetti, F. Molecular Pathology Demonstration of SARS-CoV-2 in Cytotrophoblast from Placental Tissue with Chronic Histiocytic Intervillositis, Trophoblast Necrosis and COVID-19. *J. Dev. Biol.* **2021**, *9*, 33. [CrossRef] [PubMed]
13. Patberg, E.T.; Adams, T.; Rekawek, P.; Vahanian, S.A.; Akerman, M.; Hernandez, A.; Rapkiewicz, A.V.; Ragolia, L.; Sicuranza, G.; Chavez, M.R.; et al. Coronavirus disease 2019 infection and placental histopathology in women delivering at term. *Am. J. Obstet. Gynecol.* **2021**, *224*, 382.e1–382.e18. [CrossRef] [PubMed]
14. Kreis, N.N.; Ritter, A.; Louwen, F.; Yuan, J. A Message from the Human Placenta: Structural and Immunomodulatory Defense against SARS-CoV-2. *Cells* **2020**, *9*, 1777. [CrossRef]
15. Cyprian, F.; Lefkou, E.; Varoudi, K.; Girardi, G. Immunomodulatory Effects of Vitamin D in Pregnancy and Beyond. *Front. Immunol.* **2019**, *10*, 2739. [CrossRef]

16. Sinaci, S.; Ocal, D.F.; Yucel Yetiskin, D.F.; Uyan Hendem, D.; Buyuk, G.N.; Goncu Ayhan, S.; Tanacan, A.; Ozgu-Erdinc, A.S.; Moraloglu Tekin, O.; Sahin, D. Impact of vitamin D on the course of COVID-19 during pregnancy: A case control study. *J. Steroid Biochem. Mol. Biol.* **2021**, *213*, 105964. [CrossRef]
17. Manca, A.; Cosma, S.; Palermiti, A.; Costanzo, M.; Antonucci, M.; De Vivo, E.D.; Ianniello, A.; Borella, F.; Carosso, A.R.; Corcione, S.; et al. Pregnancy and COVID-19: The Possible Contribution of Vitamin D. *Nutrients* **2022**, *14*, 3275. [CrossRef]
18. Liu, N.; Kaplan, A.T.; Low, J.; Nguyen, L.; Liu, G.Y.; Equils, O.; Hewison, M. Vitamin D Induces Innate Antibacterial Responses in Human Trophoblasts via an Intracrine Pathway. *Biol. Reprod.* **2009**, *80*, 398–406. [CrossRef]
19. Szarpak, L.; Feduniw, S.; Pruc, M.; Ciebiera, M.; Cander, B.; Rahnama-Hezavah, M.; Szarpak, Ł. The Vitamin D Serum Levels in Pregnant Women Affected by COVID-19: A Systematic Review and Meta-Analysis. *Nutrients* **2023**, *15*, 2588. [CrossRef]
20. Ganguly, A.; Tamblyn, J.A.; Finn-Sell, S.; Chan, S.Y.; Westwood, M.; Gupta, J.; Kilby, M.D.; Gross, S.R.; Hewison, M. Vitamin D, the placenta and early pregnancy: Effects on trophoblast function. *J. Endocrinol.* **2018**, *236*, R93–R103. [CrossRef]
21. Ferrer-Sánchez, N.; Díaz-Goicoechea, M.; Mayoral-Cesar, V.; García-Solbas, S.; Nievas-Soriano, B.J.; Parrón-Carreño, T.; Fernández-Alonso, A.M. Serum 25(OH) Vitamin D Levels in Pregnant Women with Coronavirus Disease 2019 (COVID-19): A Case-Control Study. *Int. J. Environ. Res. Public Health* **2022**, *19*, 3965. [CrossRef] [PubMed]
22. Moreno-Fernandez, J.; Ochoa, J.J.; De Paco Matallana, C.; Caño, A.; Martín-Alvarez, E.; Sanchez-Romero, J.; Toledano, J.M.; Puche-Juarez, M.; Prados, S.; Ruiz-Duran, S.; et al. COVID-19 during Gestation: Maternal Implications of Evoked Oxidative Stress and Iron Metabolism Impairment. *Antioxidants* **2022**, *11*, 184. [CrossRef] [PubMed]
23. Riemma, G.; De Franciscis, P.; Tesorone, M.; Coppa, E.; Schiattarella, A.; Billone, V.; Lopez, A.; Cucinella, G.; Gullo, G.; Carotenuto, R.M. Obstetric and Gynecological Admissions and Hospitalizations in an Italian Tertiary-Care Hospital during COVID-19 Pandemic: A Retrospective Analysis According to Restrictive Measures. *J. Clin. Med.* **2023**, *12*, 7097. [CrossRef] [PubMed]
24. La Rosa, V.L.; Valenti, G.; Sapia, F.; Gullo, G.; Rapisarda, A. Psychological impact of gynecological diseases: The importance of a multidisciplinary approach. *Ital. J. Gynaecol. Obstet.* **2018**, *30*, 23–26. [CrossRef]
25. Burgio, S.; Polizzi, C.; Alesi, M.; Perino, A.; Cucinella, G.; Kotlik, Y.; Lopez, A.; Vassiliadis, A.; Gullo, G. Personality Traits and Depression in Infertile Couples during the COVID-19. *J. Clin. Med.* **2024**, *13*, 4827. [CrossRef]
26. Shah, P.S.; Diambomba, Y.; Acharya, G.; Morris, S.K.; Bitnun, A. Classification system and case definition for SARS-CoV-2 infection in pregnant women, fetuses, and neonates. *Acta Obstet. Gynecol. Scand.* **2020**, *99*, 565–568. [CrossRef]
27. Valdespino-Vázquez, M.Y.; Helguera-Repetto, C.A.; León-Juárez, M.; Villavicencio-Carrisoza, O.; Flores-Pliego, A.; Moreno-Verduzco, E.R.; Díaz-Pérez, D.L.; Villegas-Mota, I.; Carrasco-Ramírez, E.; López-Martínez, I.E.; et al. Fetal and placental infection with SARS-CoV-2 in early pregnancy. *J. Med. Virol.* **2021**, *93*, 4480–4487. [CrossRef]
28. Surekha, M.V.; Suneetha, N.; Balakrishna, N.; Putcha, U.K.; Satyanarayana, K.; Geddam, J.J.B.; Sreenu, P.; Tulja, B.; Mamidi, R.S.; Rutter, G.A.; et al. Impact of COVID-19 during pregnancy on placental pathology, maternal and neonatal outcome—A cross-sectional study on anemic term pregnant women from a tertiary care hospital in southern India. *Front. Endocrinol.* **2023**, *14*, 1092104. [CrossRef]
29. Joshi, B.; Chandi, A.; Srinivasan, R.; Saini, S.S.; Prasad, G.R.V.; Puri, G.D.; Bhalla, A.; Suri, V.; Bagga, R. The placental pathology in Coronavirus disease 2019 infected mothers and its impact on pregnancy outcome. *Placenta* **2022**, *127*, 1–7. [CrossRef]
30. Sarno, L.; Locci, M.; Fulgione, C.; Perillo, F.; Dell'Isola, A.; Mantelli, D.; Sibillo, C.; Saccone, G.; Maruotti, G.M.; Terracciano, D.; et al. Characteristics of Placental Histopathology in Women with Uncomplicated Pregnancies Affected by SARS-CoV-2 Infection at the Time of Delivery: A Single-Center Experience. *Biomedicines* **2022**, *10*, 3003. [CrossRef]
31. Maranto, M.; Zaami, S.; Restivo, V.; Termini, D.; Gangemi, A.; Tumminello, M.; Culmone, S.; Billone, V.; Cucinella, G.; Gullo, G. Symptomatic COVID-19 in Pregnancy: Hospital Cohort Data between May 2020 and April 2021, Risk Factors and Medicolegal Implications. *Diagnostics* **2023**, *13*, 1009. [CrossRef] [PubMed]
32. Incognito, G.G.; Distefano, R.E.C.; Campo, G.; Gulino, F.A.; Gulisano, C.; Gullotta, C.; Gullo, G.; Cucinella, G.; Tuscano, A.; Bruno, M.T.; et al. Comparison of Maternal and Neonatal Outcomes between SARS-CoV-2 Variants: A Retrospective, Monocentric Study. *J. Clin. Med.* **2023**, *12*, 6329. [CrossRef] [PubMed]
33. Gullo, G.; Scaglione, M.; Laganà, A.S.; Perino, A.; Andrisani, A.; Chiantera, V.; Cucinella, G.; Gitas, G.; Barra, F.; Riemma, G. Assisted Reproductive Techniques and Risk of Congenital Heart Diseases in Children: A Systematic Review and Meta-analysis. *Reprod. Sci.* **2023**, *30*, 2896–2906. [CrossRef] [PubMed]
34. Maranto, M.; Gullo, G.; Bruno, A.; Minutolo, G.; Cucinella, G.; Maiorana, A.; Casuccio, A.; Restivo, V. Factors Associated with Anti-SARS-CoV-2 Vaccine Acceptance among Pregnant Women: Data from Outpatient Women Experiencing High-Risk Pregnancy. *Vaccines* **2023**, *11*, 454. [CrossRef] [PubMed]
35. Chmielewska, B.; Barratt, I.; Townsend, R.; Kalafat, E.; van der Meulen, J.; Gurol-Urganci, I.; O'Brien, P.; Morris, E.; Draycott, T.; Thangaratinam, S.; et al. Effects of the COVID-19 pandemic on maternal and perinatal outcomes: A systematic review and meta-analysis. *Lancet Glob. Health* **2021**, *9*, e759–e772. [CrossRef]
36. Gullo, G.; Scaglione, M.; Buzzaccarini, G.; Laganà, A.S.; Basile, G.; Chiantera, V.; Cucinella, G.; Zaami, S. Cell-Free Fetal DNA and Non-Invasive Prenatal Diagnosis of Chromosomopathies and Pediatric Monogenic Diseases: A Critical Appraisal and Medicolegal Remarks. *J. Pers. Med.* **2022**, *13*, 1. [CrossRef]
37. Walker, D.M.; Tolentino, V.R. COVID-19: The impact on pediatric emergency care. *Pediatr. Emerg. Med. Pract.* **2020**, *17*, 1–27.

38. Mongula, J.E.; Frenken, M.W.E.; van Lijnschoten, G.; Arents, N.L.A.; de Wit-Zuurendonk, L.D.; Schimmel-de Kok, A.P.A.; van Runnard Heimel, P.J.; Porath, M.M.; Goossens, S.M.T.A. COVID-19 during pregnancy: Non-reassuring fetal heart rate, placental pathology and coagulopathy. *Ultrasound Obstet. Gynecol.* **2020**, *56*, 773–776. [CrossRef]
39. Chen, S.; Huang, B.; Luo, D.J.; Li, X.; Yang, F.; Zhao, Y.; Nie, X.; Huang, B. Pregnancy with new coronavirus infection: Clinical characteristics and placental pathological analysis of three cases. *Zhonghua Bing Li Xue Za Zhi* **2020**, *49*, 418–423. [CrossRef]
40. Murthi, P.; Yong, H.E.; Ngyuen, T.P.; Ellery, S.; Singh, H.; Rahman, R.; Dickinson, H.; Walker, D.W.; Davies-Tuck, M.; Wallace, E.M.; et al. Role of the Placental Vitamin D Receptor in Modulating Feto-Placental Growth in Fetal Growth Restriction and Preeclampsia-Affected Pregnancies. *Front. Physiol.* **2016**, *7*, 43. [CrossRef]
41. Nguyen, T.P.; Yong, H.E.; Chollangi, T.; Borg, A.J.; Brennecke, S.P.; Murthi, P. Placental vitamin D receptor expression is decreased in human idiopathic fetal growth restriction. *J. Mol. Med.* **2015**, *93*, 795–805. [CrossRef] [PubMed]
42. Magiełda-Stola, J.; Kurzawińska, G.; Ożarowski, M.; Bogacz, A.; Wolski, H.; Drews, K.; Karpiński, T.M.; Wolek, M.; Seremak-Mrozikiewicz, A. Placental mRNA and Protein Expression of VDR, CYP27B1 and CYP2R1 Genes Related to Vitamin D Metabolism in Preeclamptic Women. *Appl. Sci.* **2021**, *11*, 11880. [CrossRef]
43. Knabl, J.; Vattai, A.; Ye, Y.; Jueckstock, J.; Hutter, S.; Kainer, F.; Mahner, S.; Jeschke, U. Role of Placental VDR Expression and Function in Common Late Pregnancy Disorders. *Int. J. Mol. Sci.* **2017**, *18*, 2340. [CrossRef] [PubMed]
44. Gullo, G.; Scaglione, M.; Cucinella, G.; Riva, A.; Coldebella, D.; Cavaliere, A.F.; Signore, F.; Buzzaccarini, G.; Spagnol, G.; Laganà, A.S.; et al. Congenital Zika Syndrome: Genetic Avenues for Diagnosis and Therapy, Possible Management and Long-Term Outcomes. *J. Clin. Med.* **2022**, *11*, 1351. [CrossRef]
45. Debelenko, L.; Katsyv, I.; Chong, A.M.; Peruyero, L.; Szabolcs, M.; Uhlemann, A.C. Trophoblast damage with acute and chronic intervillositis: Disruption of the placental barrier by severe acute respiratory syndrome coronavirus 2. *Hum. Pathol.* **2021**, *109*, 69–79. [CrossRef]

Journal of
*Clinical Medicine*

MDPI

*Article*

# Predicting Intensive Care Unit Admission in COVID-19-Infected Pregnant Women Using Machine Learning

**Azamat Mukhamediya [1], Iliyar Arupzhanov [1], Amin Zollanvari [1], Saule Zhumambayeva [2], Kamalzhan Nadyrov [2], Zaituna Khamidullina [2], Karina Tazhibayeva [2], Aigul Myrzabekova [2], Kulyash K. Jaxalykova [2], Milan Terzic [3,4], Gauri Bapayeva [4], Saltanat Kulbayeva [5], Gulzhan Narkenovna Abuova [6], Baktigali Aubayevich Erezhepov [6], Asselzhan Sarbalina [7], Aigerim Sipenova [8], Kymbat Mukhtarova [8], Ghazal Ghahramany [8] and Antonio Sarria-Santamera [8,*]**

1 Department of Electrical and Computer Engineering, School of Engineering and Digital Sciences, Nazarbayev University, Astana 010000, Kazakhstan
2 Astana Medical University, Astana 010000, Kazakhstan
3 Department of Surgery, School of Medicine, Nazarbayev University, Astana 010000, Kazakhstan
4 Clinical Academic Department of Women's Health, Corporate Fund "University Medical Center", Astana 010000, Kazakhstan
5 Department of Obstetrics and Gynecology, South Kazakhstan Medical Academy, Shymkent 160000, Kazakhstan
6 Shymkent City Infectious Disease Hospital, Shymkent 160000, Kazakhstan
7 University of Oxford, Oxford OX3 9DU, UK
8 Department of Biomedical Sciences, School of Medicine, Nazarbayev University, Astana 010000, Kazakhstan
* Correspondence: antonio.sarria@nu.edu.kz

**Abstract: Background**: The rapid onset of COVID-19 placed immense strain on many already overstretched healthcare systems. The unique physiological changes in pregnancy, amplified by the complex effects of COVID-19 in pregnant women, rendered prioritization of infected expectant mothers more challenging. This work aims to use state-of-the-art machine learning techniques to predict whether a COVID-19-infected pregnant woman will be admitted to ICU (Intensive Care Unit). **Methods**: A retrospective study using data from COVID-19-infected women admitted to one hospital in Astana and one in Shymkent, Kazakhstan, from May to July 2021. The developed machine learning platform implements and compares the performance of eight binary classifiers, including Gaussian naïve Bayes, K-nearest neighbors, logistic regression with $L_2$ regularization, random forest, AdaBoost, gradient boosting, eXtreme gradient boosting, and linear discriminant analysis. **Results**: Data from 1292 pregnant women with COVID-19 were analyzed. Of them, 10.4% were admitted to ICU. Logistic regression with $L_2$ regularization achieved the highest $F_1$-score during the model selection phase while achieving an AUC of 0.84 on the test set during the evaluation stage. Furthermore, the feature importance analysis conducted by calculating Shapley Additive Explanation values points to leucocyte counts, C-reactive protein, pregnancy week, and eGFR and hemoglobin as the most important features for predicting ICU admission. **Conclusions**: The predictive model obtained here may be an efficient support tool for prioritizing care of COVID-19-infected pregnant women in clinical practice.

**Keywords:** COVID-19; intensive care unit admission; pregnancy; machine learning; feature importance

## 1. Introduction

The rapid onset of COVID-19 placed immense strain on many already overstretched healthcare systems. As a result of the acute shortage of hospital beds and medical staff during the pandemic, various stringent patient triage protocols were introduced. The unique physiological changes during pregnancy present challenges in understanding the full scope and effects of the complexity of COVID-19 infection on pregnant women [1], rendering the clinical decision-making in these patients and risk-prioritization of expectant mothers even more challenging.

The disruption of SARS-CoV-2 not only significantly impacted societies, economies, and mental well-being but also translated into the need to accurately estimate patient prognosis based on patient-specific risk. Identifying patients at high risk of complications is critical in moments of high caseloads. In the gestational period, the presentation of COVID-19 can vary significantly, encompassing asymptomatic cases, mild respiratory symptoms that require minimal supportive treatment, and severe cases leading to hospitalization with multi-organ failure and death [2]. Given the significant changes in the immune, circulatory, respiratory, and hormonal systems in addition to specific problems that appear during this period, such as preeclampsia or gestational diabetes, the full understanding of the COVID-19 impacts on pregnant women is yet to be clarified [3]. Moreover, research exploring the influence of different pregnancy trimesters on the disease's clinical progression and complications is scarce [4].

One of the critical factors during the pandemic was prioritizing patients in need of intensive care to avoid unnecessary consumption of medical resources on low and moderate-risk patients [5]. The sudden COVID-19 outbreak intensified the shortage of hospital beds, critical care equipment, and medical professionals [6]. Proper triage systems to predict the clinical course of patients become essential for efficient management of limited medical resources, including intensive care [7].

Machine learning may classify severity and assess prognosis for COVID-19 patients across a variety of routinely collected laboratory tests and clinical data [8]. In this regard, machine learning can be viewed as a useful technique for supporting caregivers in medical decision-making, and it has been utilized in multiple COVID-19 studies to construct models that predict the severity of SARS-CoV-2 patients [9,10]. Moreover, the constructed predictive models can be used to accurately assess the risk of the outcome and will allow for individualized preventive measures in clinical settings. As a result, in this study, we aim to (i) develop a machine learning model that can predict the risk of ICU admission in COVID-19-infected pregnant women based on clinical data routinely collected during hospitalization and (ii) shed light on major factors associated with the higher risk of ICU admission for pregnant women with COVID-19 infection.

## 2. Materials and Methods

### 2.1. Study Population

This retrospective study was conducted using de-identified data from medical records of pregnant women with COVID-19 admitted at Astana Perinatal Hospital and at the Department of Obstetrics and Gynecology South Kazakhstan Medical Academy in Shymkent from 1 May 2021 to 14 July 2021. Inclusion criteria were pregnant women who were admitted to any of the previously mentioned hospitals in the period from 1 May 2021 to 14 July 2021 with SARS-CoV-2 infection confirmed through real-time polymerase chain reaction (RT-PCR). The dataset includes 46 variables, which broadly cover information about days of admission after the onset of the symptoms, length of hospital stay, obstetric history, laboratory tests, clinical symptoms, and severity of COVID-19, comorbidities, and complications (see Table 1 for detailed information about the variables). The comorbid disorders were presented as categorical variables encoded as "yes" and "no" subgroups. ICU admission was chosen as an outcome variable for prediction. The dataset is imbalanced, with the ratio of those admitted to ICU to those who are not admitted at 110:1058. Note that we did not consider using any methods to address the class imbalance directly. Instead, we used an alternative strategy to handle the class imbalance by considering the decision-making threshold as a hyperparameter and tuning it in the model selection stage.

Ethical approval was obtained from Nazarbayev University Institutional Review Ethics Committee (NU-IREC) #745/12062023. The data were extracted from electronic medical records by practicing clinicians from the hospitals and provided de-identified for conducting these analyses. All methods were carried out in accordance with the

"Reporting of studies conducted using observational routinely collected health data" (STROBE) guidelines.

**Table 1.** Baseline Demographic and Clinical Characteristics $n$ = 1168. To characterize the difference between those who were and were not admitted to ICU, $p$-values of two-sided Welch's $t$-test (for numerical features) and chi-square test (for categorical features) were calculated.

| | Trimester of Gestation | | | | | |
|---|---|---|---|---|---|---|
| **Characteristic** | **1st Trimester ($n$ = 59)** | **2nd Trimester ($n$ = 293)** | **3rd Trimester ($n$ = 813)** | **ICU Admitted ($n$ = 110)** | **Not Admitted to ICU ($n$ = 1058)** | **$p$-Value** |
| **Feature** | | | | | | |
| Age | 30.15 ± 5.92 | 30.13 ± 5.64 | 29.66 ± 5.61 | 31.52 ± 5.67 | 29.63 ± 5.59 | 0.0011 |
| Blood type | | | | | | 0.3621 |
| A | 12 | 67 | 252 | 38 | 295 | |
| AB | 3 | 28 | 67 | 9 | 90 | |
| B | 15 | 95 | 225 | 33 | 300 | |
| O | 28 | 99 | 251 | 29 | 355 | |
| Rh factor | | | | | | 0.9769 |
| − | 4 | 14 | 29 | 4 | 44 | |
| + | 54 | 275 | 765 | 105 | 995 | |
| Days of admission after symptom onset | 4.20 ± 2.44 | 4.41 ± 3.07 | 4.62 ± 3.63 | 5.83 ± 3.83 | 4.42 ± 3.38 | 0.0003 |
| Length of hospital stay | 7.64 ± 1.89 | 8.31 ± 3.36 | 6.71 ± 3.04 | 8.53 ± 5.52 | 7.02 ± 2.76 | 0.0057 |
| **Obstetric history** | | | | | | |
| Number of children | 1.29 ± 1.34 | 1.17 ± 1.06 | 1.69 ± 1.35 | 1.98 ± 1.26 | 1.50 ± 1.30 | 0.0002 |
| Number of pregnancies | 2.68 ± 1.71 | 2.66 ± 1.60 | 2.79 ± 1.69 | 2.95 ± 1.76 | 2.73 ± 1.66 | 0.2085 |
| Number of deliveries | 1.31 ± 1.36 | 1.20 ± 1.06 | 1.71 ± 1.36 | 2.02 ± 1.23 | 1.52 ± 1.31 | <0.001 |
| Multiple gestations | 0 | 4 | 4 | 1 | 7 | |
| **Laboratory tests** | | | | | | |
| Hemoglobin | 120.19 ± 19.58 | 105.79 ± 11.34 | 105.67 ± 14.79 | 97.97 ± 16.08 | 107.36 ± 14.2 | <0.001 |
| Leucocytes | 6.91 ± 2.62 | 8.25 ± 3.38 | 9.33 ± 3.65 | 12.58 ± 4.93 | 8.56 ± 3.20 | <0.001 |
| Neutrophils | 73.06 ± 9.88 | 79.50 ± 8.74 | 79.89 ± 10.3 | 86.30 ± 17.00 | 78.75 ± 8.70 | <0.001 |
| Lymphocytes | 24.50 ± 13.63 | 16.95 ± 9.11 | 16.81 ± 8.27 | 12.40 ± 8.29 | 17.73 ± 8.92 | <0.001 |
| Platelets | 205.95 ± 68.32 | 210.81 ± 77.57 | 217.69 ± 85.43 | 250.09 ± 134.92 | 211.86 ± 74.40 | 0.0043 |
| APTT | 29.08 ± 3.19 | 31.37 ± 11.08 | 31.93 ± 13.62 | 35.69 ± 13.49 | 31.22 ± 12.51 | 0.0012 |
| ALT | 29.23 ± 31.32 | 37.80 ± 58.26 | 23.46 ± 34.89 | 35.64 ± 83.34 | 26.65 ± 35.75 | 0.2808 |
| ACT | 27.47 ± 17.19 | 35.88 ± 42.0 | 29.69 ± 25.48 | 41.71 ± 59.44 | 30.10 ± 25.51 | 0.0509 |
| **Comorbidities and complications** | | | | | | |
| Preeclampsia | 0 | 3 | 23 | 10 | 16 | <0.001 |
| Small for gestational age | 0 | 1 | 18 | 2 | 17 | 1.0 |
| Intrauterine growth restriction | 0 | 0 | 17 | 3 | 14 | 0.4521 |
| Hypertension | 1 | 17 | 67 | 23 | 63 | <0.001 |
| Hyperglycemia | 3 | 53 | 121 | 29 | 148 | <0.001 |
| Gestational diabetes | 1 | 11 | 33 | 13 | 32 | <0.001 |
| Anaemia | 13 | 162 | 599 | 90 | 685 | <0.001 |
| Pneumonia | 26 | 152 | 437 | 68 | 549 | 0.05 |

**Table 1.** *Cont.*

| Characteristic | Trimester of Gestation | | | ICU Admitted ($n$ = 110) | Not Admitted to ICU ($n$ = 1058) | $p$-Value |
|---|---|---|---|---|---|---|
| | 1st Trimester ($n$ = 59) | 2nd Trimester ($n$ = 293) | 3rd Trimester ($n$ = 813) | | | |
| **Clinical symptoms and severity of COVID-19** | | | | | | |
| Fever | 34 | 125 | 231 | 31 | 359 | 0.2666 |
| Cough | 52 | 263 | 619 | 78 | 857 | 0.0156 |
| Weakness | 57 | 280 | 726 | 98 | 967 | 0.5249 |
| Sore throat | 31 | 191 | 494 | 55 | 662 | 0.0133 |
| Shortness of breath | 14 | 59 | 149 | 30 | 192 | 0.0282 |
| Myalgia | 15 | 95 | 217 | 33 | 294 | 0.7038 |
| Loss of smell and/or taste | 35 | 104 | 208 | 21 | 326 | 0.0143 |
| Runny nose | 46 | 230 | 613 | 75 | 816 | 0.0475 |
| Diarrhea | 6 | 11 | 13 | 0 | 30 | 0.1409 |
| Chest discomfort | 11 | 60 | 145 | 17 | 199 | 0.4633 |
| Sweating | 3 | 5 | 19 | 3 | 24 | 1.0 |
| ICU Admission | 0 | 13 | 96 | | | |

### 2.2. Data Pre-Processing

Several pre-processing steps were employed to prepare the dataset for the analysis. Initially, categorical variables were transformed using one-hot encoding. The dataset was randomly split into training and test sets. Missing feature values in the training and test sets were imputed based on the median of those values in the training data to prevent any data leakage between the training and test sets. The training set was normalized by applying standardization, whereas the test set was normalized based on the statistics obtained from the training set.

### 2.3. Model Selection

Eight classifiers were used: Gaussian Naïve Bayes (GNB) [11]; K-Nearest Neighbors (KNN) [11]; Logistic Regression with $L_2$ regularization (LR) [12]; Random Forest (RF) [13]; AdaBoost (ADB) [14]; Gradient Boost (GB) [15]; eXtreme Gradient Boost (XGB) [16]; and Linear Discriminant Analysis (LDA) [17]. The rationale behind selecting these predictive models is as follows: (i) the selected models represent five well-known groups: ensemble; Gaussian process; nearest neighbor; linear models; and discriminant analysis, and (ii) these models have been widely utilized in previous studies to predict ICU admission [18–20] and COVID-19 severity risk [5,8,9]. The best predictive model was selected according to the highest $F_1$-score that was estimated using a stratified 5-fold cross-validation strategy applied to the training set. Figure 1 presents the schematic diagram of the model selection procedure.

It is worth noting that the decision-making threshold was considered a hyperparameter and tuned in the model selection stage. Particularly, a classifier outputs the predicted class label for a given observation by comparing its assigned score with a predetermined threshold value. In this work, instead of using a default value (often 0 or 0.5), we treated the threshold value as an essential hyperparameter and optimized it along with other hyperparameters as a part of model selection. The hyperparameter space for threshold values includes values from 0 to 1 with a step size of 0.01. The classifier-specific hyperparameter spaces are detailed in Table 2.

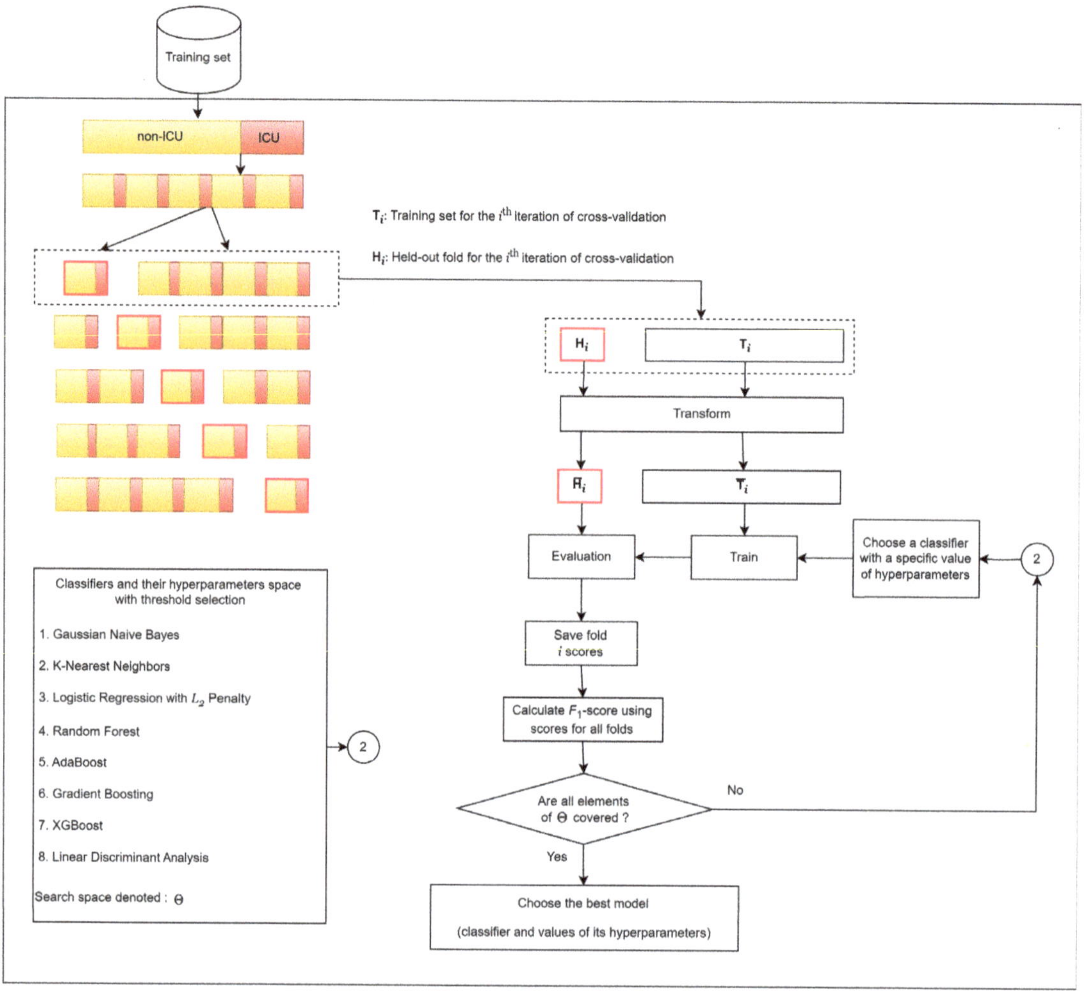


**Figure 1.** A schematic diagram of the model selection procedure.

**Table 2.** A summary of the hyperparameter spaces.

| Classifier | Hyperparameter | Hyperparameter Space |
|---|---|---|
| LR | penalty<br>regularization parameter | $L_2$<br>100, 10, 1.0, 0.1, 0.01 |
| RF | number of estimators<br>maximum depth<br>maximum features | 1, 2, 5, 10<br>2, 5, 10<br>'sqrt', 'log2' |
| LDA | solver<br>tolerance | 'svd', 'lsqr', 'eigen'<br>0.00001, 0.0001, 0.0003 |
| GB | number of estimators<br>learning rate | 10, 20, 30<br>0.001, 0.01, 0.1 |

**Table 2.** *Cont.*

| Classifier | Hyperparameter | Hyperparameter Space |
|---|---|---|
| XGB | maximum depth<br>number of estimators<br>learning rate | 5, 10<br>10, 20, 30<br>0.001, 0.01, 0.1 |
| ADB | number of estimators<br>learning rate<br>algorithm | 10, 20, 30<br>0.001, 0.01, 0.1<br>'SAMME', 'SAMME.R' |
| GNB | - | - |
| KNN | number of neighbors | 3, 5 |

### 2.4. Model Evaluation

The selected and trained predictive model was evaluated on the test set based on the following performance metrics: area under the curve (AUC); precision; sensitivity (recall); specificity; $F_1$-score; and geometric mean of sensitivity and specificity (G-mean). These metrics are defined as follows:

$$\text{precision} = \frac{\text{TP}}{\text{TP} + \text{FP}},$$

$$\text{specificity} = \frac{\text{TN}}{\text{TN} + \text{FP}},$$

$$\text{sensitivity} = \frac{\text{TP}}{\text{TP} + \text{FN}},$$

$$F_1\text{–score} = \frac{2 \times \text{precision} \times \text{recall}}{\text{precision} + \text{recall}},$$

$$\text{G–mean} = \sqrt{\text{specificity} \times \text{sensitivity}}$$

where TP, FP, TN, and FN are the number of true positives, false positives, true negatives, and false negatives, respectively.

### 2.5. SHAP Analysis

Shapley Additive exPlanations (SHAP) analysis (version 0.44.1) [21] was used to examine the effect of each feature on the prediction of the classifier and assess the importance of the feature in predicting admission to the ICU.

### 2.6. Software and Packages

The entire computational pipeline was implemented in Python (version 3.9.7) using the scikit-learn library. The computations were performed using the MacOS 13.1 (Ventura) operation system with Apple chip M1 and 8GB of RAM (Cupertino, CA, USA).

## 3. Results

### 3.1. Data Description

In this study, the initial database included 1292 cases collected from Astana Perinatal Hospital and the Department of Obstetrics and Gynecology of South Kazakhstan Medical Academy Shymkent. After eliminating those with incomplete data, 1168 pregnant women with COVID-19 were available for analysis (see Section 2.1). Specifically, the samples that contained missing values in more than 20% of their features were removed. Missing values in each feature were imputed by the median of feature values across the entire sample. The data include 22 binary, 2 categorical, and 22 numeric features (see Table S1). The training and test sets were obtained by randomly dividing entire data into two disjoint sets with a splitting ratio of 70:30. The smaller subset was used as a test set, and the larger subset was used for training purposes. Stratification was used to keep the proportion of classes that appear in the training and test splits the same as the full dataset. The training set was used to obtain the best predictive model, while the test set was used for the evaluation of the obtained model. The main characteristics of the data are shown in Table 1. 87.3% of cases were in the third trimester, and 10.4% required ICU admission.

### 3.2. Predictive Performance

As a result of model selection, the highest $F_1$-score of 0.493 ± 0.0434 was achieved by the LR model (see Figure 2). In particular, the best model is obtained based on a pipeline consisting of the hyperparameter tuning, including the decision-making threshold estimation. In Table 3, the estimate of $F_1$-scores, the estimated threshold value, and other estimated hyperparameters of each classifier are presented. Ultimately, the LR model with selected parameters and decision-making threshold value was evaluated using the test set. Table 4 presents the test-set performance metrics estimated using the best predictive LR model. The test-set confusion matrix for the LR classifier is presented in Table 5. The confusion matrix reflects a positive predictive value of 86%. Values of 87.3% of ICU admissions were in women in the third trimester. Cases with ICU admission were older, with more pregnancies and deliveries. They had lower saturation, hemoglobin, and lymphocytes, as well as more elevated leucocytes, neutrophils, platelets, and APTT. Preeclampsia, hypertension, hyperglycemia, and gestational diabetes were also frequent among these women.

**Table 3.** The $F_1$-scores, decision-making threshold value, and selected hyperparameter spaces of classifiers during the model selection. The best model is identified in bold.

| Classifier | $F_1$-Score | Threshold | Hyperparameter Space |
|---|---|---|---|
| **LR** | **0.49 ± 0.04** | **0.18** | **regularization parameter: 0.01** |
| RF | 0.48 ± 0.12 | 0.18 | maximum depth: 2; maximum features: log2; number of estimators: 10 |
| LDA | 0.47 ± 0.03 | 0.20 | solver: "svd"; tolerance: 0.00001 |
| GB | 0.47 ± 0.11 | 0.26 | learning rate: 0.1; number of estimators: 20 |
| XGB | 0.45 ± 0.08 | 0.26 | learning rate: 0.1; number of estimators: 30; maximum depth: 10 |
| ADB | 0.42 ± 0.05 | 0.34 | algorithm: "SAMME.R"; learning rate: 0.1; number of estimators: 30 |
| GNB | 0.31 ± 0.07 | 0.71 | - |
| KNN | 0.31 ± 0.04 | 0.00 | number of neighbors: 5 |

**Table 4.** Test-set performance metrics estimated using the best predictive model (logistic regression).

| Accuracy | Precision | Sensitivity | Specificity | G-Mean | $F_1$-Score | ROC AUC |
|---|---|---|---|---|---|---|
| 0.866 | 0.389 | 0.600 | 0.896 | 0.733 | 0.472 | 0.845 |

**Table 5.** Confusion matrix obtained on the test set using the best predictive model (logistic regression). Positive and negative labels represent ICU admitted and non-admitted, respectively.

| | | **Predicted** | |
|---|---|---|---|
| | | Negative | Positive |
| **Actual** | Negative | True Negative: 283 | False Positive: 33 |
| | Positive | False Negative: 14 | True Positive: 21 |

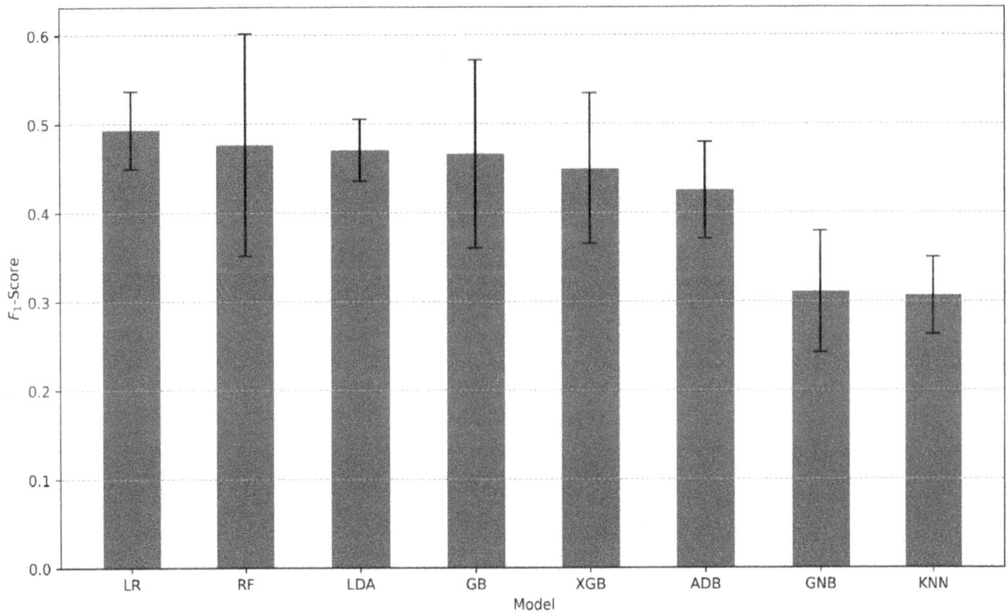


**Figure 2.** Estimated $F_1$-scores mean ± standard deviation using 5-fold cross-validation obtained on the training set.

### 3.3. *Impact Direction and Importance of Each Feature*

We utilized a SHAP analysis to assess the importance of each feature on ICU admission prediction using the trained LR classifier. Figure 3a,b depicts the bar and beeswarm plot of the ten most important features according to SHAP values. In particular, the bar plot shows the ranking of the features in terms of their importance. In this case, we can see that leukocytes, CRP, and pregnancy week are the most important features on average. On the other hand, the beeswarm plot is designed to display an information-dense summary of how the top features in a dataset impact the model's output. Each instance of the given explanation is represented by a single dot on each feature. Each position of the dot is determined by the SHAP value of that feature. Dots "pile up" along each feature row so that the width at a certain point represents the density. The color code indicates the protective (blue) or higher risk (red) of admission to the ICU. For example, the high value of leukocytes yields positive SHAP values, meaning the direct dependence between leukocytes and a higher risk of admission to the ICU. At the same time, the high value of hemoglobin decreases the risk of ICU admission as it corresponds to negative SHAP values.

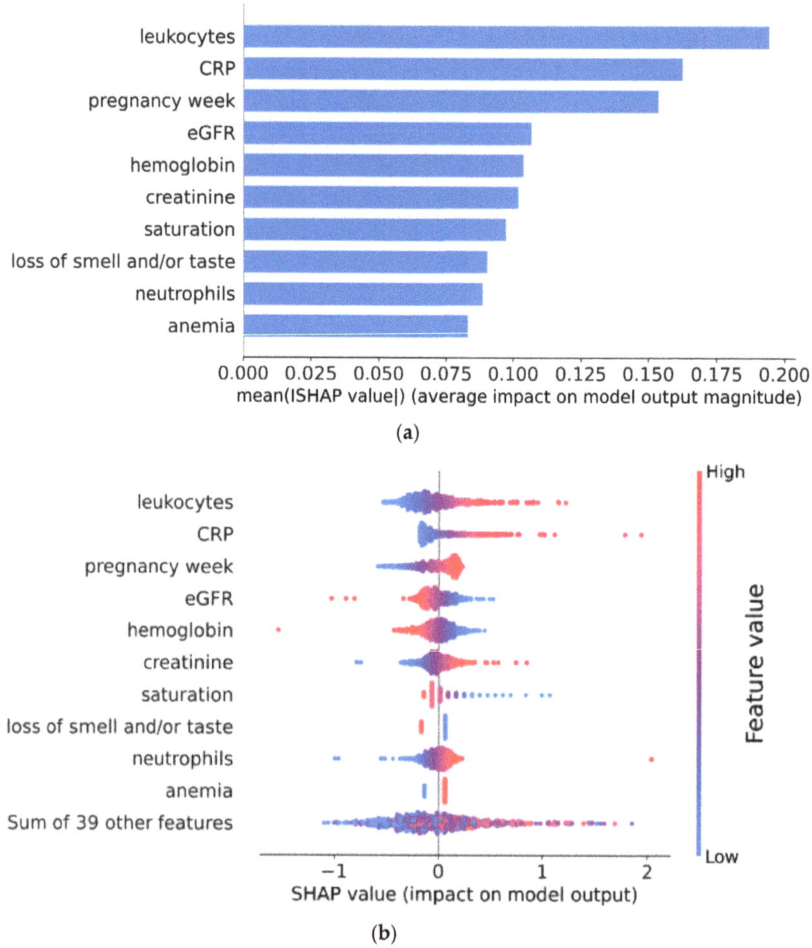


**Figure 3.** (**a**) Bar plot of top 10 features (from highest to lowest importance) based on mean SHAP value. (**b**) Beeswarm plot of top 10 features (from highest to lowest importance) based on SHAP value.

## 4. Discussion

We collected data from 1168 patients to construct predictive models of adverse outcomes related to SARS-CoV-2 infection in pregnancy. The constructed model aims to conduct higher-level risk stratification to provide efficient decision-making and advance personalized medicine upon obtaining a positive SARS-CoV2 test in pregnant patients. Our machine learning-based ICU admission predictive model can potentially be used as an auxiliary tool for supporting caregivers in medical decision-making. To construct and compare our predictive models, we leveraged a threshold-dependent metric of performance ($F_1$-score) to identify the best model.

As seen in Table 4, the best predictive model (LR) demonstrates a predictive performance in the range of 0.8–0.9 in terms of AUC. As per objective metrics of diagnostic tests, an estimated AUC in the range of 0.8–0.9 is generally considered a "good" predictive capacity for the test [22]. At the same time, LR correctly predicted 283 true negatives and 21 true positives, which correspond to a specificity of 0.896 and a sensitivity of 0.600. In addition, our model can predict cases with a low risk of developing adverse outcomes requiring ICU admission during hospitalization with a rate of 283/(283 + 33) = 0.89.

Our model achieved a moderate $F_1$-score of 0.472 with a 0.600 recall and 0.389 precision. That is to say, the model shows a satisfactory ability to identify positive cases but has lower reliability in its positive predictions. This is a natural outcome of selecting a low decision-making threshold value (the best predictive model, LR, has a threshold value of 0.18; see Table 3). It is worth noting that having high recall might be beneficial in cases where missing positives is more costly, for example, in medical diagnoses. Another possible cause of the moderate $F_1$-score is class imbalance. Recall that our dataset has a skewed class distribution (see Section 2.1).

Several studies have employed a machine learning approach to predict ICU admission for COVID-19-infected patients [18–20]. For example, Karimi et al. [18] compared different machine learning models to predict the requirements for ICU admission in COVID-19 patients. In their work, they considered six models: Support Vector Machine (SVM); Naïve Bayes; LRR; light GBM; decision tree (DT); and KNN. Among them, the best predictive model, Naïve Bayes, achieved 0.71 AUC and 0.40 $F_1$-score. Famiglini et al. [19] used four models, multi-layer perceptron, DT, SVM, and XGB, to predict ICU admission for COVID-19 patients within any of the next five days. The best predictive model, SVM, showed 0.85 AUC and 0.54 $F_1$-score. Cheng et al. [20] used the RF model as a risk prioritization tool to predict COVID-19 ICU admission within 24 h. Their model achieved 0.80 AUC and 0.18 $F_1$-score.

During the COVID-19 pandemic, the perinatal centers in Astana and Shymkent were repurposed as infectious disease hospitals. All pregnant women with a positive result for coronavirus infection in these cities were admitted to this hospital, generating the need for valid triage systems to determine the most efficient process of care for each patient within the consistently limited resources, like intensive care unit beds.

The overall proportion of ICU admissions was 10.4%, as reported by some authors [23], although some authors have reported lower values [24]. Both differences in clinical characteristics of the patients included in these analyses, as well as the period of the pandemic and circulating variants and specific healthcare-related issues like availability of ICU beds and vaccination status, may explain these differences.

SHAP analysis is an effective technique to quantify the importance of features [25]. The results of our SHAP analysis demonstrate that the most important features are leukocyte and C-reactive protein. Leukocytosis is a hematological parameter associated with more severe COVID-19 infection in pregnant women, along with neutrophilia, lymphopenia, and elevated platelet counts [26,27]. While the precise pathophysiological explanation of these hematological abnormalities in COVID-19 patients is still unclear, changes in the number of one or more blood cells have often been reported frequently in patients infected with SARS-CoV-2 [28]. Leukocytosis and neutrophilia are inflammatory responses associated with disease severity and bad outcomes. Although neutrophilia may be more specific to severe disease than leukocytosis [29], leukocyte counts have been observed more frequently, compared with neutrophil ones, in more severe cases of COVID-19-infected pregnant women [30]. C-reactive protein (CRP) is another relevant factor associated with the risk of ICU admissions for pregnant women infected with COVID-19. CRP is recognized as a robust marker of acute systemic inflammation and severe infection [31]. Elevated CRP concentrations are associated with COVID-19 severity [32] but are also typically reported in severe viral infections, including H1N1 influenza pneumonia [33,34]. Elevated CRP levels are associated with severe COVID-19 cases in pregnancy [35] and have been linked with ICU admission, preterm labor, and poor maternal outcomes [36], as they reflect underlying inflammatory responses that are heightened in severe infections [37]. We note that the "importance" of the feature indicates the "association" between the feature and the output of the model.

Lymphopenia is another indicator of severe COVID-19 infection. In pregnant women, lymphopenia often signals an impaired immune response, placing these patients at higher risk for severe infection and complications, including ICU admission and preterm delivery.

Neutrophil-to-lymphocyte ratios are valuable for detecting potentially critical and fatal cases of COVID-19 [38].

In terms of platelet counts, in cases admitted to ICU, even though they showed higher levels, they still remained in the normal range. Mild thrombocytopenia has been reported frequently in COVID-19 infection [39] as well as rebound thrombocytosis [40]; however, none of these factors were detected as major contributing elements associated with ICU admission of COVID-19-infected pregnant women by our predictive models.

Anemia and low hemoglobin levels were also associated with a higher risk of severe infection requiring ICU [41]. From an etiological standpoint, thrombosis, hemorrhage, and autoimmunity have been suggested for this association. During pregnancy, hemoglobin concentration is decreased. This is due to higher blood volume, which supplies oxygen and nutrients to the uterus, placenta, and other organs. Iron deficiency may also occur in pregnant women due to an increased need for iron, leading to further exacerbation of anemia during this period [42]. A decrease in circulating hemoglobin levels results in a reduction in oxygen availability for cells, which intensifies the hypoxia caused by COVID-19-induced acute respiratory distress syndrome [43]. In our study, anemia and hemoglobin counts had direct and inverse dependence, respectively, on the risk of ICU admissions of COVID-19-infected pregnant women. Nevertheless, none of these factors were highly associated with the risk of ICU admission for these patients.

"Loss of smell", a common symptom in COVID-19 cases, has been found primarily in the less severe cases [44,45]. The mechanism that explains "loss of smell" in COVID-19 is largely unknown, so it is unclear whether these findings may contradict previous evidence.

Gestational age at infection $\geq$ 31 weeks was an independent risk factor for severe–critical COVID-19 [46–48]. This phenomenon has also been observed in influenza infection [49], probably because of the physiological changes during pregnancy [50], such as reduced respiratory capacity, vascular and hemodynamic changes like an increased body fluid in the third space, and compromised immune system due to the need for immune tolerance for the fetus, which develop as pregnancy advances [51]. There is, however, some controversy regarding the risk that gestational age represents for COVID-19-infected pregnant women [52,53], as not all studies have identified this association.

A bidirectional relationship between kidney function and COVID-19 disease has been suggested [54]. Patients with low renal function have an increased risk of critical COVID-19 [55] and a higher risk of ICU admission [56,57] or mortality [58], although none of these studies have exclusively considered pregnant women population. Furthermore, while chronic kidney disease is associated with impairment of the immune system, it is still unknown whether their worse COVID-19 outcome can be explained by a weaker antiviral response or by systemic inflammation [59].

Other studies have identified that more advanced age, due to possible age-related immune changes, potential comorbidities, and elevated BMI, represents risk factors for more severe COVID-19 infection in pregnant women [53]. Previous research found pre-pregnancy obesity to be a strong predictor of ICU admission, as it is linked with more severe COVID-19 cases, respiratory issues, and other metabolic complications [60]. Although we found this association in the unadjusted data, the final machine learning model did not include these variables as having a relevant effect.

A similar lack of effects in the final machine learning model occurs with comorbidities like preeclampsia, hypertension, hyperglycemia, or gestational diabetes [56]. Hypertension and other cardiovascular may elevate the likelihood of ICU admission for pregnant patients with COVID-19, as these conditions exacerbate the body's inflammatory response, as well as diabetes, gestational diabetes, or preeclampsia. A possible explanation for the lack of effect of these problems is that they are actually reflected in the alterations in the inflammatory biomarkers (altered white blood cell count and elevated CRP) that, in this study, are actually associated with a higher risk of admission to ICU, since these are parameters that are also altered in these obstetric conditions.

Severe dyspnea, low oxygen saturation (<94%), and the need for mechanical ventilation are direct predictors of ICU care. Respiratory complications are often more severe in pregnant women due to reduced lung capacity as the pregnancy progresses and are linked to pneumonia and the need for ventilation. COVID-19-related pneumonia is a primary predictor of ICU admission, as it often requires mechanical ventilation to support oxygen levels [61].

Pregnant women experience unique physiological and immunological changes that differentiate their response to COVID-19 from the general population. These differences may impact the progression of the disease, clinical manifestations, management strategies, and outcomes. Pregnancy maintenance relies on finely tuned immune adaptations [57] as it must maintain tolerance to the fetus while preserving innate and adaptive immune mechanisms for protection against microbial challenges, exhibiting a shift to Th2-dominant immunity to protect the fetus, which may make them more vulnerable to viral infections, including COVID-19 [59]. CRP and other inflammatory biomarkers may be naturally elevated in pregnancy, complicating the interpretation of higher risk in pregnant women compared to the general population. These adaptations of active immunologic tolerance are precisely timed and reflect an immune clock of pregnancy in women delivering at term. The differences in susceptibility, variability in progression, and differences in the risk of COVID-19 infection severity are also associated with host genetic factors [59], like unfavorable genotypes of IFNL3/IFNL4 SNPs. Among pregnant patients with confirmed SARS-CoV-2 infection, reduced mucosal antibody responses were associated with greater infectious virus recovery and viral RNA levels [60].

Pregnancy is associated with several factors that mimic the symptoms of COVID-19, like increased blood volume, cardiac output, heart rate, shortness of breath, and fatigue, which may overlap with normal pregnancy, potentially delaying COVID-19 diagnosis. Normal changes in pregnancy are also linked to more risk of severe COVID-19 complications like reduced lung capacity due to diaphragm elevation and increased oxygen consumption or its hypercoagulable state, increasing the risk of thromboembolic events.

Our study has some limitations. It is a retrospective study that was conducted in two centers. Women included in this analysis were those who were hospitalized either through spontaneous demand or after being referred from ambulatory care, which could leave more vulnerable groups underrepresented. Because the participants were recruited from 2020 to 2021, they were unvaccinated, as vaccination was not authorized in Kazakhstan for pregnant women during that period. This period includes the second wave of COVID-19 cases in the country, which are mostly related to the Delta variant. This variant has been associated with more severe progression in pregnancy with increased ICU admissions and increased need for advanced oxygen support. The Delta variant is associated with more unfavorable maternal and neonatal outcomes, including preterm births, SGA infants, lower Apgar scores, higher maternal and fetal mortality, higher maternal admission to ICU, higher CRP levels, as well as PCT and IL-6, higher levels of lymphocytes, D-dimer, and transaminases. It is also associated with a higher rate of placental SARS-CoV-2 detection [62]. The possibility that other variants or vaccination status could alter the model's outcomes could not be derived from these data and may limit the generalizability of these findings.

During this period, there were no homogeneous protocols/ICU admission criteria for these patients, and they were treated with different drugs (corticosteroids, lopinavir/ritonavir, azithromycin, hydroxychloroquine, interferon beta, tocilizumab, and prophylactic or therapeutic heparin). We could not analyze the possible association with higher risk of ICU admission of parameters like ferritin, interleukin-6, or d-dimer as they were only available for a reduced number of cases. Ferritin, interleukin-6, or d-dimer provide insight into the immunological and inflammatory pathways involved in severe COVID-19. Although their absence limits understanding of the disease's immunological and inflammatory pathways involved in severe COVID-19 and may hinder the development of tailored management strategies, CRP is considered as the inflammatory biomarker that better mirrors the course of the disease compared to d-dimer or ferritin [63]. Excessive production of interleukin-6 is associated both with more severe COVID-19 cases [64] as well as with adverse pregnancy outcomes like preterm delivery, preterm premature rupture of the membranes, and chorioamnionitis [65]. Significantly higher interleukin-6 levels in pregnant women with no significant difference have been observed between the pregnancy trimesters [66].

This study also has some relevant strengths. First, the large number of cases was analyzed. Second, the methods that facilitate transparency and interpretability of the data were used, helping to explain not only what the model predicted but why. Third, early identifying women at higher risk of complications during pregnancy may also help to offer psychological support to couples in these stressful situations [67]. Finally, the methodological approach for this work may be extended in cases of other infectious diseases that may affect pregnancy outcomes [68] as well as in situations when excess demand requires valid triage methods to allocate patients to always limited resources, like ICU beds.

## 5. Conclusions

Routinely collected clinical and laboratory data of COVID-19-infected pregnant women may help recognize high-risk groups who are more liable for complications and more severe course or prognosis and require an ICU admission. Leucocyte counts, C-reactive protein, pregnancy week, eGFR, and hemoglobin appeared as significant predictors of high risk of severe infection requiring ICU admission. The predictive model may be an efficient support tool for prioritizing care of COVID-19-infected pregnant women in clinical practice [69]. These findings may also contribute to enhancing our understanding of the pathogenesis of the disease and subsequently improve the outcome of patients. In this work, the identified best predictive model, which was logistic regression with $L_2$ regularization, achieved an AUC of 0.845 and sensitivity and specificity of 0.600 and 0.896 on test data, respectively. This result showcases the potential usage of machine learning to serve as an efficient and supportive tool for prioritizing care of COVID-19-infected pregnant women in clinical practice, especially in resource-strained healthcare systems.

**Supplementary Materials:** The following supporting information can be downloaded at: https://www.mdpi.com/article/10.3390/jcm13247705/s1, Table S1: Description of features.

**Author Contributions:** Conceptualization, A.S.-S., A.Z., S.Z., G.B. and Z.K.; methodology, A.S.-S. and A.Z.; analysis, A.M. (Azamat Mukhamediya), I.A., A.Z., A.S. (Aigerim Sipenova) and A.S.-S.; data curation, K.T., A.M. (Aigul Myrzabekova), K.K.J., A.S. (Asselzhan Sarbalina) and A.S. (Aigerim Sipenova); writing—original draft preparation, A.S.-S., A.M. (Azamat Mukhamediya), I.A., A.Z., M.T., G.B., A.S. (Aigerim Sipenova) and G.G.; writing—review and editing, S.Z., K.N., Z.K., K.T., A.M. (Aigul Myrzabekova), K.K.J., A.S. (Asselzhan Sarbalina), S.K., G.N.A., B.A.E. and K.M.; visualization, A.M. (Azamat Mukhamediya), K.M., A.Z. and G.G.; supervision, A.S.-S., A.Z., S.Z. and Z.K.; project administration, A.S.-S.; funding acquisition, A.S.-S. All authors have read and agreed to the published version of the manuscript.

**Funding:** This research was sponsored by Nazarbayev University (Grant No. NU 021220CRP0822).

**Institutional Review Board Statement:** Ethical approval was obtained from Nazarbayev University Institutional Review Ethics Committee (NU-IREC) #745/12062023, date of approval 20 June 2024. The data were extracted from electronic medical records by practicing clinicians from the hospitals and provided de-identified for conducting these analyses.

**Informed Consent Statement:** Data analyzed here were provided by clinicians from participating hospitals extracted from medical records for analysis. Given the retrospective nature of this study, no informed consent was obtained.

**Data Availability Statement:** Data are available from the correspondence author upon request due to privacy and ethical restrictions.

**Conflicts of Interest:** The authors declare no conflicts of interest. The funders had no role in the design of this study, in the collection, analyses, or interpretation of data, in the writing of this manuscript, or in the decision to publish the results.

## References


1. McBride, O.; Murphy, J.; Shevlin, M.; Gibson-Miller, J.; Hartman, T.K.; Hyland, P.; Levita, L.; Mason, L.; Martinez, A.P.; McKay, R.; et al. Monitoring the psychological, social, and economic impact of the COVID-19 pandemic in the population: Context, design and conduct of the longitudinal COVID-19 Psychological Research Consortium (C19PRC) study. *Int. J. Methods Psychiatr. Res.* **2020**, *30*, e1861. [CrossRef]
2. Weiss, P.; Murdoch, D.R. Clinical course and mortality risk of severe COVID-19. *Lancet* **2020**, *395*, 1014–1015. [CrossRef] [PubMed]
3. Badr, A.; Mattern, J.; Carlin, A.; Cordier, A.-G.; Maillart, E.; El Hachem, L.; El Kenz, H.; Andronikof, M.; De Bels, D.; Damoisel, C.; et al. Are clinical outcomes worse for pregnant women at ≥20 weeks' gestation infected with coronavirus disease 2019? A multicenter case-control study with propensity score matching. *Am. J. Obstet. Gynecol.* **2020**, *223*, 764–768. [CrossRef] [PubMed]
4. Rizzo, G.; Mappa, I.; Maqina, P.; Bitsadze, V.; Khizroeva, J.; Makatsarya, A.; D'Antonio, F. Effect of SARS-CoV-2 infection during the second half of pregnancy on fetal growth and hemodynamics: A prospective study. *Acta Obstet. Gynecol. Scand.* **2021**, *100*, 1034–1039. [CrossRef] [PubMed]
5. Hwangbo, S.; Kim, Y.; Lee, C.; Lee, S.; Oh, B.; Moon, M.K.; Kim, S.W.; Park, T. Machine learning models to predict the maximum severity of COVID-19 based on initial hospitalization record. *Front. Public Health* **2022**, *10*, 1007205. [CrossRef] [PubMed]
6. Artiga-Sainz, L.M.; Sarria-Santamera, A.; Martínez-Alés, G.; Quintana-Díaz, M. New Approach to Managing the COVID-19 Pandemic in a Complex Tertiary Care Medical Center in Madrid, Spain. *Disaster Med. Public Health Prep.* **2022**, *16*, 2097–2102. [CrossRef] [PubMed]
7. Sabitova, A.K.; Ortega, M.-A.; Ntegwa, M.J.; Sarria-Santamera, A. Impact of the COVID-19 pandemic on access to and delivery of maternal and child healthcare services in low-and middle-income countries: A systematic review of the literature. *Front. Public Health* **2024**, *12*, 1346268. [CrossRef]
8. Laatifi, M.; Douzi, S.; Bouklouz, A.; Ezzine, H.; Jaafari, J.; Zaid, Y.; El Ouahidi, B.; Naciri, M. Machine learning approaches in COVID-19 severity risk prediction in Morocco. *J. Big Data* **2022**, *9*, 5. [CrossRef] [PubMed]
9. Xiong, Y.; Ma, Y.; Ruan, L.; Li, D.; Lu, C.; Huang, L. Comparing different machine learning techniques for predicting COVID-19 severity. *Infect. Dis. Poverty* **2022**, *11*, 19. [CrossRef]
10. Wendland, P.; Schmitt, V.; Zimmermann, J.; Häger, L.; Göpel, S.; Schenkel-Häger, C.; Kschischo, M. Machine learning models for predicting severe COVID-19 outcomes in Hospitals. *Inform. Med. Unlocked* **2023**, *37*, 101188. [CrossRef] [PubMed]
11. Duda, R.O.; Hart, P.E.; Stork, D.G. *Pattern Classification*; Wiley: New York, NY, USA, 2001.
12. Hastie, T.; Tibshirani, R.; Friedman, J.H. *The Elements of Statistical Learning*; Springer Series in Statistics; Springer: Berlin/Heidelberg, Germany, 2009.
13. Breiman, L. Random Forests. *Mach. Learn.* **2001**, *45*, 5–32. [CrossRef]
14. Freund, Y.; Schapire, R.E. A decision-theoretic generalization of on-line learning and an application to boosting. *J. Comput. Syst. Sci.* **1997**, *55*, 119–139. [CrossRef]
15. Friedman, J.H. Greedy function approximation: A gradient boosting machine. *Ann. Stat.* **2001**, *29*, 1189–1232. [CrossRef]
16. Chen, T.; Guestrin, C. XGBoost. In Proceedings of the 22nd ACM SIGKDD International Conference on Knowledge Discovery and Data Mining 2016, San Francisco, CA, USA, 13–17 August 2016. [CrossRef]
17. Anderson, T.W. Classification by multivariate analysis. *Psychometrika* **1951**, *16*, 31–50. [CrossRef]
18. Karimi, Z.; Malak, J.S.; Aghakhani, A.; Najafi, M.S.; Ariannejad, H.; Zeraati, H.; Yekaninejad, M.S. Machine learning approaches to predict the need for intensive care unit admission among Iranian COVID-19 patients based on ICD-10: A cross-sectional study. *Health Sci. Rep.* **2024**, *7*, e70041. [CrossRef] [PubMed]
19. Famiglini, L.; Campagner, A.; Carobene, A.; Cabitza, F. A robust and parsimonious machine learning method to predict ICU admission of COVID-19 patients. *Med. Biol. Eng. Comput.* **2022**, 1–13. [CrossRef] [PubMed]
20. Cheng, F.Y.; Joshi, H.; Tandon, P.; Freeman, R.; Reich, D.L.; Mazumdar, M.; Kohli-Seth, R.; Levin, M.A.; Timsina, P.; Kia, A. Using machine learning to predict ICU transfer in hospitalized COVID-19 patients. *J. Clin. Med.* **2020**, *9*, 1668. [CrossRef]
21. Lundberg, S.M.; Lee, S.I. A unified approach to interpreting model predictions. *Adv. Neural Inf. Process. Syst.* **2017**, *30*, 4765–4774.
22. Pines, J.M.; Raja, A.S.; Bellolio, F.; Carpenter, C.R. (Eds.) *Evidence-Based Emergency Care: Diagnostic Testing and Clinical Decision Rules*; John Wiley & Sons: Hoboken, NJ, USA, 2023.
23. Kılıç, İ.; Ankaralı, H.; Aydın, G.A.; Ünal, S.; Özsoy, H.G.T. A prediction model for severe COVID-19 infection and intensive care unit admission in pregnant women. *Turk. J. Intensive Care* **2024**, *22*, 50–61. [CrossRef]
24. Álvarez Bartolomé, A.; Abdallah Kassab, N.A.; Cruz Melguizo, S.; de la Cruz Conty, M.L.; Forcen Acebal, L.; Abascal Saiz, A.; Pintado Recarte, P.; Martinez Varea, A.; Cerrillos Gonzalez, L.; García Fernández, J.; et al. Critical Care in SARS-CoV-2 infected pregnant women: A prospective multicenter study. *Biomedicines* **2022**, *10*, 475. [CrossRef] [PubMed]
25. El-Kady, A.M.; Aldakheel, F.M.; Allemailem, K.S.; Almatroudi, A.; Dbas, A.R.; Al Hamed, H.; Alsulami, M.; Alshehri, W.A.; El-Ashram, S.; Kreys, E.; et al. Clinical characteristics, outcomes and prognostic factors for critical illness in hospitalized COVID-19 patients in Saudi Arabia: A retrospective cohort study. *Int. J. Gen. Med.* **2022**, *15*, 6945–6963. [CrossRef] [PubMed]
26. Sun, G.; Zhang, Y.; Liao, Q.; Cheng, Y. Blood test results of pregnant COVID-19 patients: An updated case-control study. *Front. Cell. Infect. Microbiol.* **2020**, *10*, 560899. [CrossRef]
27. Gajendra, S. Spectrum of hematological changes in COVID-19. *Am. J. Blood Res.* **2022**, *12*, 43–53. [PubMed]
28. Huang, G.; Kovalic, A.J.; Graber, C.J. Prognostic value of leukocytosis and lymphopenia for coronavirus disease severity. *Emerg. Infect. Dis.* **2020**, *26*, 1839–1841. [CrossRef] [PubMed]

29. Yazdani, A.N.; Abdi, A.; Velpuri, P.; Patel, P.; DeMarco, N.; Agrawal, D.K.; Rai, V. A review of hematological complications and treatment in COVID-19. *Hematol. Rep.* **2023**, *15*, 562–577. [CrossRef] [PubMed]
30. Wool, G.D.; Miller, J.L. The impact of COVID-19 disease on platelets and coagulation. *Pathobiology* **2020**, *88*, 15–27. [CrossRef]
31. Vasileva, D.; Badawi, A. C-reactive protein as a biomarker of severe H1N1 influenza. *Inflamm. Res.* **2018**, *68*, 39–46. [CrossRef]
32. Plebani, M. Why C-reactive protein is one of the most requested tests in clinical laboratories? *Clin. Chem. Lab. Med. CCLM* **2023**, *61*, 1540–1545. [CrossRef] [PubMed]
33. Yamamoto, R.; Asano, H.; Umazume, T.; Takaoka, M.; Noshiro, K.; Saito, Y.; Nakagawa, K.; Chiba, K.; Nakakubo, S.; Nasuhara, Y.; et al. C-reactive protein level predicts need for medical intervention in pregnant women with SARS-CoV-2 infection: A retrospective study. *J. Obstet. Gynaecol. Res.* **2022**, *48*, 938–945. [CrossRef]
34. Smith, R.; Oakley, E.; Grandner, G.W.; Rukundo, G.; Farooq, F.; Ferguson, K.; Baumann, S.; Adams Waldorf, K.M.; Afshar, Y.; Ahlberg, M.; et al. Clinical risk factors of adverse outcomes among women with COVID-19 in the pregnancy and postpartum period: A sequential, prospective meta-analysis. *Am. J. Obstet. Gynecol.* **2023**, *228*, 161–177. [CrossRef]
35. Chen, M.; Zeng, J.; Liu, X.; Sun, G.; Gao, Y.; Liao, J.; Yu, J.; Luo, X.; Qi, H. Changes in physiology and immune system during pregnancy and coronavirus infection: A Review. *Eur. J. Obstet. Gynecol. Reprod. Biol.* **2020**, *255*, 124–128. [CrossRef] [PubMed]
36. Abu-Ismail, L.; Taha, M.J.; Abuawwad, M.T.; Al-Bustanji, Y.; Al-Shami, K.; Nashwan, A.; Yassin, M. COVID-19 and anemia: What do we know so far? *Hemoglobin* **2023**, *47*, 122–129. [CrossRef] [PubMed]
37. Aziz, M.; Goyal, H.; Haghbin, H.; Lee-Smith, W.M.; Gajendran, M.; Perisetti, A. The association of "Loss of smell" to COVID-19: A systematic review and meta-analysis. *Am. J. Med. Sci.* **2021**, *361*, 216–225. [CrossRef] [PubMed]
38. Giannis, D.; Ziogas, I.A.; Gianni, P. Coagulation disorders in coronavirus infected patients: COVID-19, SARS-CoV-1, MERS-COV and lessons from the past. *J. Clin. Virol.* **2020**, *127*, 104362. [CrossRef]
39. Li, F.; He, M.; Zhou, M.; Lai, Y.; Zhu, Y.; Liu, Z.; Wang, Y.; Wang, Y. Association of C-reactive protein with mortality in COVID-19 patients: A secondary analysis of a cohort study. *Sci. Rep.* **2023**, *13*, 20361. [CrossRef]
40. Ikeagwulonu, R.C.; Ugwu, N.I.; Ezeonu, C.T.; Ikeagwulonu, Z.C.; Uro-Chukwu, H.C.; Asiegbu, U.V.; Obu, D.C.; Briggs, D.C. C-Reactive Protein and COVID-19 Severity: A Systematic Review. *West Afr. J. Med.* **2021**, *38*, 1011–1023.
41. Purja, S.; Shin, H.; Lee, J.-Y.; Kim, E.Y. Is loss of smell an early predictor of COVID-19 severity: A systematic review and meta-analysis. *Arch. Pharmacal Res.* **2021**, *44*, 725–740. [CrossRef] [PubMed]
42. Berumen-Lechuga, M.G.; Leaños-Miranda, A.; Molina-Pérez, C.J.; García-Cortes, L.R.; Palomo-Piñón, S. Risk factors for severe–critical COVID-19 in pregnant women. *J. Clin. Med.* **2023**, *12*, 5812. [CrossRef]
43. Kalafat, E.; Prasad, S.; Birol, P.; Tekin, A.B.; Kunt, A.; Di Fabrizio, C.; Alatas, C.; Celik, E.; Bagci, H.; Binder, J.; et al. An internally validated prediction model for critical COVID-19 infection and intensive care unit admission in symptomatic pregnant women. *Am. J. Obstet. Gynecol.* **2022**, *226*, 403.e1–403.e13. [CrossRef]
44. Abdelmola, A.; Albasheer, O.; Kariri, A.; Akkam, F.; Hakami, R.; Essa, S.; Jali, F.M. Characteristics and outcomes of coronavirus disease- 2019 among pregnant women in Saudi Arabia; a retrospective study. *Int. J. Women's Health* **2024**, *16*, 475–490. [CrossRef] [PubMed]
45. Dawood, F.S.; Garg, S.; Fink, R.V.; Russell, M.L.; Regan, A.K.; Katz, M.A.; Booth, S.; Chung, H.; Klein, N.P.; Kwong, J.C.; et al. Epidemiology and clinical outcomes of hospitalizations for acute respiratory or febrile illness and laboratory-confirmed influenza among pregnant women during six influenza seasons, 2010–2016. *J. Infect. Dis.* **2019**, *221*, 1703–1712. [CrossRef] [PubMed]
46. Vouga, M.; Favre, G.; Martinez-Perez, O.; Pomar, L.; Acebal, L.F.; Abascal-Saiz, A.; Hernandez, M.R.V.; Hcini, N.; Lambert, V.; Carles, G.; et al. Maternal outcomes and risk factors for COVID-19 severity among pregnant women. *Sci. Rep.* **2021**, *11*, 13898. [CrossRef] [PubMed]
47. Shoji, K.; Tsuzuki, S.; Akiyama, T.; Matsunaga, N.; Asai, Y.; Suzuki, S.; Iwamoto, N.; Funaki, T.; Yamada, M.; Ozawa, N.; et al. Clinical characteristics and outcomes of coronavirus disease 2019 (COVID-19) in pregnant women: A propensity score–matched analysis of data from the COVID-19 Registry Japan. *Clin. Infect. Dis.* **2022**, *75*, e397–e402. [CrossRef]
48. Ghosh, R.; Gutierrez, J.P.; de Jesús Ascencio-Montiel, I.; Juárez-Flores, A.; Bertozzi, S.M. SARS-CoV-2 infection by trimester of pregnancy and adverse perinatal outcomes: A Mexican retrospective cohort study. *BMJ Open* **2024**, *14*, e075928. [CrossRef]
49. Arakaki, T.; Hasegawa, J.; Sekizawa, A.; Ikeda, T.; Ishiwata, I.; Kinoshita, K. Risk factors for severe disease and impact of severity on pregnant women with COVID-19: A case–control study based on data from a nationwide survey of maternity services in Japan. *BMJ Open* **2022**, *12*, e068575. [CrossRef]
50. Schiffl, H.; Lang, S.M. Long-term interplay between COVID-19 and chronic kidney disease. *Int. Urol. Nephrol.* **2023**, *55*, 1977–1984. [CrossRef] [PubMed]
51. Cei, F.; Chiarugi, L.; Brancati, S.; Montini, M.S.; Dolenti, S.; Di Stefano, D.; Beatrice, S.; Sellerio, I.; Messiniti, V.; Gucci, M.M.; et al. Early reduction of estimated glomerular filtration rate (EGFR) predicts poor outcome in acutely ill hospitalized COVID-19 patients firstly admitted to medical regular wards (EGFR-Cov19 Study). *Biomed. Pharmacother.* **2022**, *153*, 113454. [CrossRef]
52. Mirijello, A.; Piscitelli, P.; de Matthaeis, A.; Inglese, M.; D'Errico, M.M.; Massa, V.; Greco, A.; Fontana, A.; Copetti, M.; Florio, L.; et al. Low EGFR is a strong predictor of worse outcome in hospitalized COVID-19 patients. *J. Clin. Med.* **2021**, *10*, 5224. [CrossRef] [PubMed]
53. Li, W.-X.; Xu, W.; Huang, C.-L.; Fei, L.; Xie, X.-D.; Li, Q.; Chen, L. Acute cardiac injury and acute kidney injury associated with severity and mortality in patients with COVID-19. *Eur. Rev. Med. Pharmacol. Sci.* **2021**, *25*, 2114–2122. [CrossRef]

54. Mikami, T.; Miyashita, H.; Yamada, T.; Harrington, M.; Steinberg, D.; Dunn, A.; Siau, E. Risk factors for mortality in patients with COVID-19 in New York City. *J. Gen. Intern. Med.* **2020**, *36*, 17–26. [CrossRef]
55. Blazquez-Navarro, A.; Mittmann, L.; Thieme, C.J.; Anft, M.; Paniskaki, K.; Doevelaar, A.; Seibert, F.S.; Hoelzer, B.; Konik, M.J.; Berger, M.M.; et al. Impact of low EGFR on the immune response against COVID-19. *J. Nephrol.* **2022**, *36*, 199–202. [CrossRef]
56. Tossetta, G.; Fantone, S.; delli Muti, N.; Balercia, G.; Ciavattini, A.; Giannubilo, S.R.; Marzioni, D. Preeclampsia and severe acute respiratory syndrome coronavirus 2 infection: A systematic review. *J. Hypertens.* **2022**, *40*, 1629–1638. [CrossRef]
57. Aghaeepour, N.; Ganio, E.A.; Mcilwain, D.; Tsai, A.S.; Tingle, M.; Van Gassen, S.; Gaudilliere, D.K.; Baca, Q.; McNeil, L.; Okada, R.; et al. An immune clock of human pregnancy. *Sci. Immunol.* **2017**, *2*, eaan2946. [CrossRef] [PubMed]
58. Kinder, J.M.; Turner, L.H.; Stelzer, I.A.; Miller-Handley, H.; Burg, A.; Shao, T.-Y.; Pham, G.; Way, S.S. Cd8+ T cell functional exhaustion overrides pregnancy-induced fetal antigen alloimmunization. *Cell Rep.* **2020**, *31*, 107784. [CrossRef] [PubMed]
59. Zahid, W.; Farooqui, N.; Zahid, N.; Ahmed, K.; Anwar, M.F.; Rizwan-ul-Hasan, S.; Hussain, A.R.; Sarría-Santamera, A.; Abidi, S.H. Association of Interferon lambda 3 and 4 gene snps and their expression with COVID-19 disease severity: A cross-sectional study. *Infect. Drug Resist.* **2023**, *16*, 6619–6628. [CrossRef]
60. St Clair, L.A.; Eldesouki, R.E.; Sachithanandham, J.; Yin, A.; Fall, A.; Morris, C.P.; Norton, J.M.; Abdullah, O.; Dhakal, S.; Barranta, C.; et al. Reduced control of SARS-CoV-2 infection associates with lower mucosal antibody responses in pregnancy. *mSphere* **2024**, *9*, e0081223. [CrossRef]
61. Chinn, J.; Sedighim, S.; Kirby, K.A.; Hohmann, S.; Hameed, A.B.; Jolley, J.; Nguyen, N.T. Characteristics and Outcomes of Women with COVID-19 Giving Birth at US Academic Centers During the COVID-19 Pandemic. *JAMA Netw. Open* **2021**, *4*, e2120456. [CrossRef]
62. Incognito, G.G.; Distefano, R.E.C.; Campo, G.; Gulino, F.A.; Gulisano, C.; Gullotta, C.; Gullo, G.; Cucinella, G.; Tuscano, A.; Bruno, M.T.; et al. Comparison of Maternal and Neonatal Outcomes between SARS-CoV-2 Variants: A Retrospective, Monocentric Study. *J. Clin. Med.* **2023**, *12*, 6329. [CrossRef]
63. Lombardi, A.; Duiella, S.; Li Piani, L.; Comelli, A.; Ceriotti, F.; Oggioni, M.; Muscatello, A.; Bandera, A.; Gori, A.; Ferrazzi, E. Inflammatory biomarkers in pregnant women with COVID-19: A retrospective cohort study. *Sci. Rep.* **2021**, *11*, 13350. [CrossRef]
64. Qiu, X.; Zhang, L.; Tong, Y.; Qu, Y.; Wang, H.; Mu, D. Interleukin-6 for early diagnosis of neonatal sepsis with premature rupture of the membranes: A meta-analysis. *Medicine* **2018**, *97*, e13146. [CrossRef]
65. Castelli, V.; Cimini, A.; Ferri, C. Cytokine Storm in COVID-19. When You Come Out of the Storm, You Won't Be the Same Person Who Walked. *Front. Immunol.* **2020**, *11*, 2132. [CrossRef] [PubMed]
66. Tanacan, A.; Yazihan, N.; Erol, S.A.; Anuk, A.T.; Yucel Yetiskin, F.D.; Biriken, D.; Ozgu-Erdinc, A.S.; Keskin, H.L.; Moraloglu Tekin, O.; Sahin, D. The impact of COVID-19 infection on the cytokine profile of pregnant women: A prospective case-control study. *Cytokine* **2021**, *140*, 155431. [CrossRef] [PubMed]
67. Burgio, S.; Cucinella, G.; Perino, A.; Baglio, G.; Crifasi, L.; Krysiak, R.; Kowalcze, K.; Gullo, G. Effectiveness of Psychological Counseling Intervention in High-Risk Pregnancies in Italy. *J. Pers. Med.* **2024**, *14*, 976. [CrossRef] [PubMed]
68. Gullo, G.; Scaglione, M.; Cucinella, G.; Riva, A.; Coldebella, D.; Cavaliere, A.F.; Signore, F.; Buzzaccarini, G.; Spagnol, G.; Laganà, A.S.; et al. Congenital Zika Syndrome: Genetic Avenues for Diagnosis and Therapy, Possible Management and Long-Term Outcomes. *J. Clin. Med.* **2022**, *11*, 1351. [CrossRef]
69. Riemma, G.; De Franciscis, P.; Tesorone, M.; Coppa, E.; Schiattarella, A.; Billone, V.; Lopez, A.; Cucinella, G.; Gullo, G.; Carotenuto, R.M. Obstetric and Gynecological Admissions and Hospitalizations in an Italian Tertiary-Care Hospital during COVID-19 Pandemic: A Retrospective Analysis According to Restrictive Measures. *J. Clin. Med.* **2023**, *12*, 7097. [CrossRef] [PubMed]

Journal of
*Clinical Medicine*

MDPI

*Article*

# Incidence of Spontaneous Abortions During the COVID-19 Pandemic in a Regional County Hospital in Romania: A Retrospective Cohort Study

**Diana Burlacu [1,2,*], Agnes Burlacu [1], Emmanuel Ladanyi [1,3], Bela Szabo [1,3] and Tibor Mezei [1,2]**

1 George Emil Palade University of Medicine, Pharmacy, Science, and Technology of Targu Mures, 540142 Targu Mures, Romania; agnesburlacu.endo@yahoo.com (A.B.); ladanyiemmanuel@gmail.com (E.L.); bela.szabo@umfst.ro (B.S.)
2 Department of Pathology, County Emergency Clinical Hospital of Targu Mures, 54000 Targu Mures, Romania; tibor.mezei@umfst.ro
3 Department of Obstetrics and Gynecology, County Emergency Clinical Hospital of Targu Mures, 54000 Targu Mures, Romania
* Correspondence: dianaburlacu@yahoo.com

## Abstract

**Background**: The first trimester of pregnancy is known for its proinflammatory state, so it is considered a challenging period due to increased maternal vulnerability to viral infections. The main purpose of the current study was to evaluate the incidence trend of early miscarriages and whether there was any possible influence of the COVID-19 pandemic on pregnancy outcomes. **Materials and Methods**: We conducted a retrospective cohort study in which we included all pregnant women who had been admitted to our hospital between January 2018 and December 2022. Our aim was to compare the percentage of early miscarriages occurring in the pre-pandemic period (January 2018–February 2020) and during the pandemic (March 2020–December 2022). We decided to measure the total number and percentage of early pregnancy outcomes, including all viable pregnancies, ectopic pregnancies, and both medical and spontaneous abortions. **Results**: The annual incidence of registry-identified early miscarriages declined from 5.4% of 12–46-year-old women in 2018 to 3.6% in 2022 ($p = 0.008$). An overall incidence rate of 3.66% [95% C.I. 3.26–4.05] was calculated, with 4.25% [95% C.I. 3.35–4.41] in the pre-pandemic period and 3.24% [95% C.I. 2.82–3.57] during the pandemic. The highest incidence rate ($p < 0.0001$) was identified among nulliparous women (36.9%). **Conclusions**: To conclude, this study proved that the increase in the early miscarriage incidence rate could be assigned to an advanced maternal age, irrespective of one's reproductive history. This study proved that no significant increase in the incidence rate of early miscarriage during the COVID-19 pandemic was noted, suggesting that this viral infection does not alter the risk of miscarriages. We hope that these findings help women deal with emotional stress and offer them reassurance about bearing children during pandemic periods.

**Keywords:** pregnancy; miscarriage; stress; COVID-19 pandemic; viral infection

## 1. Introduction

Spontaneous abortion or miscarriage is defined as the loss of a pregnancy before viability, with less than 20 weeks of gestation and a birthweight of less than 500 g. Approximately 23 million miscarriages are registered annually around the world [1].

Pregnant women are considered a vulnerable category to viral infections, especially during the first trimester, due to its well-known proinflammatory state [2]. Previous Coronavirus pandemics have been associated with adverse feto-maternal outcomes [3]. There are also other pandemics with a documented effect on pregnancy outcomes. A study published in 2016 provided evidence regarding adverse pregnancy outcomes in the case of the Zika virus pandemic. An increased incidence in the birth of newborns with microcephaly and maternal febrile rash illness was registered during 2015–2016. This may highlight the vertical transmission of the virus, but no linkage between Zika virus infection in pregnant women and abortion was encountered [4,5].

Prenatal diagnostic tests (chorionic villous sampling, amniocentesis, cordocentesis) primarily focus on the identification of genetic abnormalities in the fetus; however, they may also have a role in the identification of infectious diseases that may have an adverse effect on fetal development [6]. These tests aim to detect specific pathogens, including rubella, cytomegalovirus, toxoplasmosis, varicella, parvovirus, Zika virus, and many others, as these may cause the postpartum TORCH syndrome or other long-term complications [7,8].

The COVID-19 (Coronavirus disease) pandemic led to self-isolation during the first few months, causing fear, stress, and uncertainty regarding both the medical implications and unknown consequences deriving from this viral infection [9]. Although, at the present moment, there is a growing body of evidence regarding the impact of COVID-19 on maternal and perinatal outcomes, data on the real impact of the pandemic on the obstetric population in European countries still need to be made available.

The purpose of this study was to assess the possible adverse effects of the COVID-19 pandemic on early pregnancies in terms of miscarriage. Furthermore, it aimed to determine the change in the incidence of spontaneous abortions during the COVID-19 pandemic. We wanted to evaluate whether pregnancy outcomes had been influenced by epidemic-associated chronic stress.

## 2. Materials and Methods

Our retrospective cohort study included all pregnant women who had been admitted to the Obstetrics and Gynecology Clinic in the Targu-Mures Emergency Clinical Hospital, Romania, between 2018 and 2022. We compared the incidence of spontaneous abortions registered during the pre-pandemic and pandemic periods as follows: January 2018–February 2020 and March 2020–December 2022. The 11th of March 2020 was officially declared the beginning of the COVID-19 pandemic [10]. We decided to measure the total number and percentage of early pregnancy outcomes, including all viable pregnancies, ectopic pregnancies, and both medical and spontaneous abortions. We also categorized pregnant women into three groups: nulliparous women, women with a history of one viable delivery, and women with more than one viable delivery.

We defined early pregnancy as a pregnancy under 36 gestational weeks, after which we considered it an at-term pregnancy.

## 3. Results

Between 2018 and 2022, we identified 5624 women who had been admitted to the Obstetrics and Gynecology Clinic. Of these, 2326 had been admitted pre pandemic, while 3298 had been admitted during the pandemic.

The annual incidence of registry-identified spontaneous abortions declined from 5.44% in 2018 to 3.57% in 2022. Moreover, the trend showed a significant decrease over these years ($p = 0.008$), with an $R^2$ value of 0.036 (see Figure 1).

An overall incidence rate of 3.66% [95% CI 3.26–4.05] was calculated, with 4.25% [95% CI 3.35–4.41] in the pre-pandemic period and 3.24% [95% CI 2.82–3.57] during the pandemic.

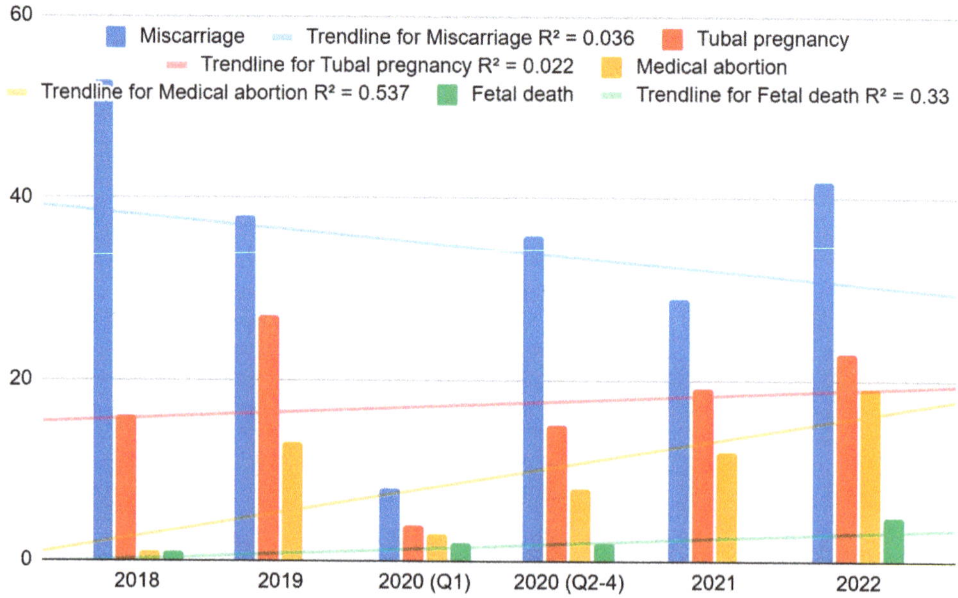


**Figure 1.** Trend of annual incidence rate of pathological pregnancies.

Extreme maternal age groups also showed a decrease in the rate of spontaneous miscarriages. A total of 18.2% (pre-pandemic period) and 16.8% (pandemic period) of pregnant women suffered spontaneous abortions in the age group <20 years old, while 10.1% (pre-pandemic period) and 8.4% (pandemic period) women suffered spontaneous abortions in the age group >40 years old ($p = 0.001$).

Maternal age was significantly associated with miscarriage ($p = 0.018$). In 2018, pregnant women aged 25–29 years had the highest percentage of miscarriages (29.9%). During 2019, 2020, 2021, and 2022, the highest percentage of miscarriages occurred in the maternal group 30–34 years old: 28.9% (2019), 27.9% (2020), 31.1% (2021), and 28.4% (2022) (see Figures 1 and 2).

Our data indicated a higher incidence rate of miscarriages occurring among nulliparous women, compared to parous women, after categorizing all pregnant women in this study into the three groups. Hence, the proportion of all miscarriages among registry-identified pregnancies during the first study period was as follows: 32.3% were attributed to nulliparous women, 22.2% to primiparous women with a history of one viable delivery, and 45.5% to multiparous women with a history of more than one viable delivery. During the second study period, these proportions increased to 41.1% among nulliparous women ($p < 0.001$) and 31.8% among primiparous women with a history of one viable delivery, while they decreased to 27.1% among multiparous women with a history of more than one viable delivery ($p < 0.001$) (see Figure 3).

During 2018–2022, a total of 20.4% registry-identified early pregnancies were noted, with 18.9% in 2018, 23.5% in 2019, 19.8% in 2020, 18.0% in 2021, and 21.8% in 2022 ($p = 0.012$). A total of 19.5% and 20.1% of early pregnancies occurred during the pre-pandemic and pandemic periods, respectively.

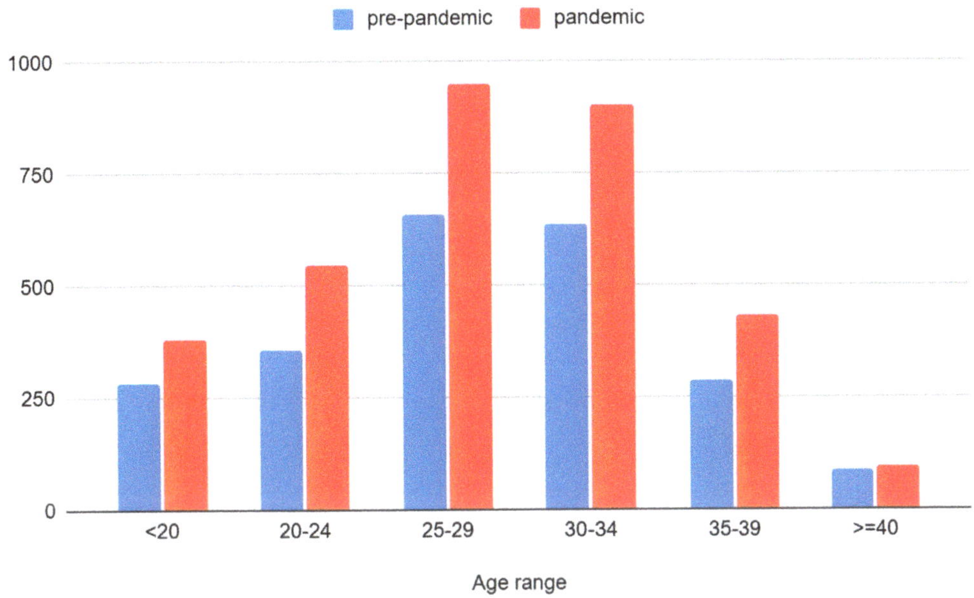


**Figure 2.** Miscarriages associated with maternal group age during the entire study period.

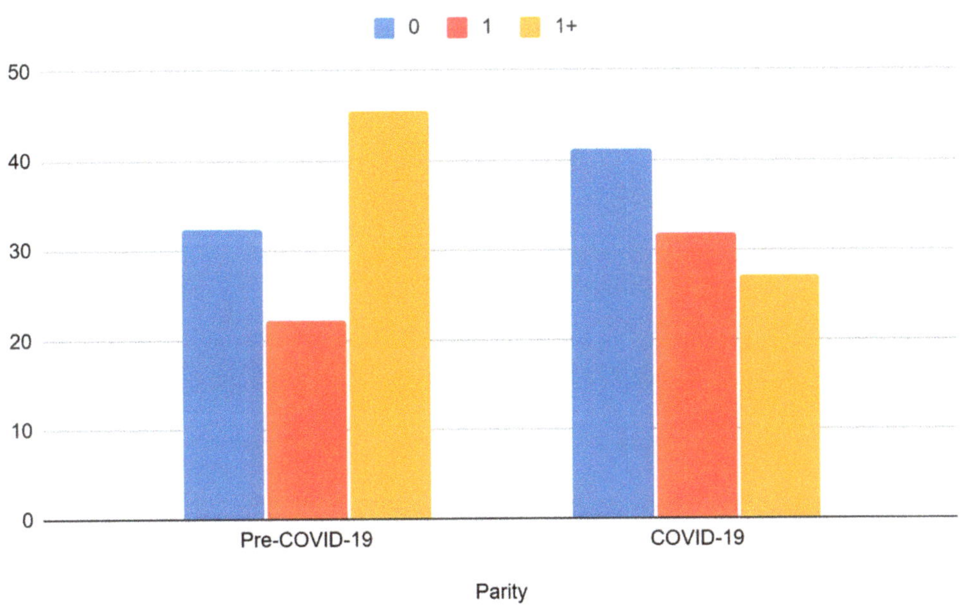


**Figure 3.** Comparison of miscarriage trend correlated with women's parity between the two study periods.

During the pandemic period, we observed a significant association between parity and gestational age at the time of delivery, with 30.9% of nulliparous women, 20.1% of primiparous women, and 19.5% of multiparous women having early pregnancies ($p = 0.044$).

Of all registered pregnancies during the study interval, 377 (6.7% of all pregnancies) were considered pathological. These included ectopic pregnancies (104, 1.84%), medically justified abortions (57, 1.01%), spontaneous abortions (206, 3.66%), and fetal demise (10, 0.19%) ($p = 0.002$), as shown in Figure 4.

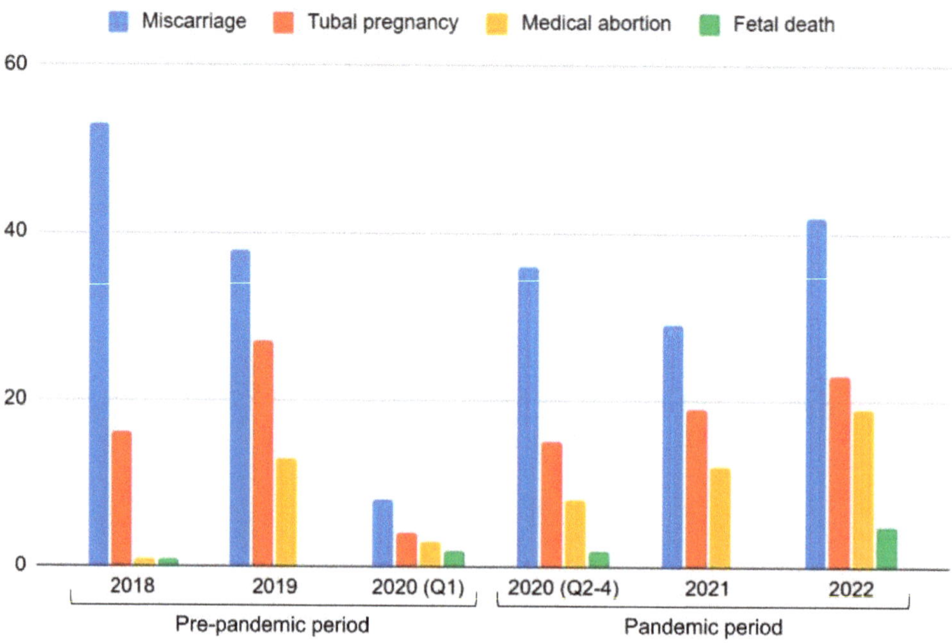


**Figure 4.** Incidence of pathological pregnancies before and during the pandemic.

During the pandemic, no statistical association was noted between spontaneous abortions and SARS-CoV-2 active infection ($p = 0.978$). Only 0.9% of spontaneous abortions and one maternal death were associated with viral infection.

## 4. Discussion

Miscarriage has been intensively studied, since it is among the commonest adverse pregnancy outcomes. More than 15% of clinically recognized pregnancies may have this outcome [11,12]. As some recently published data indicate, our study demonstrated a higher incidence of miscarriages with an increasing maternal age, specifically in women aged 30 years or more [13,14].

Two register-based studies presented evidence regarding the highest risk of miscarriage in women aged 45 years or more, proving that the rate of miscarriage increased with women's parity [15]. In contrast, we noted that the biggest proportion of all registry-identified miscarriages was mostly seen among nulliparous women. When comparing nulliparous and parous women, more than half of all registry-identified miscarriages occurred in nulliparous women.

It has been previously theorized that women facing miscarriages lack certain factors that would lead to full-term pregnancy development and not recurrent spontaneous abortions. Several hypotheses have been proposed to support such an "absent factor" mechanism. In previous studies, an IG antibody that could lead to total blockage of the mixed lymphocyte reaction was thought to be either absent or present in low titers in samples from women with recurrent spontaneous abortions [16,17].

The more HLA antigens are shared between partners, the higher the risk of spontaneous abortion. Consequently, women who share a variable amount of HLA types with their partners might experience an adverse pregnancy outcome, depending on the segregation of their genotype [18,19]. Still, these immunological theories were not fully reinforced by the clinical studies that followed [20,21].

On the other hand, another theory proposed by Clarke et al. postulated that any residual material in the uterine cavity after a miscarriage might jeopardize future pregnancies. According to this hypothesis, any possible "rest" from trophoblastic cells would influence the outcome of a pregnancy, since anencephaly or spina bifida were documented in women whose last pregnancy ended in miscarriage compared to controls whose outcome was a typical baby [18,22]. Prospective studies are needed to identify which factors could determine whether a first pregnancy will result in success or failure, thus offering prophylactic pre-conceptual counseling to nulligravid women.

In many instances, however, the exact cause of a miscarriage remains unknown. Multiple risk factors are considered, such as maternal age, genetics, and hormonal and environmental factors. A recent study suggested that parental chromosomal rearrangements could determine more than 50% of all recurrent miscarriages [23]. An advanced maternal age has been found to be one of the most significant risk factors. Consequently, in approximately half of spontaneous abortions before a gestational age of 12 weeks, fetal chromosomal abnormalities due to meiotic errors are found, caused by an advanced maternal age at the time of conception [15,24,25]. Another study found that autosomal trisomies are the most common genetic anomalies (52% of all miscarriages), followed by polyploidy (21%) and, finally, monosomy X (13% of cases) [26].

Although common, affecting one in ten women throughout their lifetime, miscarriage also has common risk factors, such as increasing age in both partners. In our study, this risk factor was also highlighted as being related to miscarriage. Furthermore, permanent stress as an adjustment to the lifestyle that modern life entails, along with daily habits (alcohol consumption and cigarette smoking included), outlines the typical portrait of a woman who is more prone to suffer a miscarriage [26]. In the general population, patients diagnosed with COVID-19 were more susceptible to developing thromboembolism due to excessive inflammation, hypoxia, and immobilization [26].

This misconception, postulating that miscarriages are often inevitable and that a woman who has suffered such a loss should keep trying to become pregnant until, eventually, she is able to carry at least one pregnancy to term, should belong to the past. This thinking can lead to psycho-emotional damage for the families in question. Regarding the possibility of a subsequent successful pregnancy, miscarriage is often associated with several fetal risk factors, namely preterm birth and fetal growth restriction [26]. This supposed increase in preterm delivery risk has been preliminary reported as varying up to 47%. Although insufficient, the correlation between COVID-19 infection, miscarriage, and a subsequent preterm delivery has been suggested based on some reported cases due to the premature rupture of membranes [26].

Moreover, spontaneous abortion can be a significant trigger for depression and anxiety in women, representing a significant psychological burden for them [27]. Mostly, they may struggle with feelings of guilt over what they have done wrong or what they could have done differently to prevent the loss of the pregnancy. Many studies have discovered an impressive percentage of women prone to psychiatric symptoms in the weeks to months after a pregnancy loss, most of them not having children [28,29]. The majority of women suffering a miscarriage are willing to know whether there is anything they can do to prevent a future miscarriage. These couples usually seek health care advice on how long they should be waiting before trying to conceive again [30]. Still, a consensus on an appropriate interpregnancy interval after suffering a pregnancy loss is lacking. The World

Health Organization (WHO) only recommends waiting at least six months, this limitation being based on a single cross-sectional study [31,32].

The beginning of the COVID-19 pandemic caused the self-isolation of community members, leading to stress, fear, and economic instability, alongside other already known factors. The chronic stress associated with this situation might have had a significant influence on pregnancy outcomes. A systematic review from 2017 suggested this hypothesis when studying the exposure of pregnant women to armed conflict [33]. Another study addressed a possible linkage between pregnancy outcomes and exposure to stress caused by rocket-attack alarms, showing a high risk of spontaneous abortion [34].

The Middle East Respiratory Syndrome (MERS) and Severe Acute Respiratory Syndrome (SARS) pandemics have both been studied regarding their possible impact on adverse pregnancy outcomes. Indeed, these two pandemics have been associated with increased maternal morbidity and mortality. Despite the small number of reported cases confirmed with MERS and SARS infection during pregnancy, the data revealed a feto-maternal fatality rate of almost 30% [30].

Infection with SARS-CoV during the 2002–2003 epidemic determined more than 50% of spontaneous abortions. During this pandemic from the early 2000s, an increased fatality rate was studied among pregnant patients. With a fatality rate of 25%, this outcome could be attributed to several physiological changes in pulmonary function usually occurring during advanced pregnancy [35].

No vertical transmission of the virus was detected, as no viral particles were discovered in the products of conception or after the histopathological examination of the placenta. Instead, the main causes of miscarriages during this pandemic period were severe maternal respiratory failure and hypoxemia. A more comprehensive description was published after the placentas of patients infected with SARS-CoV were examined: multiple cases of placental infection suggesting maternal vascular malperfusion (MVM) lesions and avascular villi suggesting fetal thrombosis were reported, alongside numerous cases of significant placental weight reduction. These histopathological changes were more likely related to hypoxemia and feto-maternal circulatory insufficiency as a direct result of SARS-CoV infection. Furthermore, in other studies, severe adverse pregnancy outcomes have also been associated with Middle East Respiratory Syndrome Coronavirus (MERS-CoV) [36,37].

There is growing evidence related to COVID-19's association with miscarriage [38–40]. Pregnant women belong to a category of people known to be at risk for numerous comorbidities. Although no increased risk related to COVID-19 infection was encountered among pregnant women compared to the remaining population in Ref. [40], almost 85% of pregnant women were thought to experience mild COVID-19 infection symptoms, 10% more severe disease, and 5% critical disease. The most commonly reported symptoms were shortness of breath, fever, and dry cough [40].

Vertical maternal–fetal transmission has been previously documented when maternal infection with TORCH syndrome and Zika virus was serologically confirmed, causing important fetal consequences. The first trimester of pregnancy has a critical importance, since fetal organs develop during this time. Hence, any maternal infection at this point could have an adverse impact on fetal development, compared to later gestational weeks [36,37].

Vertical transmission of this viral infection can occur during fetal intrauterine life through the placenta, during delivery through the aspiration of cervical–vaginal secretions, and through breastfeeding postpartum [40]. No evidence of transplacental transmission of COVID-19 exists [41], although several observational studies regarding this possibility have been published [40].

No significant increase in the risk of miscarriage in patients infected with COVID-19 during the first trimester has been observed [3,42]. Rather, studies related to miscarriage in pregnant women bearing this infection have shown that most miscarriages occur due to placental insufficiency, preterm delivery, and intrauterine growth restriction [37,43].

Solid evidence regarding the effect of COVID-19 infection on placental pathology is still limited, but given the amount of vascular maternal adverse outcomes, more frequent maternal vascular malperfusion (MVM) and fetal vascular malperfusion (FVM) have been observed [40]. On the other hand, many studies reported so far have revealed the absence of any particular connection regarding COVID-19 infection and most placental pathologies, when compared with controls [44–46].

The maternal organism's homeostasis has a physiological reaction to stress, with hypothalamic–pituitary–adrenal (HPA) axis activation as the first mechanism. The activation of this axis determines the release of the corticotropin-releasing hormone (CRH), which activates the adrenocorticotropic hormone, eventually leading to cortisol release from the adrenal gland. The latter, referred to as the stress hormone, then negatively impacts physiological mechanisms, thus becoming unable to properly restore homeostasis [47].

The literature reveals numerous studies that have determined a linkage between adverse pregnancy outcomes and levels of cortisol [48]. Lower birth weight, prematurity, and miscarriage have also been encountered in said studies. It is worth mentioning that not only high levels of cortisol have been discovered to be associated with adverse outcomes, but also a decrease in cortisol levels [49]. The vasoconstriction caused by a high level of norepinephrine has been found to be related to adverse pregnancy outcomes, since it may impair the uterine arteries, which could lead to inappropriate placental perfusion.

Angiotensin-converting enzyme 2 (ACE2) has been studied as the cellular entry receptor for SARS-CoV-2. During pregnancy, the feto-maternal interface is represented by both the placenta and the decidua. Hence, viral receptor expression at the level of the placenta or decidua represents the viral infection promoter. In a previous study of a placenta at 14 gestational weeks, four main cell types were shown to reveal ACE2 expression during single-cell transcriptome genomic data sequencing: stromal cells, villous cytotrophoblast, and syncytiotrophoblasts from the placenta and perivascular cells from the decidua. A high expression of ACE2 at the level of these cells implies adverse feto-maternal outcomes, given the possibility of placental dysfunction, insufficiency, and subsequent pregnancy complications [40].

At the present moment, there are few publications on the outcomes of pregnant women with COVID-19, most of them related to women in the second or third trimester [42]. Many viral infections can be harmful to the fetus during the first trimester of pregnancy, and whether Severe Acute SARS-Cov-2 is one of them is yet to be determined. Data on COVID-19 during pregnancy remain limited, mostly acquired from limited sample studies [44–46].

During the pandemic, both positive and negative aspects were experienced by pregnant patients and their families. As expected, a sense of loss of the birthing experience under normal circumstances was felt, since the hospital policies limited family members' visits. Panic and overall emotional stress were encountered upon positive Sar-Cov-2 testing. On the other hand, such strict policies led to a more profound and intimate feto-maternal connection, without the presence of other family members [47–49].

Our study had some limitations. Firstly, this was a single-center study that used registry data to identify miscarriages. We only had access to information for miscarriages diagnosed and treated within the public specialized health care sector. Thus, women with early pregnancy loss who possibly never sought medical attention were likely not included in this study.

It is also worthwhile to note that the pandemic could have potentially changed women's willingness to visit hospital environments regularly. As such, pregnant women might have had doubts about their safety in the hospital environment and, some of them, might have decided to put an end to their prenatal medical visit routine, presenting to the hospital only when the viability of the pregnancy could no longer be helped.

The retrospective nature of this study prevented us from using tools to compare stress levels between women who had experienced miscarriages and those who did not. However, we believe that the pandemic had an impact on almost every aspect of people's lives, serving as a unique stressor.

Early pregnancy was not exempt from such stress, and our study aimed to explore some of the effects of this situation. The full impact of the recent pandemic on reproduction is a complex issue, and many aspects are yet to be determined.

## 5. Conclusions

To conclude, this study proved that the observed increase in the early miscarriage incidence rate could be assigned to an advanced maternal age, irrespective of patients' reproductive history. This study proved that no significant increase in the incidence rate of early miscarriage during the COVID-19 pandemic was noted, suggesting that this viral infection did not alter the risk of miscarriages. Meanwhile, the increased average age of primiparous women could have been another reason for the higher proportion of miscarriages among nulliparous women.

We hope that these findings help women deal with emotional stress and offer reassurance about bearing children during pandemic periods. The present study is the first Eastern European study to investigate the overall declining incidence rate of early miscarriage during the COVID-19 pandemic.

**Author Contributions:** Conceptualization, D.B. and T.M.; methodology, B.S.; formal analysis, A.B.; investigation, E.L.; data curation, A.B. and E.L.; writing—original draft preparation, D.B.; writing—review and editing, T.M. All authors have read and agreed to the published version of the manuscript.

**Funding:** This research received no external funding.

**Institutional Review Board Statement:** The study was performed with the approval of the hospital's Ethics Committee (registration number 29680/22 November 2022).

**Informed Consent Statement:** Informed consent was obtained from all subjects involved in the study.

**Data Availability Statement:** Data available on reasonable request due to ethical restrictions.

**Conflicts of Interest:** The authors declare no conflict of interest.

## References

1. The Lancet. The Lancet Miscarriage: Worldwide Reform of Care Is Needed. *Lancet* **2021**, *397*, 1597. [CrossRef] [PubMed]
2. Liu, H.; Wang, L.-L.; Zhao, S.-J.; Kwak-Kim, J.; Mor, G.; Liao, A.-H. Why Are Pregnant Women Susceptible to COVID-19? An Immunological Viewpoint. *J. Reprod. Immunol.* **2020**, *139*, 103122. [CrossRef] [PubMed]
3. la Cour Freiesleben, N.; Egerup, P.; Hviid, K.V.R.; Severinsen, E.R.; Kolte, A.M.; Westergaard, D.; Fich Olsen, L.; Prætorius, L.; Zedeler, A.; Christiansen, A.-M.H.; et al. SARS-CoV-2 in First Trimester Pregnancy: A Cohort Study. *Hum. Reprod.* **2021**, *36*, 40–47. [CrossRef] [PubMed]
4. Kleber de Oliveira, W.; Cortez-Escalante, J.; De Oliveira, W.T.G.H.; do Carmo, G.M.I.; Henriques, C.M.P.; Coelho, G.E.; Araújo de França, G.V. Increase in Reported Prevalence of Microcephaly in Infants Born to Women Living in Areas with Confirmed Zika Virus Transmission during the First Trimester of Pregnancy—Brazil, 2015. *MMWR Morb. Mortal. Wkly. Rep.* **2016**, *65*, 242–247. [CrossRef]
5. Sookaromdee, P.; Wiwanitkit, V. Abortion and Zika Virus Congenital Infection. *Rev. Bras. Ginecol. Obstet.* **2018**, *40*, 497. [CrossRef]
6. Carlson, L.M.; Vora, N.L. Prenatal Diagnosis: Screening and Diagnostic Tools. *Obstet. Gynecol. Clin. N. Am.* **2017**, *44*, 245–256. [CrossRef]
7. Rana, A.; Sharma, K.A. Diagnosis of Infections in Fetus: Ultrasound and Invasive Techniques. *J. Fetal Med.* **2020**, *07*, 243–252. [CrossRef]

8. Auriti, C.; De Rose, D.U.; Santisi, A.; Martini, L.; Piersigilli, F.; Bersani, I.; Ronchetti, M.P.; Caforio, L. Pregnancy and Viral Infections: Mechanisms of Fetal Damage, Diagnosis and Prevention of Neonatal Adverse Outcomes from Cytomegalovirus to SARS-CoV-2 and Zika Virus. *Biochim. Biophys. Acta Mol. Basis Dis.* **2021**, *1867*, 166198. [CrossRef]
9. Rotshenker-Olshinka, K.; Volodarsky-Perel, A.; Steiner, N.; Rubenfeld, E.; Dahan, M.H. COVID-19 Pandemic Effect on Early Pregnancy: Are Miscarriage Rates Altered, in Asymptomatic Women? *Arch. Gynecol. Obstet.* **2021**, *303*, 839–845. [CrossRef]
10. Hui, D.S.; Azhar, E.I.; Madani, T.A.; Ntoumi, F.; Kock, R.; Dar, O.; Ippolito, G.; Mchugh, T.D.; Memish, Z.A.; Drosten, C.; et al. The Continuing 2019-nCoV Epidemic Threat of Novel Coronaviruses to Global Health—The Latest 2019 Novel Coronavirus Outbreak in Wuhan, China. *Int. J. Infect. Dis.* **2020**, *91*, 264–266. [CrossRef]
11. Sundermann, A.C.; Hartmann, K.E.; Jones, S.H.; Torstenson, E.S.; Velez Edwards, D.R. Interpregnancy Interval After Pregnancy Loss and Risk of Repeat Miscarriage. *Obstet. Gynecol.* **2017**, *130*, 1312–1318. [CrossRef] [PubMed]
12. Ventura, S.J.; Curtin, S.C.; Abma, J.C.; Henshaw, S.K. Estimated Pregnancy Rates and Rates of Pregnancy Outcomes for the United States, 1990–2008. *Natl. Vital Stat. Rep.* **2012**, *60*, 1–21. [PubMed]
13. Nybo Andersen, A.M.; Wohlfahrt, J.; Christens, P.; Olsen, J.; Melbye, M. Maternal Age and Fetal Loss: Population Based Register Linkage Study. *BMJ* **2000**, *320*, 1708–1712. [CrossRef]
14. Feodor Nilsson, S.; Andersen, P.K.; Strandberg-Larsen, K.; Nybo Andersen, A.-M. Risk Factors for Miscarriage from a Prevention Perspective: A Nationwide Follow-up Study. *BJOG* **2014**, *121*, 1375–1384. [CrossRef]
15. Magnus, M.C.; Wilcox, A.J.; Morken, N.-H.; Weinberg, C.R.; Håberg, S.E. Role of Maternal Age and Pregnancy History in Risk of Miscarriage: Prospective Register Based Study. *BMJ* **2019**, *364*, l869. [CrossRef]
16. Rocklin, R.E.; Kitzmiller, J.L.; Carpenter, C.B.; Garovoy, M.R.; David, J.R. Maternal-Fetal Relation. Absence of an Immunologic Blocking Factor from the Serum of Women with Chronic Abortions. *N. Engl. J. Med.* **1976**, *295*, 1209–1213. [CrossRef]
17. Stimson, W.H.; Strachan, A.F.; Shepherd, A. Studies on the Maternal Immune Response to Placental Antigens: Absence of a Blocking Factor from the Blood of Abortion-Prone Women. *Br. J. Obstet. Gynaecol.* **1979**, *86*, 41–45. [CrossRef]
18. Regan, L.; Braude, P.R.; Trembath, P.L. Influence of Past Reproductive Performance on Risk of Spontaneous Abortion. *BMJ* **1989**, *299*, 541–545. [CrossRef]
19. Power, D.A.; Catto, G.R.; Mason, R.J.; MacLeod, A.M.; Stewart, G.M.; Stewart, K.N.; Shewan, W.G. The Fetus as an Allograft: Evidence for Protective Antibodies to HLA-Linked Paternal Antigens. *Lancet* **1983**, *2*, 701–704. [CrossRef]
20. Caudle, M.R.; Rote, N.S.; Scott, J.R.; DeWitt, C.; Barney, M.F. Histocompatibility in Couples with Recurrent Spontaneous Abortion and Normal Fertility. *Fertil. Steril.* **1983**, *39*, 793–798. [CrossRef]
21. Jazwinska, E.C.; Kilpatrick, D.C.; Smart, G.E.; Liston, W.A. Feto-Maternal HLA Compatibility Does Not Have a Major Influence on Human Pregnancy except for Lymphocytotoxin Production. *Clin. Exp. Immunol.* **1987**, *69*, 116–122. [PubMed]
22. Clarke, C.; Hobson, D.; McKendrick, O.M.; Rogers, S.C.; Sheppard, P.M. Spina Bifida and Anencephaly: Miscarriage as Possible Cause. *Br. Med. J.* **1975**, *4*, 743–746. [CrossRef] [PubMed]
23. Garrido-Gimenez, C.; Alijotas-Reig, J. Recurrent Miscarriage: Causes, Evaluation and Management. *Postgrad. Med. J.* **2015**, *91*, 151–162. [CrossRef] [PubMed]
24. Wilcox, A.J.; Weinberg, C.R.; O'Connor, J.F.; Baird, D.D.; Schlatterer, J.P.; Canfield, R.E.; Armstrong, E.G.; Nisula, B.C. Incidence of Early Loss of Pregnancy. *N. Engl. J. Med.* **1988**, *319*, 189–194. [CrossRef]
25. Almeida, N.D.; Basso, O.; Abrahamowicz, M.; Gagnon, R.; Tamblyn, R. Risk of Miscarriage in Women Receiving Antidepressants in Early Pregnancy, Correcting for Induced Abortions. *Epidemiology* **2016**, *27*, 538–546. [CrossRef]
26. Goddijn, M.; Leschot, N.J. Genetic Aspects of Miscarriage. *Best Pract. Res. Clin. Obstet. Gynaecol.* **2000**, *14*, 855–865. [CrossRef]
27. Griebel, C.P.; Halvorsen, J.; Golemon, T.B.; Day, A.A. Management of Spontaneous Abortion. *Am. Fam. Physician* **2005**, *72*, 1243–1250.
28. Neugebauer, R.; Kline, J.; O'Connor, P.; Shrout, P.; Johnson, J.; Skodol, A.; Wicks, J.; Susser, M. Determinants of Depressive Symptoms in the Early Weeks after Miscarriage. *Am. J. Public Health* **1992**, *82*, 1332–1339. [CrossRef]
29. Thapar, A.K.; Thapar, A. Psychological Sequelae of Miscarriage: A Controlled Study Using the General Health Questionnaire and the Hospital Anxiety and Depression Scale. *Br. J. Gen. Pract.* **1992**, *42*, 94–96.
30. Bardos, J.; Hercz, D.; Friedenthal, J.; Missmer, S.A.; Williams, Z. A National Survey on Public Perceptions of Miscarriage. *Obstet. Gynecol.* **2015**, *125*, 1313–1320. [CrossRef]
31. Conde-Agudelo, A.; Belizán, J.M.; Breman, R.; Brockman, S.C.; Rosas-Bermudez, A. Effect of the Interpregnancy Interval after an Abortion on Maternal and Perinatal Health in Latin America. *Int. J. Gynaecol. Obstet.* **2005**, *89* (Suppl. S1), S34–S40. [CrossRef] [PubMed]
32. Marston, C.; Conde-Agudelo, A.; World Health Organization. Department of Making Pregnancy Safer; World Health Organization. Reproductive Health and Research. In *Report of a WHO Technical Consultation on Birth Spacing, Geneva, Switzerland, 13–15 June 2005*; WHO: Geneva, Switzerland, 2007.
33. Keasley, J.; Blickwedel, J.; Quenby, S. Adverse Effects of Exposure to Armed Conflict on Pregnancy: A Systematic Review. *BMJ Glob. Health* **2017**, *2*, e000377. [CrossRef] [PubMed]

34. Wainstock, T.; Lerner-Geva, L.; Glasser, S.; Shoham-Vardi, I.; Anteby, E.Y. Prenatal Stress and Risk of Spontaneous Abortion. *Psychosom. Med.* **2013**, *75*, 228–235. [CrossRef] [PubMed]
35. Wong, S.F.; Chow, K.M.; Leung, T.N.; Ng, W.F.; Ng, T.K.; Shek, C.C.; Ng, P.C.; Lam, P.W.Y.; Ho, L.C.; To, W.W.K.; et al. Pregnancy and Perinatal Outcomes of Women with Severe Acute Respiratory Syndrome. *Am. J. Obstet. Gynecol.* **2004**, *191*, 292–297. [CrossRef]
36. Wong, T.C.; Lee, Z.Y.; Sia, T.L.L.; Chang, A.K.W.; Chua, H.H. Miscarriage Risk in COVID-19 Infection. *SN Compr. Clin. Med.* **2020**, *2*, 1449–1452. [CrossRef]
37. Rana, M.S.; Usman, M.; Alam, M.M.; Khalid, A.; Ikram, A.; Salman, M.; Zaidi, S.S.Z.; Faryal, R.; Qadir, M.; Umair, M.; et al. First Trimester Miscarriage in a Pregnant Woman Infected with COVID-19 in Pakistan. *J. Infect.* **2021**, *82*, e27–e28. [CrossRef]
38. Kazemi, S.N.; Hajikhani, B.; Didar, H.; Hosseini, S.S.; Haddadi, S.; Khalili, F.; Mirsaeidi, M.; Nasiri, M.J. COVID-19 and Cause of Pregnancy Loss during the Pandemic: A Systematic Review. *PLoS ONE* **2021**, *16*, e0255994. [CrossRef]
39. Hosier, H.; Farhadian, S.F.; Morotti, R.A.; Deshmukh, U.; Lu-Culligan, A.; Campbell, K.H.; Yasumoto, Y.; Vogels, C.B.; Casanovas-Massana, A.; Vijayakumar, P.; et al. SARS-CoV-2 Infection of the Placenta. *J. Clin. Investig.* **2020**, *130*, 4947–4953. [CrossRef]
40. Shmakov, R.G.; Prikhodko, A.; Polushkina, E.; Shmakova, E.; Pyregov, A.; Bychenko, V.; Priputnevich, T.V.; Dolgushin, G.O.; Yarotskaya, E.; Pekarev, O.; et al. Clinical Course of Novel COVID-19 Infection in Pregnant Women. *J. Matern. Fetal. Neonatal Med.* **2022**, *35*, 4431–4437. [CrossRef]
41. Muhidin, S.; Behboodi Moghadam, Z.; Vizheh, M. Analysis of Maternal Coronavirus Infections and Neonates Born to Mothers with 2019-nCoV; a Systematic Review. *Arch. Acad. Emerg. Med.* **2020**, *8*, e49.
42. Cosma, S.; Carosso, A.R.; Cusato, J.; Borella, F.; Carosso, M.; Bovetti, M.; Filippini, C.; D'Avolio, A.; Ghisetti, V.; Di Perri, G.; et al. Coronavirus Disease 2019 and First-Trimester Spontaneous Abortion: A Case-Control Study of 225 Pregnant Patients. *Am. J. Obstet. Gynecol.* **2021**, *224*, 391.e1–e391.e7. [CrossRef] [PubMed]
43. Ryan, G.A.; Purandare, N.C.; McAuliffe, F.M.; Hod, M.; Purandare, C.N. Clinical Update on COVID-19 in Pregnancy: A Review Article. *J. Obstet. Gynaecol. Res.* **2020**, *46*, 1235–1245. [CrossRef] [PubMed]
44. Yan, J.; Guo, J.; Fan, C.; Juan, J.; Yu, X.; Li, J.; Feng, L.; Li, C.; Chen, H.; Qiao, Y.; et al. Coronavirus Disease 2019 in Pregnant Women: A Report Based on 116 Cases. *Am. J. Obstet. Gynecol.* **2020**, *223*, 111.e1–e111.e14. [CrossRef]
45. Cao, D.; Yin, H.; Chen, J.; Tang, F.; Peng, M.; Li, R.; Xie, H.; Wei, X.; Zhao, Y.; Sun, G. Clinical Analysis of Ten Pregnant Women with COVID-19 in Wuhan, China: A Retrospective Study. *Int. J. Infect. Dis.* **2020**, *95*, 294–300. [CrossRef]
46. Ferrazzi, E.; Frigerio, L.; Savasi, V.; Vergani, P.; Prefumo, F.; Barresi, S.; Bianchi, S.; Ciriello, E.; Facchinetti, F.; Gervasi, M.T.; et al. Vaginal Delivery in SARS-CoV-2-Infected Pregnant Women in Northern Italy: A Retrospective Analysis. *BJOG* **2020**, *127*, 1116–1121. [CrossRef]
47. Ajayi, K.V.; Harvey, I.S.; Panjwani, S.; Uwak, I.; Garney, W.; Page, R.L. Narrative Analysis of Childbearing Experiences during the COVID-19 Pandemic. *MCN Am. J. Matern./Child Nurs.* **2021**, *46*, 284–292. [CrossRef]
48. Hicks, L.E. Multiple Case Study Exploring the Impact of Visitor Restrictions in Hospitals on Childbirth Support during the COVID-19 Pandemic. *Reprod. Female Child Health* **2023**, *2*, 271–278. [CrossRef]
49. Bolgeo, T.; Gambalunga, F.; Di Matteo, R.; Gatti, D.; Roberti, E.; Dealberti, D.; Fadda, B.; Grassi, E.; Gambarini, L.; Iacorossi, L.; et al. Becoming a Mother during the COVID-19 Pandemic: The Lived Experience as Told by Birthing Mothers: A Qualitative Study. *J. Nurs. Manag.* **2022**, *30*, 4138–4144. [CrossRef]

Journal of
*Clinical Medicine*

MDPI

*Article*

# SARS-CoV-2 Infection and Its Association with Maternal and Fetal Redox Status and Outcomes: A Prospective Clinical Study

**Marija Bicanin Ilic [1,2,*], Tamara Nikolic Turnic [3,4,5], Igor Ilic [6], Aleksandar Nikolov [1,2], Srdjan Mujkovic [1,2], Dejana Rakic [1,2], Nikola Jovic [1,2], Neda Arsenijevic [1,2], Slobodanka Mitrovic [7,8], Marija Spasojevic [7,8], Jelena Savic [7,8], Katarina Mihajlovic [3,5], Nevena Jeremic [3,5,9], Jovana Joksimovic Jovic [5,10], Bozidar Pindovic [3,5], Goran Balovic [11,12] and Aleksandra Dimitrijevic [1,2]**

1 Faculty of Medical Sciences, Department of Gynecology and Obstetrics, University of Kragujevac, 34000 Kragujevac, Serbia; aleksandar.nikolov2@gmail.com (A.N.); drsrdjanmujkovic@gmail.com (S.M.); dejavulovic@gmail.com (D.R.); docctorny@gmail.com (N.J.); velickovicneda@gmail.com (N.A.); saskadkg@gmail.com (A.D.)
2 Clinic of Gynecology and Obstetrics, University Clinical Center Kragujevac, 34000 Kragujevac, Serbia
3 Faculty of Medical Sciences, Department of Pharmacy, University of Kragujevac, 34000 Kragujevac, Serbia; tnikolict@gmail.com (T.N.T.); katarina.mih17@gmail.com (K.M.); nbarudzic@hotmail.com (N.J.); pindovic.bozidar@gmail.com (B.P.)
4 N.A. Semashko Public Health and Healthcare Department, F.F. Erismann Institute of Public Health, I.M. Sechenov First Moscow State Medical University (Sechenov University), 119435 Moscow, Russia
5 Center of Excellence for Redox Balance Research in Cardiovascular and Metabolic Disorders, 34000 Kragujevac, Serbia; jovana_joksimovic@yahoo.com
6 Department of Radiology, University Clinical Center Kragujevac, 34000 Kragujevac, Serbia
7 Faculty of Medical Sciences, Department of Pathology, University of Kragujevac, 34000 Kragujevac, Serbia; smitrovic@fmn.kg.ac.rs (S.M.); spasojevicmarija89@gmail.com (M.S.); jecasavic998@gmail.com (J.S.)
8 Department of Pathology, University Clinical Center Kragujevac, 34000 Kragujevac, Serbia
9 Federal State Autonomous Educational Institution of Higher Education I.M. Sechenov First, Moscow State Medical University of the Ministry of Health of the Russian Federation (Sechenov University), 119991 Moscow, Russia
10 Faculty of Medical Sciences, Department of Physiology, University of Kragujevac, 34000 Kragujevac, Serbia
11 Faculty of Medical Sciences, Department of Surgery, University of Kragujevac, 34000 Kragujevac, Serbia; gbalovic@gmail.com
12 Center of Pediatric Surgery, University Clinical Center Kragujevac, 34000 Kragujevac, Serbia
* Correspondence: malaabahelica@gmail.com

## Abstract

**Background:** The impact of the SARS-CoV-2 viral infection during pregnancy on the fetus can be direct—transmitted through the placenta—and indirect—creating unfavorable conditions for the development of the fetus because of inflammation, micro-thrombosis, and hypercoagulation. Our study aimed to determine the types and frequency of pathohistological changes in placental tissue in SARS-CoV-2-positive pregnant women and to examine the possible role of oxidative stress in the prognosis of the delivery and its maternal and fetal complications. **Methods:** This prospective clinical study included 50 pregnant women divided into two groups, SARS-CoV-2 positive (COVID-19 group) and SARS-CoV-2 negative (control group), from who we collected demographic, clinical, obstetric, biochemical and pathologic data. Data about the newborn characteristics were also collected, which included anamnestic, clinical, and biochemical data. **Results:** The values of the superoxide anion radical and index of lipid peroxidation were significantly different in mothers concerning the presence of the SARS-CoV-2 infection, while the levels of the nitric oxide, index of lipid peroxidation, reduced glutathione, and superoxide dismutase were significantly different in the newborns depending on the SARS-CoV-2 infection. Newborn characteristics were similar between groups except for concentrations of IgM antibody. The incidence of pathohistological changes of the FVM type in the COVID-19 group of pregnant women was 46%, while in the control group, the incidence was 18%. **Conclusions**: This study confirmed the significant impact of the SARS-CoV-2 viral infection on maternal and fetal biochemical parameters and oxidative stress-mediated placental dysfunction. Future studies should be performed with more participants and follow-up neonatal development.

**Keywords:** COVID 19; pregnancy; placental pathological lesions; neonatal oxidative stress; SARS-CoV-2 fetal transmission

## 1. Introduction

WHO data show that the number of patients with COVID-19 from the beginning of the pandemic to August 2024 exceeds 776 million, with more than 6.95 million deaths [1,2].

Even after the WHO declared the end of the pandemic on 11 May 2023, COVID-19 remains one of the biggest challenges facing the health system and world economy because of its rapid spreading and unpredictable course.

SARS-CoV-2 is the pathogen responsible for the onset of COVID-19, belonging to the group of beta-type Coronaviridae [3,4]. Based on the structure, it is an enveloped RNA virus that shares a genetic sequence with some SARS viruses identified in bats and pangolins, indicating a zoogenic origin [5]. SARS-CoV-2 components are RNA and four structural proteins: spike (S) protein, nucleocapsid (N) protein, envelope (E) protein, and membrane (M) protein with a specific role in the pathogenesis of the disease [6].

The RNA of the virus is a template for the multiplication of viral RNA and proteins that are further released infecting new cells. The release of the virus into the bloodstream leads to an inflammatory reaction mediated by the release of cytokines and the consequent activation of the coagulation system [7,8]. The activation of monocytes as part of the acute phase response leads to damage to the endothelium, which is crucial for activating the procoagulant system within the body and forming immune-thrombosis.

Based on the severity of symptoms, COVID-19 can be asymptomatic, mild, moderate, severe, and critical [9]. The viral load, inflammation, and the state of the immune system also influence the severity of the clinical course [1]. Factors such as age, gender, associated diseases, and obesity are related to the severity of the disease and increased mortality [10]. SARS-CoV-2 infection also interferes with a woman's reproductive health, negatively affecting ovarian function [11]. The physiological changes that accompany pregnancy could theoretically contribute to the development of more severe forms of COVID-19 in this group of patients [12]. Based on clinical experience and the conclusions of studies conducted during previous epidemics caused by coronaviruses such as Severe Acute Respiratory Syndrome (SARS) and Middle Eastern Respiratory Syndrome (MERS), patients infected during pregnancy are classified as patients with an increased risk of developing severe forms of disease and mortality [13,14]. There is a growing concern about possible neonatal and perinatal complications based on experience with ZIKA infection that is capable of crossing the placenta and causing fetal development damage [15]. Data from the US Centers for Disease Control and Prevention show that pregnant women have the same risk of death, but an increased risk of developing complications that require hospitalization and admission to the ICU compared to patients who are not pregnant [7].

Direct cytotoxicity of the virus and endothelial injury led to inflammatory changes in the complex functioning of the pregnant woman's immune system. This system constantly changes to satisfy the demands of the growing embryo and, thus, the time of infection can be of great importance for the prognosis of the course of the disease, maternal immune response, release from the virus, and perinatal outcome [16].

The impact of viral infection on the fetus can be direct—transmitted through the placenta—and indirect—creating unfavorable conditions for the development of the fetus because of inflammation, micro-thrombosis, and hypercoagulation.

There are three modes of transmission of the virus to the fetus/neonate: direct/intrauterine transmission, intrapartum, and postpartum transmission.

Oxidative stress is one of the key factors in the pathogenesis of COVID-19 infection [17–19]. Oxidative stress is an impaired homeostasis in the body between oxidants and antioxidants, which leads to further disruption of the redox system and damage to molecules. Free radicals are highly reactive molecules with an excess of one or more electrons that easily interact with other molecules and lead to disruptions in the physiologically tuned system of a healthy organism. Excessive production of free radicals: reactive oxygen species (ROS), reactive nitrogen species (RNS), and reactive chlorine species (CRS) lead to direct peroxidation of membranes, structural proteins, enzymes, and nucleic acids, and can be neutralized under physiological conditions via an interaction with enzymatic and non-enzymatic antioxidants. In addition to endogenous (enzymatic and non-enzymatic antioxidants), there is also a group of exogenous (natural or synthetic antioxidants) that also have a role in binding unpaired electrons of free radicals and stabilizing them, and their cumulative effect is defined as total antioxidant capacity (TAS) [20–23].

During scientific attempts to determine the level of oxidative stress in the body, a whole panel of biochemical markers of OS were created, which, based on their origin, were divided into:

Molecules that interact with free radicals, such as:

- Products of lipid peroxidation: malondialdehyde, acrolein, isoprostanes),
- Protein oxidation products: (carbonyl protein, tyrosine group),
- DNA oxidation products (8-hydroxy-2deoxyguanosine),
- Protein stress reactions, new biomarkers (microRNAs)

Molecules that belong to the antioxidant protection system, such as

- Enzymes (myeloperoxidase),
- Glutathione level
- Circulating antioxidants (CAT, GPX, SOD) [22,24–26]

Pregnancy itself represents a state of increased oxidative stress due to the intense metabolic and immunological alterations necessary for the complex process of growth and development of conception products. The main source of ROS in pregnancy is the placenta, where these molecules are key factors in the complex system responsible for intercellular signaling, transcription, adaptive homeostasis, apoptosis, and host defense through phagocytosis [27–30]. Viral infections affect the excitation of oxidative stress of the host through numerous mechanisms such as excessive cytokine production, activation of the complement system, release of lipid mediators, and lipid peroxidation during the interaction of the body's defense cells with viral pathogens [31,32].

Examining the changes in the placenta provides us with a unique opportunity to uncover the mechanisms by which the virus affects pregnancy and the fetus. In addition to its nutritional, excretory, oxygenation, and hormonal function, the placenta has an important protective role and is the main barrier to bacterial and viral infections in the fetus. This role predisposes the placenta to pathological changes under the direct influence of the SARS-CoV-2 virus and the consequences of systemic disease and coagulation changes. Based on the Amsterdam classification system, placental lesions could be defined as maternal vascular malperfusions, fetal vascular malperfusions, acute chorioamnionitis, and villitis of unknown etiology [33].

We hypothesized that:

1. There is a statistically significant difference in the frequency of pathohistological changes in placental tissue in patients with confirmed SARS-CoV-2 infection during pregnancy compared to the control group.
2. Vertical transmission of SARS CoV-2 from mother to fetus is possible.
3. Compared to the control group, there is a statistically significant increase in maternal and umbilical cord blood biomarkers of oxidative stress in patients infected with SARS-CoV-2 during pregnancy.
4. Patients with more pronounced pathohistological changes in placental tissue have significantly elevated levels of oxidative stress markers.
5. There is a statistically significant difference in the neonatal outcome of newborns of mothers with COVID-19 compared to the control group.
6. Certain clinical parameters such as gestational age, sex of the newborn, and maternal age significantly affect the level of oxidative stress markers in the newborn.

This study aims to:

1. To determine the types and frequency of pathohistological changes in placental tissue in patients in whom SARS-CoV-2 infection was confirmed during pregnancy and compare them with the control group
2. Determine from the plasma and lysate of erythrocytes of the mother's blood immediately before delivery and the blood of the newborn from the umbilical cord the values of the parameters of the antioxidant protection system, as well as pro-oxidants: lipid peroxide index measured as TBARS, nitric oxide in the form of nitrite ($NO_2^-$), superoxide anion radical ($O_2^-$) and hydrogen peroxide ($H_2O_2$), catalase (CAT), superoxide dismutase (SOD), reduced glutathione (GSH).
3. Determine the neonatal outcome: Apgar score, body weight of the newborn, admission to the intensive care unit, and length of stay in the neonatology department and ICU

## 2. Materials and Methods

### 2.1. Ethical Concerns

Following the Good Clinical Practice and revised Helsinki Declaration, this study was designed as a case-series clinical study. The Ethical Committee of Clinical Center Kragujevac approved the study number: 01/21-18 from 28 January 2021. Written informed consent was obtained from all participants for research and publication before inclusion in the study.

### 2.2. Participants

This prospective clinical study included pregnant women who gave birth from February 2021 to March 2022 at the at the Gynecology Clinic at University Clinical Center Kragujevac, aged between 18 and 43 years old, from Central West Serbia, followed during the period from the diagnosis of a positive SARS-CoV-2 test to discharge from the obstetrics department after delivery and discharge of the newborn from the Department of Neonatology at University Clinical Center Kragujevac, Serbia.

### 2.3. Protocol of Study

Two cohorts were derived from the population of pregnant women who were delivered at the OB/GYN Clinic of the University Clinical Center in Kragujevac: women who had a positive result for SARS-CoV-2 (by RT-PCR method and/or rapid antigen test) during the pregnancy. The control cohort were woman who had a negative result on a rapid antigen or RT-PCR SARS-CoV-2 test on their admission day to the Obstetric Clinic for delivery, who were asymptomatic during hole pregnancy, and who had no IgG and IgM

SARS-CoV-2 antibodies detected on serological blood test. The main inclusion criteria were positive RT-PCR and/or rapid antigen tests for SARS-CoV-2 during the pregnancy. Exclusion criteria were positive personal history of thromboembolic diseases, thrombophilia, antiphospholipid syndrome, diabetes mellitus, systemic lupus erythematosus, hypertensive disorders in pregnancy, Rhesus factor incompatibility, ongoing anticoagulant therapy, tobacco smoking during pregnancy, and vaccination against COVID 19. Within the cohort of pregnant women who tested positive for the presence of SARS-CoV-2 during pregnancy concerning the time of gestation in which the infection occurred, three subgroups of patients were distinguished, within whom the impact of COVID-19 on placental tissue was monitored in parallel:

1. Patients who were diagnosed with SARS-CoV-2 in the first trimester of pregnancy (from pregnancy to the end of week 13 of gestation)
2. Patients who were diagnosed with SARS-CoV-2 in the second trimester of pregnancy (from 14 to the end of week 27 of gestation)
3. Patients diagnosed with SARS-CoV-2 in the third trimester of pregnancy (28 to 42 weeks of gestation)

### 2.4. *Sampling and Collecting Data*

We reviewed the electronic medical record for each subject and recorded demographic, clinical, obstetric, laboratory, and pathological data. At that time, none of the patients in either group were vaccinated against COVID-19. Blood samples were collected from those two groups following delivery, namely: maternal peripheric blood and the umbilical cord blood for oxidative stress biomarkers testing, and placental tissue (a section of the entire thickness of the placenta with the membranes and one section of the umbilical cord for pathohistological analysis, fixed for 48 h in a formalin solution to eliminate the infectivity).

### 2.5. *Determination of Oxidative Stress Markers*

We collected venous blood from each participant, maternal peripheric blood, and umbilical cord blood for oxidative stress biomarkers testing within 3 min following delivery. Oxidative stress biomarkers were assessed spectrophotometrically from plasma samples (Shimadzu UV 1800, Tokyo, Japan), the index of lipid peroxidation, determined as thiobarbituric acid-reactive substances (TBARS), nitrites ($NO_2^-$), levels of superoxide anion radical ($O_2^-$), and hydrogen peroxide ($H_2O_2$).

#### 2.5.1. Determination of TBARS

The plasma sample was incubated with 1% thiobarbituric acid in 0.05 NaOH for 15 min at 100 °C and measured as TBARS at 530 nm. As a control, distilled water was used as a blind probe [34].

#### 2.5.2. Nitrite Determination ($NO_2^-$)

Rapidly breaking down nitric oxide (NO) produces stable nitrite/nitrate compounds determined spectrophotometrically at 543 nm using Griess's reagent according to Green's method. Sodium nitrite was used as the reference standard to calculate the nitrite levels [35].

#### 2.5.3. Superoxide Anion Radical Determination ($O_2^-$)

Superoxide anion radical quantities were determined using an assay mixture containing nitroblue tetrazolium. The measurement was carried out at 530 nm on the wavelength. The blank control was performed using distilled water [36].

2.5.4. Hydrogen Peroxide Determination ($H_2O_2$)

Horseradish peroxidase was utilized to accelerate the oxidation of phenol red by $H_2O_2$, which was used as a basis for the $H_2O_2$ measurement. 800 μL of freshly created phenol red solution was used to precipitate 200 μL of perfusate, and 10 μL of freshly made (1:20) horseradish peroxidase was added next. Distilled water was utilized as the blank probe. At 610 nm, the level of $H_2O_2$ was detected [37].

2.5.5. Catalase Activity Determination (CAT)

The analysis of catalase activity was carried out based on the Aebi method [38].

First, we diluted the hemolysate with distilled water in a ratio of 1:7. An amount of 100 μL of the hemolysate sample was then mixed with an equal volume of ethanol along with 50 μL of CAT buffer and 1000 μL of 10 mM $H_2O_2$. The catalase activity was then determined spectrophotometrically at a wavelength of 230 nm [38].

2.5.6. Superoxide Dismutase Activity Determination (SOD)

The activity of superoxide dismutase was carried out using the Beutler method. In Eppendorf, we first mixed [39] 100 μL of hemolysate with 1 mL of carbonate buffer, then processed the sample into a vortex and finally added 100 μL of adrenaline. Spectrophotometry was performed at a wavelength of 470 nm [39,40].

2.5.7. Reduced Glutathione Concentration Determination (GSH)

The concentration of reduced glutathione (GSH) was determined using the Beutler method. The method principle is based on the oxidation reaction of GSH with 5,5-dithio-bis-6,2-nitrobenzoic acid. Spectrophotometric measurements were made at a wavelength of 412 nm [39].

*2.6. Pathohistological Analysis of Placental Tissue*

Samples were also collected according to the recommendations of the Amsterdam Consensus [41]. Six samples were taken: first a sample of the amniotic sheath from the rupture site to the edge of the placenta; a sample of the cross-section of the umbilical cord, one from the fetal and the other about 5 cm from the uterine insertion; and three more sections of the full-thickness placental disc cut with a scalpel, covering the uterine and fetal sides, taken from the central two-thirds of the surface of the placenta and one from the insertion site.

Tissue processing: dehydration, rinsing, and impregnation were carried out using a tissue processor and then molded into paraffin blocks. Then, using a rotating microtome (Leica RM2135, Tokyo, Japan), we cut the tissue into samples 5 μm thick, at room temperature, which were then immersed in a water bath at a temperature of 400 °C. The cross-sections processed in this way were applied to the subject glasses (Superfrost-OT Plus microscope slides) for microscopy.

Staining Hematoxylin–Eosin Technique

To de-paraffin the tissues, it was necessary to first subject the glasses to heating to +56 °C and then to spontaneous cooling. After that, we immersed them in xylol consecutively twice for 5 min each. Once we deparaffinated the tissues, we proceeded to rehydrate the tissues by immersing the glasses in solutions with decreasing concentrations of ethyl alcohol and then evaporating them with distilled water. The next step was staining with Mayer solution (Sigma Aldrich, St. Louis, MO, USA) for 10 min, after rinsing with distilled water and staining with an alcohol solution of eosin (Sigma Aldrich, USA) for the next 2 min. A dehydration process was then carried out, which involved submerging the glass by increasing concentrations of ethyl alcohol and then illuminating it with two xylol solutions, each for 5 min [42]. The tiles prepared in this way were then protected by cover glass after treatment with a medium covering and dried at room temperature. The analysis was carried out independently by two experienced pathologists on an Olympus BX51 light microscope, Tokyo, Japan. In the case of inconsistent results, the attitude of the third pathologist was decisive.

### 2.7. Statistical Analysis

All data are presented in the form of tables and graphs. Statistical analysis was done using the descriptive (mean, standard deviations and errors, and analytical tests, frequency, range) and analytical tests (Student *t*-test, Chi-square test). The statistical threshold was set at 0.05. All analysis was done in SPSS version 26 for Apple. Inc. (Cupertino, CA, USA).

## 3. Results

### 3.1. Basic Demographic and Anamnestic Data of Study Group

This study included 50 pregnant women divided into two groups, SARS-CoV-2 positive (COVID-19 group) and SARS-CoV-2 negative (control group). In the first group, the mean age was 30.61 ± 4.72, and in the negative groups, the mean age was 31.41 ± 4.65. The mean gestational week at delivery was 39.19 ± 0.98 in SARS-CoV-2 positive women, and 39.42 ± 1.26 in the group SARS-CoV-2 negative. Based on the severity of symptoms 41.38% of patients had mild symptoms, and 58.62% had moderate symptoms.

### 3.2. Characteristics of the Newborns at Delivery According to the Presence of SARS-CoV-2 Infection in Mothers

Table 1 presents the mean values of the newborn characteristics at delivery. Most of them were similar in both groups, except for the concentrations of IgM antibody, where we found that newborns from the COVID group of mothers had significantly higher levels of these inflammatory markers in comparison with the SARS-CoV-2 negative group (as shown in Table 1).

**Table 1.** The mean values of the parameters related to the newborn at delivery according to the presence of SARS-CoV-2 infection. Results are presented as mean plus standard deviations. Statistical analysis was done using the Student *t* test.

| Parameters | | Gestational Age in Weeks at Delivery | APGAR Score 1′ | APGAR Score 5′ | Baby Body Weight (g) | Baby Body Length (cm) | Head Circumference (cm) | IgM Antibody (g/L) | Placenta Weight (g) |
|---|---|---|---|---|---|---|---|---|---|
| SARS-CoV-2+ | Mean | 39.19 | 8.96 | 9.10 | 3359.17 | 48.75 | 34.38 | 3.42 | 608.26 |
| | SD | 0.98 | 0.62 | 0.62 | 491.69 | 2.25 | 1.58 | 3.25 | 129.81 |
| SARS-CoV-2− | Mean | 39.42 | 9.23 | 9.19 | 3534.09 | 50.27 | 35.23 | 0.30 | 577.37 |
| | SD | 1.26 | 0.61 | 0.60 | 404.35 | 2.12 | 1.38 | 0.27 | 143.37 |
| *p* value | | $p = 0.676$ | $p = 0.556$ | $p = 0.780$ | $p = 0.465$ | $p = 0.681$ | $p = 0.899$ | $p = 0.000$ * | $p = 0.322$ |

A symbol asterisk (*) represents the *p* values less than 0.05.

### 3.3. Analysis of the Oxidative Stress Levels According to the Presence of SARS-CoV-2 Infection

According to the presence of the SARS-CoV-2 infection, the mean values of redox status parameters are presented in the form of Figures 1a–d and 2a–c. The values of the superoxide anion radical and index of lipid peroxidation were significantly different in mothers concerning the presence of the SARS-CoV-2 infection, while the levels of the nitric oxide, index of lipid peroxidation, reduced glutathione, and superoxide dismutase were significantly different in the newborns depending on the SARS-CoV-2 infection (Figures 1 and 2, Table 2). Other parameters were not significantly changed (Figures 1 and 2, Table 2).

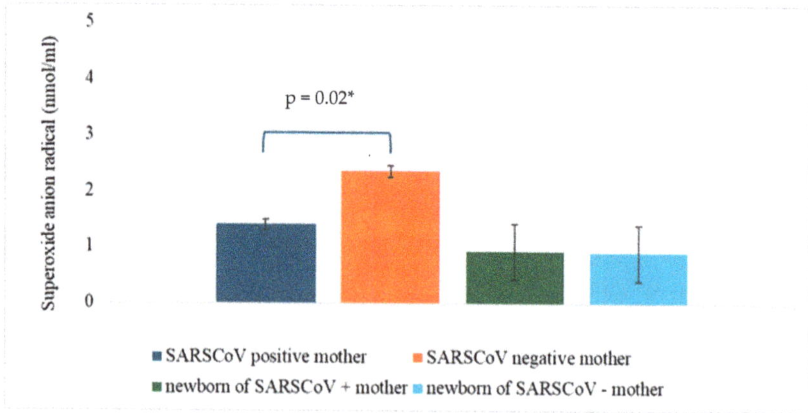


(a)

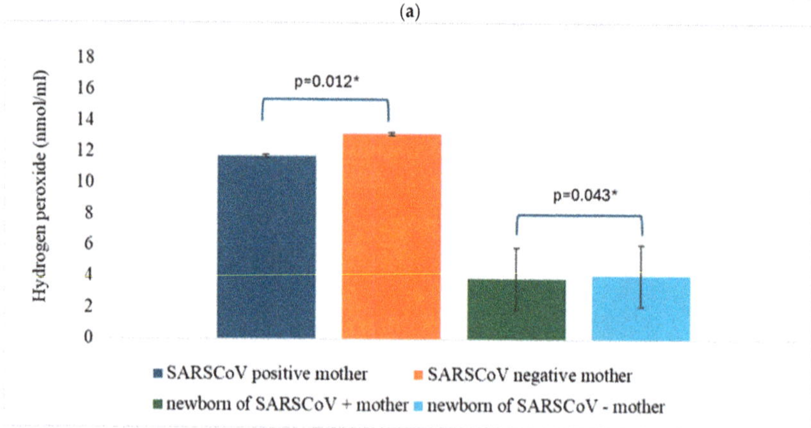


(b)

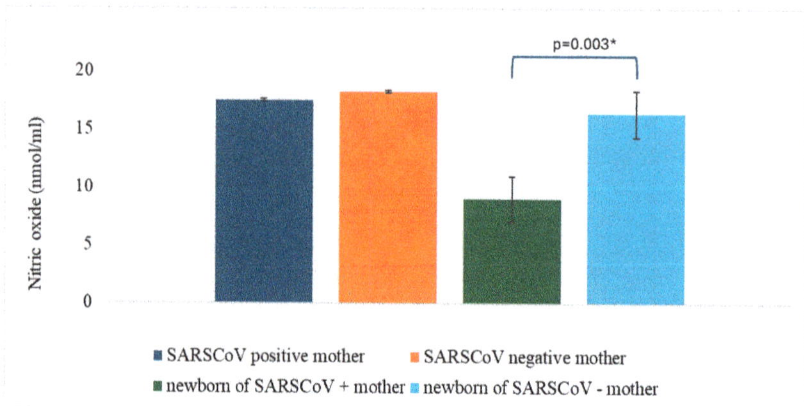


(c)

**Figure 1.** *Cont.*

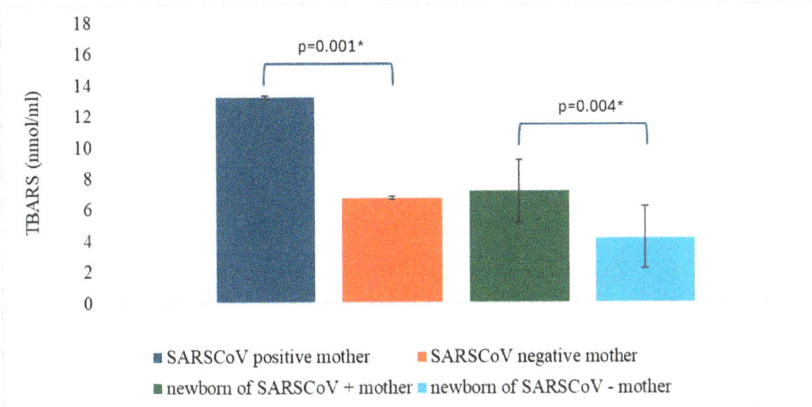


(d)

**Figure 1.** (**a**) The mean concentration of the plasma superoxide anion radical ($O_2^-$). Results are presented as the mean plus standard deviations. Statistical analysis was done using the Student *t* test. The asterisk (*) represents the statistically significant value ($p < 0.05$). (**b**) The mean concentration of the plasma hydrogen peroxide ($H_2O_2^-$). Results are presented as mean plus standard deviations. Statistical analysis was done using the student *t* test. The asterisk (*) represents the statistically significant value ($p < 0.05$). (**c**) The mean concentration of the plasma nitric oxide ($NO^-$). Results are presented as mean plus standard deviations. Statistical analysis was done using the Student *t* test. The asterisk (*) represents the statistically significant value ($p < 0.05$). (**d**) The mean concentration of the plasma index of lipid peroxidation (TBARS). Results are presented as mean plus standard deviations. Statistical analysis was done using the Student *t* test. The asterisk (*) represents the statistically significant value ($p < 0.05$).

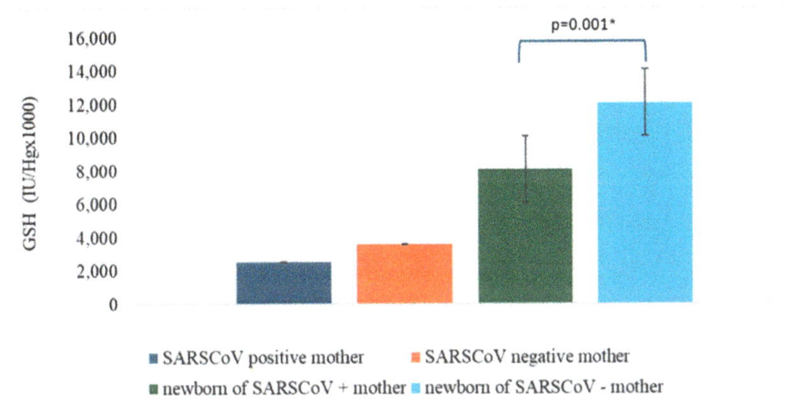


(a)

**Figure 2.** *Cont.*

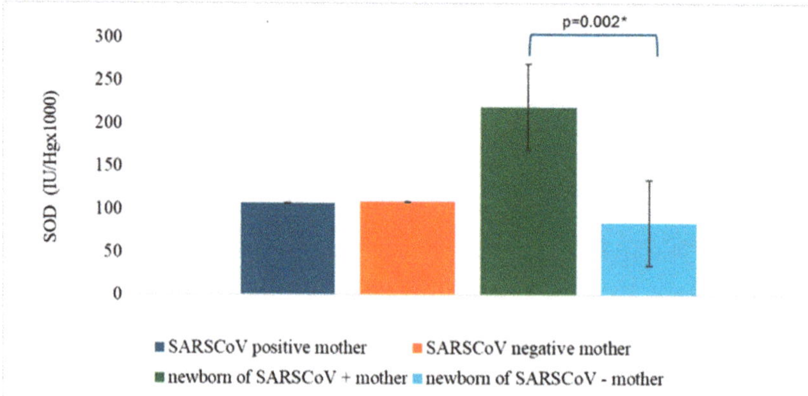


(**b**)

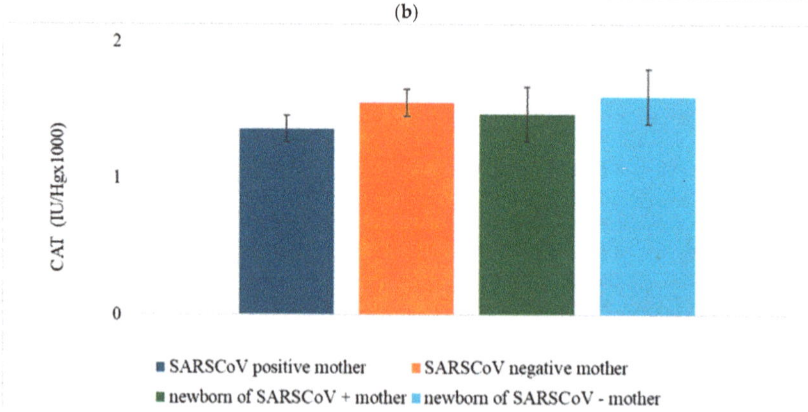


(**c**)

**Figure 2.** (**a**) The mean activity of the hemolysate reduced glutathione (GSH). Results are presented as the mean plus standard deviations. Statistical analysis was done using the Student $t$ test. Asterisk (*) represents the statistically significant value ($p < 0.05$). (**b**) The mean activity of the hemolysate superoxide dismutase (SOD). Results are presented as mean plus standard deviations. Statistical analysis was done using the Student $t$ test. Asterisk (*) represents the statistically significant value ($p < 0.05$). (**c**) The mean activity of the hemolysate catalase (CAT). Results are presented as mean plus standard deviations. Statistical analysis was done using the Student $t$ test.

**Table 2.** Data from statistical analysis using the Student T test in comparison with two groups of concentrations of pro-oxidative markers antioxidative enzymes. Asterisk (*) represents the statistically significant value ($p < 0.05$).

| Comparison | Mothers | Newborns |
|---|---|---|
| | **SARS-CoV-2+ vs. SARS-CoV-2−** | **SARS-CoV-2+ vs. SARS-CoV-2−** |
| $O_2^-$ | $p = 0.002$ * | $p = 0.113$ |
| $H_2O_2$ | $p = 0.012$ * | $p = 0.043$ * |
| $NO^-$ | $p = 0.509$ | $p = 0.003$ * |
| TBARS | $p = 0.001$ * | $p = 0.004$ * |
| GSH | $p = 0.322$ | $p = 0.001$ * |
| SOD | $p = 0.488$ | $p = 0.002$ * |
| CAT | $p = 0.566$ | $p = 0.623$ |

### 3.4. The Histopathologic Lesions in the Placenta Concerning the Presence of SARS-CoV-2 Infection and the Timing of Infection

The incidence of pathohistological changes of the FVM type in the COVID-19 group of pregnant women was 46%. In contrast, in the control group, they were represented in 18% of placentas, and the incidence of MVM in the COVID group was 32%, and in the experimental group, this was 18%. According to the moment of infection in the first trimester, pathohistological changes were registered in only 3% of patients infected in the first trimester. In contrast, they were more prevalent when the infection occurred during the second and third trimesters in 44.4% and 47% of patients in the COVID group. Inflammatory lesions in placental tissue were detected in 14.81% of placentas in the COVID group and only 4.5% of subjects in the control group. A total of 70% of all placental lesions were detected in patients with a moderate/severe presentation of COVID-19. Table 3 presents mothers' main morphometrical placental characteristics regarding the presence of COVID-19. The results are presented as the frequency of the observed entity as a percentage (%) (Table 3).

### 3.5. Neonatal Outcome

In the COVID-19 group, 62% of newborns were girls, 38% were boys, and in the control group, 41% were girls and 59% were boys.

The mode of delivery was vaginal birth in 68%, and C-section in 32% in the COVID-19 group, and vaginal birth in 45%, and C-section in 55% in the control group. Newborns of mothers from the COVID group had a similar mid-length of hospitalization—4.37 $\pm$ 1.1 days—as newborns from the control group, who had a mid-length of hospitalization 4.22 $\pm$ 2.72 days.

The length of newborn stay in the neonatal ICU was 3.51 $\pm$ 1.08 days in the COVID group and 2.22 $\pm$ 1.39 days in the control group. Using a t-test for two independent samples we noticed a significant difference in the length of hospitalization in the NICU between the two groups ($p \leq 0.0006$).

Newborns from COVID-positive mothers were tested with nasopharyngeal swabs for RT-PCR SARS-CoV-2 test in the first 24 h post-delivery. Only one positive result was registered in newborns.). A total of 42.8% of newborns from the COVID group mothers had positive SARS-CoV-2 IgM antibody results, and in the control group there were no positive SARS-CoV-2 IgM antibody results.

**Table 3.** Morphometrical Placental characteristics of mothers regarding the presence of COVID-19. Results are presented as the frequency of the observed entity in percentage (%).

| Placental Characteristics | Thrombosis | Avascular Villi | Deposits of Fibrines | Villous Stromal Vascular Karyorrhexis | Obliteration of Blood Vessels | Vascular Ectasia | Delayed Villous Maturation | Placental Infarction | Retroplacental Hemorrhage | Hypoplasia of Distal Villus | Accelerated Villous Maturation | Decidual Arteriopathy | Inflammatory Changes |
|---|---|---|---|---|---|---|---|---|---|---|---|---|---|
| COVID-19 participants | + [6/28] [21.4%] | ++ [9/28] [32.1%] | + [1/28] [3.57%] | [0/28] [0%] | +++ [12/28] [42.8%] | ++ [8/28] [28.5%] | [0/28] [0%] | + [3/28] [10.7%] | ++ [7/28] [25%] | + [2/28 [7.14%] | ++ [8/28] [28.5%] | [0/28] [0%] | + [4/28] [14.3%] |
| Non-COVID-19 participants | + [1/22] [4.54%] | + [1/22] [4.54%] | [0/22] [0%] | [0/22] [0%] | + [1/22] [4.54%] | - [0/22] [0%] | + [1/22] [4.54%] | [0/22] [0%] | - [0/22] [0%] | [0/22] [0%] | ++ [4/22] [18.1%] | [0/22] [0%] | [0/22] [0%] |

+ = presence of entity in 10%. ++ = presence of entity in 25%. +++ = presence of an entity in 40% and more.

## 4. Discussion

This prospective clinical study aimed to analyze the differences between basic, clinical, anamnestic, and biochemical data among pregnant women who were affected by COVID-19 or not affected. The special purpose of this research lies in the evaluation of the effects of the SARS-CoV-2 infection on fetal and newborn characteristics. Based on previous findings and literature data, for the first time, this study evaluated the pathohistological changes in placental tissue among COVID-19 women who gave birth.

In the COVID group predominant mode of delivery was vaginal birth, except in a group of pregnant women with active COVID infection during delivery. Although the C-section birth rate was high (32%) it was significantly lower than previous studies showed [43–45]. The leading indications for C-section in the COVID group were previous delivery completed by C-section, fetal distress during labor, and malpresentation, similar to the control group. Our study showed that there was no statistically significant increase in the number of cesarean sections in patients with COVID-19 during pregnancy. Studies dealing with this issue had contradictory results, and some investigators have shown an increased risk of operative termination of labor in COVID-19 patients [46–48], but others have shown that the mode of delivery does not depend on COVID-19 infection in pregnancy [49].

No significant differences in neonatal outcomes were found between COVID-19 and the control group regarding birth weight, length, and head circumference. Some similar studies showed associations between COVID-19 symptoms and birth weight, the risk of prematurity, and ventilation in the early neonatal period [50]. The hospitalization length for newborns was similar in both groups. No significant decrease in hospitalizations was noted in our study, despite expectations because of the suspension of elective admissions, similarly as Gaetano's study has shown [51].

Neonatal ICU hospitalization length was $3.51 \pm 1.08$ days in the COVID group and $2.22 \pm 1.39$ days in the control group. Our findings support expert recommendations about the necessity of multidisciplinary teams available in hospitals that take care of COVID-19-positive and suspected mothers and their infants [52]. Additionally, a neonatal intensive care unit is mandatory for hospitals that take care of the delivery of those patients, and there is no clear evidence about possible direct transmission of SARS-CoV-2 from mother to infant.

Pregnancy and placental growth and development are accompanied by numerous changes due to the balance of the ROS and the antioxidant protection system, which is also involved in the complex mechanisms of cell signaling. The development of the placenta begins with the insertion of a fertilized blastocyst and the primary mode of transport through the placenta is diffusion conditions of low partial pressure of $O_2$, which is necessary for the normal growth and development of the embryo and the prevention of the formation of ROS [53]. As pregnancy progresses from the periphery of the placenta to the center, there is a gradual opening of the occluding blood vessels and a gradual increase in the partial pressure of oxygen within the intervillous space due to the continuous flow of oxygenated blood. This process takes place at the end of the first trimester and is responsible for the shift in the partial pressure of oxygen in the intervillous space [54]. When there is a disturbance at any level of placentation, the result is a sudden increase in oxygen pressure within the intervillous space and the consequent formation of ROS [55]. A gradual increase in $O_2$ pressure allows the placenta to adapt to the new conditions of ROS formation by developing an antioxidant protection system (primarily by producing GPx and CAT) [56]. To counteract the effect of ROS ($O_2^-$, NO, $H_2O_2$, $ONOO^-$) in the cells of the cytotrophoblast and stroma, a protection system is developed that includes the enzymes MnSOD, CuSOD, ZnSOD. However, when the level of ROS production exceeds the antioxidative capacity of the placenta, protein, lipids, and DNA damage occurs with consecutive cell damage and death [53,56].

The determination of individual biomarkers of oxidative stress in placental pathology has no scientific or clinical significance, but a comparative examination at birth showed a positive correlation between elevated values of OS biomarkers in the mother's blood and blood from the umbilical cord of the newborn [57]. Placental ischemia, resulting from SARS-CoV-2 infection, or systemic hypoxia and inflammation, leads to a disturbance in the balance of ROS and antioxidant protection and the onset of oxidative stress. OS is responsible for damage to proteins, lipids, and DNA. The placenta has mechanisms to counteract oxidative stress to reduce tissue damage, such as the production of NO, a potent vasodilator and antioxidant [58].

Our study showed that levels of TBARS were significantly increased in mothers of the COVID-19 group ($p = 0.002$) compared with mothers of the control group, possibly because of lipid membrane damage caused by the SARS-CoV-2 virus. $O_2^-$ levels were significantly higher in mothers from a control group and $H_2O_2$ levels were significantly higher in mothers and neonates from a control group, which corresponds with the mode of delivery. SC was more frequent in the control group 55% and 32% in the COVID-19 group. The method of delivery could significantly affect the elevated level of biomarkers OS in the newborn, where these values are significantly increased in prolonged vaginal delivery and emergency cesarean section, as well as in stimulated oxytocin delivery. [20,59–61]. Additionally, the leading indication for C-section in the control group was non-reassuring fetal status and previous C-section.

Levels of NO were significantly lower in newborns of the COVID-19 group in our study, indicating that the placentas of COVID mothers could not sufficiently counterbalance the production of ROS after and during SARS-CoV-2 infection. Increased levels of SOD in COVID-19 group newborns suggested that the placenta developed an enzymatic oxidative damage defense system.

The effect of the oxidative stress of the mother on the oxidative stress of the fetus depends on the antioxidant capacity of the newborn, which is determined genetically, depending on the sex of the fetus, the maturity of the fetus, and the age of the mother [20].

Studies focused on the effect of oxidative stress on placental tissue depending on the timing of infection in pregnancy have shown that changes within the scinciotroblast dominate the first trimester compared to the cytotrophoblast. This is reflected in a decrease in the surface area of microvilli and a decrease in mitochondria, with a very low amount of antioxidants detected [62]. A factor responsible for the onset of oxidative stress during the second and third trimesters is the intermittent flow of maternal blood within the villus, which produces ischemic reperfusion damage [63]

Some studies have proposed that the determination of different types of OS biomarkers from the umbilical cord, placenta, and maternal blood could have implications in the prediction of placental pathology and clinical symptomatology [58,64]. Our study showed that TBARS could have clinical implications in identifying high-risk COVID-19 pregnancies requiring closer monitoring and neonatal care with pediatric follow-ups watching neonatal development. Other OS biomarkers in our study were more dependent on the mode of delivery and placental ability to counterbalance the oxidative stress.

Besides oxidative stress damage, a potential pregnancy hazard is the transmission of the virus to the fetus. There are a few possible maternal/fetal (neonatal) infection methods. Fetal infection can occur in utero by direct transplacental transmission. The other possible way is intrapartum infection (neonatal contact with cervical or vaginal secretions or blood), and the third way is after birth via breastfeeding or direct maternal-neonatal contact [65]. All patients with active COVID newborns were tested with a SARS-CoV-2 RT PCR test, only one was positive. Our study found that 42.8% of newborns from the COVID group mothers had positive IgM antibody findings. A similar study performed by Maranto showed IgM positive in 2.4% of newborns [50]. Initial studies focused on direct transmission showed that there was no convincing evidence of this mode of infection; however, at the end of the pandemic, worldwide pandemic meta-analyses showed that about 8.8% of newborns of COVID-19-positive mothers at birth had a positive SARS-CoV-2 PCR or serological test obtained after taking a nasopharyngeal swab [66,67]. The method of determining direct transmission to the fetus is also a subject of scientific doubt. In adults, the respiratory tract is the primary site of infection and the highest concentration of the virus, and the analysis of samples is performed through a nasopharyngeal or oropharyngeal swab. In a newborn, in addition to this method, it is proposed to do the serological determination of the concentration of specific IgM antibodies to SARS-CoV-2, concerning the unknown site of primary infection [68,69]. IgM antibodies as part of the immune response to a specific viral infection, unlike IgG antibodies, cannot cross the placental barrier and can be useful in determining potential direct transmission to the fetus, but the weakness of this method is the existence of a cross-reaction and a false positive result, and the PCR test of the nasopharyngeal/oropharyngeal mucosa is the gold standard for determining the presence of SARS-CoV-2 infection in the newborns [70]. Studies focused on direct transmission have also used RNA Scope and in-situ hybridization in scinciciotrophoblast cells, but the main problem with interpreting the results is the inconsistency of the results of the available tests. The sensitivity of the RT-PCR test is highest from the bronchial lavage sample (93%), and significantly lower from the nasopharyngeal swab and feces (63% and 29%, respectively), but as it is invasive, this method is not suitable for testing pregnant women and newborns [71].

Investigating routes of possible fetal or neonatal transmission should provide sufficient information for future decisions considering the obstetric way of delivery, neonatal care, isolation of neonates, or safety of breastfeeding [72].

During this interaction of viruses and the host, if the overproduction of ROS exceeds the antioxidant capacity of the placenta, tissue damage may occur [31,73]. Maternal vascular malperfusions (MVM) were the most frequent finding of some studies, while others have reported fetal vascular malperfusions (FVM) as a predominant finding, diagnosed according to the Amsterdam criteria based, on the side of the placenta on which they occurred [45,74–77]. (FVM) Fetal vascular malperfusions are specific lesions of the placenta that arise from the obstruction of fetal blood flow. They can originate from the umbilical cord (hyperkoyling of the umbilical cord), from hypercoagulability, hypoxia, and inflammation-mediated endothelial damage (acute chorioamnionitis with chorionic vasculitis or funisitis and chronic villitis) [78–82].

According to the Amsterdam criterion, FVM is represented by the following findings: thrombosis, segmental avascular villi, villous stromal-vascular karyorexa, vascular intramural fibrin deposition, blood vessel obliteration/fibromuscular sclerosis and vascular ectasia [79]. MVM encompasses a spectrum of macroscopic and microscopic changes in the placenta. These changes are the result of ischemic (hypoxic) damage and oxidative stress [83]. Macroscopic changes are placental hypoplasia (weight < 10th percentile), narrowed umbilical cord (diameter less than 0.8 cm at term), infarction, and retroplacental hemorrhage [41,79,84]. Microscopic lesions of the placenta include distal villi hypoplasia and accelerated villi maturation [41,79,84].

In addition to vascular changes, some studies have also proven the presence of inflammatory histopathological changes within the placentas of patients infected with COVID. Chronic villitis can be a consequence of viral infections, but in most cases, the etiology has not been identified [85]. Several studies have examined macroscopic and microscopic histopathological changes within the placental tissue in patients infected during pregnancy, but the results are incoherent [86–92]. Some studies even demonstrated no specific placental pathological findings in COVID patients regardless of the timing or severity of the disease [93,94]. The weaknesses of these studies are represented by the small number of samples, the inconsistency in the classification of histopathological changes, confounding factors such as chronic diseases in pregnancy and lifestyle habits that can have a significant impact on the result, as well as the choice of the control group.

Our study showed that placental pathology findings differ significantly between COVID-19 and the control group. We have found MVM lesions in 32% of the placentas of the COVID group and 18% of patients in the control group (Figure 3a,b). FVM lesions were present in 46% of the placentas of patients in the COVID group and 18% of patients in the control group (Figure 3c–e). Previous studies showed unequivocal results of placental findings, some demonstrated FVM in 30% and the other only 8% of placentas examined [76,95]. The most frequent findings in placental pathology of COVID patients in our study were: the obliteration of blood vessels, avascular villi, retroplacental hemorrhage, and accelerated villus maturation. Other studies' most frequent pathophysiological findings were fibrin deposition, microcalcification, thrombus (Figure 3d), avascular villi (Figure 3e), infraction, and villous edema (Figure 3f) [96].

Previous observational studies dealing with the problem of MVM have shown that these changes were asymptomatic, but the cumulative effect was reflected in placental hypoperfusion leading to adverse perinatal outcome and fetal complications and is associated with preeclampsia and intrauterine growth retardation (IUGR) [97–100]. IUGR is a fetus that does not reach its genetic potential during intrauterine growth and development and is present in as many as 15% of pregnancies [101].

FVM lesions are associated with abnormalities of the neonatal central nervous system, IUGR, fetal cardiac abnormalities, intrauterine fetal death, and stillbirth [65,74,82,102].

Impaired placental function is responsible for short and long-term adverse outcomes for the child and mother. Short-term consequences require urgent intervention in the antepartum or peripartum period. Placental pathologic lesions could be a valuable clue in discovering long-term consequences that require special attention [103]. However, pathological reports of placental tissue should be available not only to obstetricians but more importantly to pediatricians who should be aware of potential risks for a child's long-term developmental consequences [104].

Besides the evident difference in the frequency of placental lesions between SARS-CoV-2 and the control group in our study, there was no evidence of a significant difference in fetal and neonatal outcomes except in the newborns' length of stay in the NICU. There is evidence that fetuses exposed to SARS-CoV-2 influence intrauterine have a tenfold increased risk for neurodevelopmental delay [105], so further follow-up should be warranted for those neonates. Neurodevelopmental disorders are not easily recognizable so an adequate timeframe should be set to follow development through early childhood, preschool, and school-age [103]. Given that the growth and development of the placenta is a dynamic process controlled by genetics and immunology, the moment when COVID-19 infection occurs during pregnancy can be an important factor in histopathological changes and maternal and fetal outcomes. Some studies showed that the timing of infection is crucial for developing pathophysiological placental lesions [74].

Genetic abnormalities are associated with placental lesions and no favorable neonatal outcome, so future studies should take into consideration the performance of non-invasive prenatal diagnosis tests as a reliable alternative to invasive methods in reviling genetic abnormalities in participants' offspring [106].

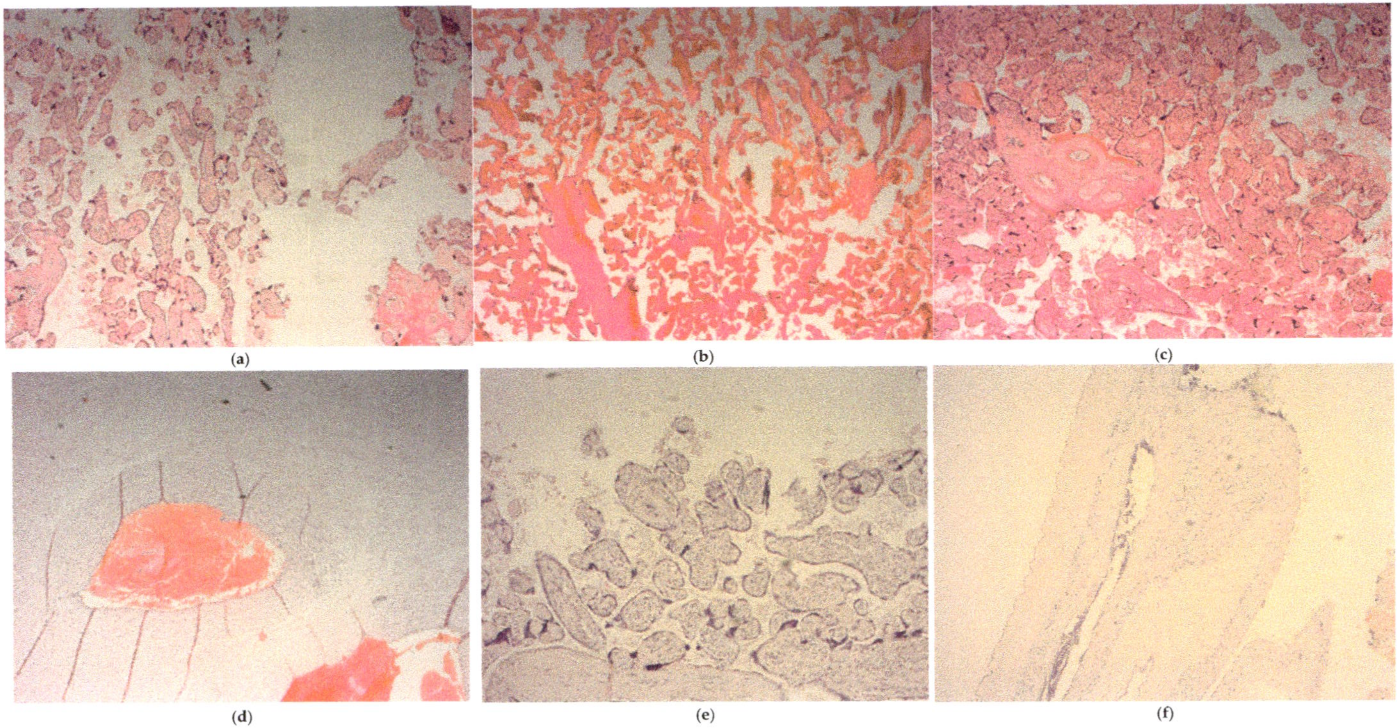


**Figure 3.** The representative pathohistological findings in placental tissue samples among the study population; (**a**,**b**) distal villous hypoplasia-long villi with a wide intervillous space; (**c**) the vascular ectasia-enlarged luminal diameter of the chorionic vessel; (**d**) villus vessel thrombosis-organized intraluminal thrombus; (**e**) avascular villus-lose of vessels with preservation of trophoblast; (**f**) chorioamnionitis-numerous polymorphonuclear leukocytes infiltrate edematous fetal membranes; magnification 100×.

At the beginning of our study, COVID-19 vaccines were not available in our county, and during the study when vaccination started there were no clear recommendations for vaccination during pregnancy. Serbian Government Health Department recommended vaccination during pregnancy in March 2022 when the collection of material for our study was completed. They recommended the vaccination of all women of fertility age without the need to postpone pregnancy and vaccination during the whole period of pregnancy with the Pfizer-BioNTech vaccine [107] Even then, there was a low vaccine acceptance in the population of pregnant women in Serbia. Vaccination acceptance is dependable on the patient's education level, perception of barriers to vaccines, but also gynecologist advice [108], so future studies should provide more adequate information for doctors and patients.

Future studies should consider the vaccinal status against SARS-CoV-2, and the possible influence of vaccines on placental changes and neonatal and maternal outcomes. Future studies should also determine the variant of the SARS-CoV-2 virus because some studies showed differences in fetal and maternal outcomes depending on the presence of variant Alpha, Delta, or Omicron [109].

Besides potential pregnancy hazards originating from placental pathological lesions and increased oxidative stress, there is also increased psychological stress influencing the mental health of pregnant women during the COVID-19 pandemic. The increased number of suicides and self-harming was noticed during the pandemic [13] Some studies showed a relationship between neuroticism and a fear of COVID-19, and neuroticism is also a predictor of depression [110]. Patients from this group of high-risk pregnant require continuous psychological support during this delicate lifetime moment that should even extend beyond childbirth [111].

Our study's limitations include the small number of participants and the fact that it was unblinded for pathologists, so there is potential bias.

## 5. Conclusions

Based on the previous observation, in the summary we can conclude the following issues:

1. The types and frequency of pathohistological changes in placental tissue in patients with SARS-CoV-2 confirmed infection during pregnancy differs from the control group. FVM is found to be the most frequent placental lesion in the COVID-19 group. Additionally, there were no significant differences noticed in neonatal outcomes, and delayed consequences are possible for those neonates, so more frequent follow-ups should be warranted for children whose mothers were SARS-CoV positive during pregnancy.
2. Neonates of SARS-CoV-2 mothers had a longer NICU hospitalization length, so the approach to those high-risk pregnancies should be multidisciplinary with mandatory NICU in hospitals that provide medical care and delivery for SARS-CoV-2 positive patients.
3. Values of the parameters of the antioxidant protection system, as well as pro-oxidants: (lipid peroxide index measured as TBARS, nitric oxide in the form of nitrite ($NO_2^-$), superoxide anion radical ($O_2^-$), hydrogen peroxide $H_2O_2$, superoxide dismutase (SOD), reduced glutathione (GSH)) significantly differed between the COVID-19 and control group samples. T-BARS is a valuable biomarker of possible SARS-CoV-2 placental damage. It could help to identify high-risk COVID-19 pregnancies that require special attention regarding delivery and neonatal care.
4. Other OS biomarkers in our study were more dependent on the mode of delivery and placental ability to counterbalance oxidative stress.

5. Neonatal outcome: Apgar score and body weight of the newborn did not differ significantly between newborns from mothers of COVID-19 and the control group. COVID-19 patients do not have higher obstetrics potential for a C-section or instrumental delivery.
6. Placental pathology reports should be available to pediatricians because they could be valuable in identifying neonates with a risk for long-term developmental consequences.

COVID-19 pregnancies exhibited an increase in histopathological abnormalities of the placenta, namely vascular and inflammatory changes of unknown etiology, as well as disturbing the redox status of mothers and newborns. Future studies investigating the specific influence of SARS-CoV-2 on placental tissue and newborn outcomes are needed, with more participants considering the vaccinal status of the patient, variant of SARS-CoV-2, with longer follow-ups for newborns, following neonatal and child development through early childhood, preschool, and school age.

**Author Contributions:** Conceptualization, M.B.I. and A.D.; methodology N.J. (Nevena Jeremic); software, B.P. and I.I.; validation, G.B., N.A. and J.J.J.; formal analysis, A.N.; investigation, K.M., S.M. (Slobodanka Mitrovic); M.S., S.M. (Srdjan Mujkovic) and J.S. resources, N.A.; data curation, D.R.; writing—original draft preparation, M.B.I.; writing—review and editing, T.N.T.; visualization, T.N.T.; supervision, A.N.; project administration, N.J. (Nikola Jovic); funding acquisition, A.D. All authors have read and agreed to the published version of the manuscript.

**Funding:** This research was funded by the Faculty of Medical Sciences, University of Kragujevac, Junior Project, grant number 13/21.

**Institutional Review Board Statement:** This study was designed as a case-series clinical study following the Good Clinical Practice and revised Helsinki Declaration. This study was approved by the Ethical Committee of University Clinical Center Kragujevac number: 01/21-18, approval date: 28 January 2021.

**Informed Consent Statement:** Written informed consent has been obtained from the patient(s) to publish this paper.

**Data Availability Statement:** All data is available at the request of the corresponding author.

**Conflicts of Interest:** The authors declare no conflicts of interest.

## Abbreviations

The following abbreviations are used in this manuscript:

| | |
|---|---|
| COVID-19 | Coronavirus disease 2019 |
| NICU | Neonatal Intensive care unit |
| SARS-CoV-2 | Severe Acute Respiratory Syndrome Coronavirus 2 |
| FVM | Fetal Vascular Malperfusion |
| MVM | Maternal Vascular Malperfusion |
| VTR | Venous Thrombosis |
| ROS | Reactive Oxygen Species |
| RNS | Reactive Nitric Species |
| CRS | Chlorine Reactive Species |
| TAS | Total Antioxidative Status |
| CAT | Catalase |
| GPX | Glutathione peroxidase |
| SOD | Superoxide dismutase |
| IUGR | Intrauterine Grow Restriction |
| TBARS | Thiobarbituric acid Reactive Substances |
| GSH | Glutathione |
| RT-PCR | Reverse Transcription Polymerase Chain Reaction |

## References


1. Zhu, Y.; Sharma, L.; Chang, D. Pathophysiology and clinical management of coronavirus disease (COVID-19): A mini-review. *Front. Immunol.* **2023**, *14*, 1116131. [CrossRef]
2. World Health Organization 2023 data.who.int, WHO Coronavirus (COVID-19) Dashboard > Cases [Dashboard]. Available online: https://data.who.int/dashboards/covid19/cases (accessed on 16 September 2024).
3. Macáková, K.; Pšenková, P.; Šupčíková, N.; Vlková, B.; Celec, P.; Záhumenský, J. Effect of SARS-CoV-2 Infection and COVID-19 Vaccination on Oxidative Status of Human Placenta: A Preliminary Study. *Antioxidants* **2023**, *12*, 1403. [CrossRef]
4. CCDC Weekly. Protocol for Prevention and Control of COVID-19 (Edition 6). *China CDC Wkly* **2020**, *2*, 321–326. [CrossRef] [PubMed]
5. Asselah, T.; Durantel, D.; Pasmant, E.; Lau, G.; Schinazi, R.F. COVID-19: Discovery, diagnostics and drug development. *J. Hepatol.* **2021**, *74*, 168–184. [CrossRef]
6. Zhang, Z.; Nomura, N.; Muramoto, Y.; Ekimoto, T.; Uemura, T.; Liu, K.; Yui, M.; Kono, N.; Aoki, J.; Ikeguchi, M.; et al. Structure of SARS-CoV-2 membrane protein essential for virus assembly. *Nat. Commun.* **2022**, *13*, 1–12. [CrossRef] [PubMed]
7. D'souza, R.; Malhamé, I.; Teshler, L.; Acharya, G.; Hunt, B.J.; McLintock, C. A critical review of the pathophysiology of thrombotic complications and clinical practice recommendations for thromboprophylaxis in pregnant patients with COVID-19. *Acta Obstet. Gynecol. Scand.* **2020**, *99*, 1110–1120. [CrossRef] [PubMed]
8. Xiong, T.-Y.; Redwood, S.; Prendergast, B.; Chen, M. Coronaviruses and the cardiovascular system: Acute and long-term implications. *Eur. Hear. J.* **2020**, *41*, 1798–1800. [CrossRef]
9. Chan, J.F.-W.; To, K.K.-W.; Tse, H.; Jin, D.Y.; Yuen, K.Y. Interspecies transmission and emergence of novel viruses: Lessons from bats and birds. *Trends Microbiol.* **2013**, *21*, 544–555. [CrossRef]
10. Zu, Z.Y.; Di Jiang, M.; Xu, P.P.; Chen, W.; Ni, Q.Q.; Lu, G.M.; Zhang, L.J. Coronavirus Disease 2019 (COVID-19): A Perspective from China. *Radiology* **2020**, *296*, E15–E25. [CrossRef] [PubMed]
11. Gullo, G.; Lopez, A.; Loreto, C.; Cucinella, G.; La Verde, M.; Andrisani, A.; Burgio, S.; Carotenuto, R.; Ganduscio, S.; Baglio, G.; et al. COVID-19 and Female Fertility: An Observational Prospective Multicenter Cohort Study: Upholding Reproductive Rights in Emergency Circumstances. *Diagnostics* **2024**, *14*, 2118. [CrossRef] [PubMed]
12. Bende, M.; Gredmark, T. Nasal Stuffiness During Pregnancy. *Laryngoscope* **1999**, *109*, 1108–1110. [CrossRef] [PubMed]
13. Wastnedge, E.A.N.; Reynolds, R.M.; van Boeckel, S.R.; Stock, S.J.; Denison, F.C.; Maybin, J.A.; Critchley, H.O.D. Pregnancy and COVID-19. *Physiol Rev.* **2021**, *101*, 303–318. [CrossRef]
14. Di Mascio, D.; Khalil, A.; Saccone, G.; Rizzo, G.; Buca, D.; Liberati, M.; Vecchiet, J.; Nappi, L.; Scambia, G.; Berghella, V.; et al. Outcome of coronavirus spectrum infections (SARS, MERS, COVID-19) during pregnancy: A systematic review and meta-analysis. *Am. J. Obstet. Gynecol. MFM* **2020**, *2*, 100107. [CrossRef] [PubMed]
15. Gullo, G.; Scaglione, M.; Cucinella, G.; Riva, A.; Coldebella, D.; Cavaliere, A.F.; Signore, F.; Buzzaccarini, G.; Spagnol, G.; Laganà, A.S.; et al. Congenital Zika Syndrome: Genetic Avenues for Diagnosis and Therapy, Possible Management and Long-Term Outcomes. *J. Clin. Med.* **2022**, *11*, 1351. [CrossRef]
16. Narang, K.; Enninga, E.A.L.; Gunaratne, M.D.S.K.; Ibirogba, E.R.; Trad, A.T.A.; Elrefaei, A.; Theiler, R.N.; Ruano, R.; Szymanski, L.M.; Chakraborty, R.; et al. SARS-CoV-2 Infection and COVID-19 During Pregnancy: A Multidisciplinary Review. *Mayo Clin. Proc.* **2020**, *95*, 1750–1765. [CrossRef] [PubMed]
17. Sies, H.; Berndt, C.; Jones, D.P. Oxidative Stress. *Annu. Rev. Biochem.* **2017**, *6*, 715–748. [CrossRef] [PubMed]
18. Sies, H. Oxidative stress: A concept in redox biology and medicine. *Redox Biol.* **2015**, *4*, 180–183. [CrossRef] [PubMed]
19. Sies, H. Oxidative Stress: Concept and Some Practical Aspects. *Antioxidants* **2020**, *9*, 852. [CrossRef] [PubMed]
20. Chitra, M.; Mathangi, D.C.; Priscilla, J. Oxidative stress during spontaneous vaginal delivery: Comparison between maternal and neonatal oxidative status. *Int. J. Med. Res. Rev.* **2016**, *4*, 60–66.
21. Marín, R.; Abad, C.; Rojas, D.; Chiarello, D.I.; Alejandro, T.G. Biomarkers of oxidative stress and reproductive complications. *Adv. Clin. Chem.* **2023**, *113*, 157–233.
22. Simon-Szabo, Z.; Fogarasi, E.; Nemes-Nagy, E.; Denes, L.; Croitoru, M.; Szabo, B. Oxidative stress and peripartum outcomes (Review). *Exp. Ther. Med.* **2021**, *22*, 1–6. [CrossRef] [PubMed]
23. Ghiselli, A.; Serafini, M.; Natella, F.; Scaccini, C. Total antioxidant capacity as a tool to assess redox status: Critical view and experimental data. *Free. Radic. Biol. Med.* **2000**, *29*, 1106–1114. [CrossRef] [PubMed]
24. Perrone, S.; Laschi, E.; Buonocore, G. Biomarkers of oxidative stress in the fetus and in the newborn. *Free. Radic. Biol. Med.* **2019**, *142*, 23–31. [CrossRef] [PubMed]
25. Fogarasi, E.; Croitoru, M.D.; Fülöp, I.; Muntean, D.L. Is the Oxidative Stress Really a Disease? *Acta Med. Marisiensis.* **2016**, *62*, 112–120. [CrossRef]
26. Ibrahim, A.; Khoo, M.I.; Ismail, E.H.E.; Hussain, N.H.N.; Zin, A.A.M.; Noordin, L.; Abdullah, S.; Mahdy, Z.A.; Lah, N.A.Z.N. Oxidative stress biomarkers in pregnancy: A systematic review. *Reprod. Biol. Endocrinol.* **2024**, *22*, 1–12. [CrossRef] [PubMed]
27. Davies, K.J.A. Adaptive homeostasis. *Mol. Asp. Med.* **2016**, *49*, 1–7. [CrossRef] [PubMed]

28. Burton, G.J.; Jauniaux, E. Oxidative stress. *Best Pract. Res Clin Obs. Gynaecol.* **2011**, *25*, 287–299. [CrossRef]
29. Valenzuela, F.J.; Vera, J.; Venegas, C.; Pino, F.; Lagunas, C. Circadian System and Melatonin Hormone: Risk Factors for Complications during Pregnancy. *Obstet. Gynecol. Int.* **2015**, *2015*, 1–10. [CrossRef] [PubMed]
30. Cha, J.; Sun, X.; Dey, S.K. Mechanisms of implantation: Strategies for successful pregnancy. *Nat. Med.* **2012**, *18*, 1754–1767. [CrossRef]
31. Marín, R.; Pujol, F.H.; Rojas, D.; Sobrevia, L. SARS- CoV-2 infection and oxidative stress in early-onset preeclampsia. *Biochim. Biophys. Acta (BBA)-Mol. Basis Dis.* **2021**, *1868*, 166321. [CrossRef]
32. Peterhans, E. Sendai virus stimulates chemiluminescence in mouse spleen cells. *Biochem. Biophys. Res. Commun.* **1979**, *91*, 383–392. [CrossRef]
33. Redline, R.W.; Ravishankar, S.; Bagby, C.M.; Saab, S.T.; Zarei, S. Four major patterns of placental injury: A stepwise guide for understanding and implementing the 2016 Amsterdam consensus. *Mod. Pathol.* **2021**, *34*, 1074–1092. [CrossRef] [PubMed]
34. Ohkawa, H.; Ohishi, N.; Yagi, K. Assay for lipid peroxides in animal tissues by thiobarbituric acid reaction. *Anal. Biochem.* **1979**, *95*, 351–358. [CrossRef] [PubMed]
35. Green, L.C.; Wagner, D.A.; Glogowski, J.; Skipper, P.L.; Wishnok, J.S.; Tannenbaum, S.R. Analysis of nitrate, nitrite, and [15N]nitrate in biological fluids. *Anal. Biochem.* **1982**, *126*, 131–138. [CrossRef]
36. *Handbook Methods for Oxygen Radical Research*; CRC Press: Boca Raton, FL, USA, 2018.
37. Pick, E.; Keisari, Y. A simple colorimetric method for the measurement of hydrogen peroxide produced by cells in culture. *J. Immunol. Methods* **1980**, *38*, 161–170. [CrossRef] [PubMed]
38. Aebi, H. Catalase in vitro. *Methods Enzymol.* **1984**, *105*, 121–126. [CrossRef] [PubMed]
39. Beutler, E. *Red Blood Cell Metabolism, A Manual of Biochemical Methods*, 2nd ed.; Bergmeyen, H.V.E., Ed.; Grune and Stratton: New York, NY, USA, 1975; pp. 112–114.
40. Beutler, E. *Red Cell Metabolism: A Manual of Biochemical Methods*, 3rd ed.; Grune and Stratton: New York, NY, USA, 1982; 105p.
41. Khong, T.Y.; Mooney, E.E.; Ariel, I.; Balmus, N.C.M.; Boyd, T.K.; Brundler, M.-A.; Derricott, H.; Evans, M.J.; Faye-Petersen, O.M.; Gillan, J.E.; et al. Sampling and Definitions of Placental Lesions: Amsterdam Placental Workshop Group Consensus Statement. *Arch. Pathol. Lab. Med.* **2016**, *140*, 698–713. [CrossRef] [PubMed]
42. Fischer, A.H.; Jacobson, K.A.; Rose, J.; Zeller, R. Hematoxylin and Eosin Staining of Tissue and Cell Sections. *Cold Spring Harb. Protoc.* **2008**, *2008*, pdb.prot4986. [CrossRef] [PubMed]
43. Knight, M.; Bunch, K.; Vousden, N.; Morris, E.; Simpson, N.; Gale, C.; O'Brien, P.; Quigley, M.; Brocklehurst, P.; Kurinczuk, J.J.; et al. Characteristics and outcomes of pregnant women admitted to hospital with confirmed SARS-CoV-2 infection in UK: National population based cohort study. *BMJ* **2020**, *8*, m2107. [CrossRef] [PubMed]
44. Chen, L.; Li, Q.; Zheng, D.; Jiang, H.; Wei, Y.; Zou, L.; Feng, L.; Xiong, G.; Sun, G.; Wang, H.; et al. Clinical Characteristics of Pregnant Women with COVID-19 in Wuhan, China. *N. Engl. J. Med.* **2020**, *382*, e100. [CrossRef]
45. Prabhu, M.; Cagino, K.; Matthews, K.C.; Friedlander, R.L.; Glynn, S.M.; Kubiak, J.M.; Yang, Y.J.; Zhao, Z.; Baergen, R.N.; DiPace, J.I.; et al. Pregnancy and postpartum outcomes in a universally tested population for SARS-CoV-2 in New York City: A prospective cohort study. *BJOG Int. J. Obstet. Gynaecol.* **2020**, *127*, 1548–1556. [CrossRef] [PubMed]
46. Giaxi, P.; Maniatelli, E.; Vivilaki, V. Evaluation of mode of delivery in pregnant women infected with COVID-19. *Eur. J. Midwifery* **2020**, *4*, 28. [CrossRef]
47. Liu, H.; Liu, F.; Li, J.; Zhang, T.; Wang, D.; Lan, W. Clinical and CT imaging features of the COVID-19 pneumonia: Focus on pregnant women and children. *J. Infect.* **2020**, *80*, e7–e13. [CrossRef] [PubMed]
48. Chen, H.; Guo, J.; Wang, C.; Luo, F.; Yu, X.; Zhang, W.; Li, J.; Zhao, D.; Xu, D.; Gong, Q.; et al. Clinical characteristics and intrauterine vertical transmission potential of COVID-19 infection in nine pregnant women: A retrospective review of medical records. *Lancet* **2020**, *395*, 809–815. [CrossRef]
49. Miyamoto, M.; Perreand, E.; Mangione, M.; Patel, M.; Cojocaru, L.; Seung, H.; Chua, J.; Turan, O.M.; Turan, S. Mode of Delivery in Patients with COVID-19. *Am. J. Obstet. Gynecol.* **2021**, *226*, S582–S583. [CrossRef]
50. Maranto, M.; Zaami, S.; Restivo, V.; Termini, D.; Gangemi, A.; Tumminello, M.; Culmone, S.; Billone, V.; Cucinella, G.; Gullo, G. Symptomatic COVID-19 in Pregnancy: Hospital Cohort Data between May 2020 and April 2021, Risk Factors and Medicolegal Implications. *Diagnostics* **2023**, *13*, 1009. [CrossRef] [PubMed]
51. Riemma, G.; De Franciscis, P.; Tesorone, M.; Coppa, E.; Schiattarella, A.; Billone, V.; Lopez, A.; Cucinella, G.; Gullo, G.; Carotenuto, R.M. Obstetric and Gynecological Admissions and Hospitalizations in an Italian Tertiary-Care Hospital during COVID-19 Pandemic: A Retrospective Analysis According to Restrictive Measures. *J. Clin. Med.* **2023**, *12*, 7097. [CrossRef] [PubMed]
52. de Carvalho, W.B.; Gibelli, M.A.B.C.; Krebs, V.L.J.; Calil, V.M.L.T.; Johnston, C. Expert recommendations for the care of newborns of mothers with COVID-19. *Clinics* **2020**, *75*, e1932. [CrossRef] [PubMed]
53. Burton, G.J.; Hempstock, J.; Jauniaux, E. Oxygen, early embryonic metabolism and free radical-mediated embryopathies. *Reprod. Biomed.* **2003**, *6*, 84–96. [CrossRef] [PubMed]

54. Jauniaux, E.; Hempstock, J.; Greenwold, N.; Burton, G.J. Trophoblastic Oxidative Stress in Relation to Temporal and Regional Differences in Maternal Placental Blood Flow in Normal and Abnormal Early Pregnancies. *Am. J. Pathol.* **2003**, *162*, 115–125. [CrossRef]
55. Jauniaux, E.; Zaidi, J.; Jurkovic, D.; Campbell, S.; Hustin, J. Pregnancy: Comparison of colour Doppler features and pathological findings in complicated early pregnancy. *Hum. Reprod.* **1994**, *9*, 2432–2437. [CrossRef]
56. Jauniaux, E.; Watson, A.L.; Hempstock, J.; Bao, Y.P.; Skepper, J.N.; Burton, G.J. Onset of Maternal Arterial Blood Flow and Placental Oxidative Stress: A Possible Factor in Human Early Pregnancy Failure. *Am. J. Pathol.* **2000**, *157*, 2111–2122. [CrossRef] [PubMed]
57. Fogel, I.; Pinchuk, I.; Kupferminc, M.J.; Lichtenberg, D.; Fainaru, O. Oxidative stress in the fetal circulation does not depend on mode of delivery. *Am. J. Obstet. Gynecol.* **2005**, *193*, 241–246. [CrossRef] [PubMed]
58. Schoots, M.H.; Gordijn, S.J.; Scherjon, S.A.; van Goor, H.; Hillebrands, J.-L. Oxidative stress in placental pathology. *Placenta* **2018**, *69*, 153–161. [CrossRef] [PubMed]
59. Hracsko, Z.; Safar, Z.; Orvos, H.; Novak, Z.; Pal, A.; Varga, I.S. Evaluation of oxidative stress markers after vaginal delivery or Caesarean section. *In Vivo* **2007**, *21*, 703–706.
60. Chiba, T.; Omori, A.; Takahashi, K.; Tanaka, K.; Kudo, K.; Manabe, M.; Mariya, Y.; Kashiwakura, I. Correlations between the detection of stress-associated hormone/oxidative stress markers in umbilical cord blood and the physical condition of the mother and neonate. *J. Obstet. Gynaecol. Res.* **2010**, *36*, 958–964. [CrossRef] [PubMed]
61. Karaçor, T.; Sak, S.; Başaranoğlu, S.; Peker, N.; Ağaçayak, E.; Sak, M.E.; Turgut, A.; Evsen, M.S.; Evliyaoğlu, O.; Gül, T. Assessment of oxidative stress markers in cord blood of newborns to patients with oxytocin-induced labor. *J. Obstet. Gynaecol. Res.* **2017**, *43*, 860–865. [CrossRef] [PubMed]
62. Watson, A.; Skepper, J.; Jauniaux, E.; Burton, G. Changes in concentration, localization and activity of catalase within the human placenta during early gestation. *Placenta* **1998**, *19*, 27–34. [CrossRef]
63. Hung, T.-H.; Skepper, J.N.; Burton, G.J. In Vitro Ischemia-Reperfusion Injury in Term Human Placenta as a Model for Oxidative Stress in Pathological Pregnancies. *Am. J. Pathol.* **2001**, *159*, 1031–1043. [CrossRef] [PubMed]
64. Rolfo, A.; Cosma, S.; Nuzzo, A.M.; Salio, C.; Moretti, L.; Sassoè-Pognetto, M.; Carosso, A.R.; Borella, F.; Cutrin, J.C.; Benedetto, C. Increased Placental Anti-Oxidant Response in Asymptomatic and Symptomatic COVID-19 Third-Trimester Pregnancies. *Biomedicines* **2022**, *10*, 634. [CrossRef]
65. Caparros-Gonzalez, R.A.; Pérez-Morente, M.A.; Hueso-Montoro, C.; Álvarez-Serrano, M.A.; de la Torre-Luque, A. Congenital, Intrapartum and Postnatal Maternal-Fetal-Neonatal SARS-CoV-2 Infections: A Narrative Review. *Nutrients* **2020**, *12*, 3570. [CrossRef] [PubMed]
66. Chi, H.; Chiu, N.-C.; Tai, Y.-L.; Chang, H.-Y.; Lin, C.-H.; Sung, Y.-H.; Tseng, C.-Y.; Liu, L.Y.-M.; Lin, C.-Y. Clinical features of neonates born to mothers with coronavirus disease-2019: A systematic review of 105 neonates. *J. Microbiol. Immunol. Infect.* **2020**, *54*, 69–76. [CrossRef]
67. Cruz, N.A.N.; Stoll, D.; Casarini, D.E.; Bertagnolli, M. Role of ACE2 in pregnancy and potential implications for COVID-19 susceptibility. *Clin. Sci.* **2021**, *135*, 1805–1824. [CrossRef]
68. Martin, M.A.; Keith, M.; Pace, R.M.; Williams, J.E.; Ley, S.H.; Barbosa-Leiker, C.; Caffé, B.; Smith, C.B.; Kunkle, A.; Lackey, K.A.; et al. SARS-CoV-2 specific antibody trajectories in mothers and infants over two months following maternal infection. *Front Immunol.* **2022**, *13*, 1015002. [CrossRef]
69. Flannery, D.D.; Gouma, S.; Dhudasia, M.B.; Mukhopadhyay, S.; Pfeifer, M.R.; Woodford, E.C.; Triebwasser, J.E.; Gerber, J.S.; Morris, J.S.; Weirick, M.E.; et al. Assessment of Maternal and Neonatal Cord Blood SARS-CoV-2 Antibodies and Placental Transfer Ratios. *JAMA Pediatr.* **2021**, *175*, 594. [CrossRef]
70. Schwartz, D.A.; Morotti, D.; Beigi, B.; Moshfegh, F.; Zafaranloo, N.; Patanè, L. Confirming Vertical Fetal Infection With Coronavirus Disease 2019: Neonatal and Pathology Criteria for Early Onset and Transplacental Transmission of Severe Acute Respiratory Syndrome Coronavirus 2 From Infected Pregnant Mothers. *Arch. Pathol. Lab. Med.* **2020**, *144*, 1451–1456. [CrossRef]
71. Lamouroux, A.; Attie-Bitach, T.; Martinovic, J.; Leruez-Ville, M.; Ville, Y. Evidence for and against vertical transmission for severe acute respiratory syndrome coronavirus 2. *Am. J. Obstet. Gynecol.* **2020**, *223*, 91.e1–91.e4. [CrossRef] [PubMed]
72. Schwartz, D.A.; Thomas, K.M. Characterizing COVID-19 maternal-fetal transmission and placental infection using comprehensive molecular pathology. *EBioMedicine* **2020**, *60*, 102983. [CrossRef] [PubMed]
73. Rani, N.; Dhingra, R.; Arya, D.S.; Kalaivani, M.; Bhatla, N.; Kumar, R. Role of oxidative stress markers and antioxidants in the placenta of preeclamptic patients. *J. Obstet. Gynaecol. Res.* **2010**, *36*, 1189–1194. [CrossRef] [PubMed]
74. Glynn, S.M.; Yang, Y.J.; Thomas, C.; Friedlander, R.L.; Cagino, K.A.; Matthews, K.C.; Riley, L.E.; Baergen, R.N.; Prabhu, M. SARS-CoV-2 and Placental Pathology. *Am. J. Surg. Pathol.* **2022**, *46*, 51–57. [CrossRef] [PubMed]
75. Mulvey, J.J.; Magro, C.M.; Ma, L.X.; Nuovo, G.J.; Baergen, R.N. Analysis of complement deposition and viral RNA in placentas of COVID-19 patients. *Ann. Diagn. Pathol.* **2020**, *46*, 151530. [CrossRef] [PubMed]

76. Patberg, E.T.; Adams, T.; Rekawek, P.; Vahanian, S.A.; Akerman, M.; Hernandez, A.; Rapkiewicz, A.V.; Ragolia, L.; Sicuranza, G.; Chavez, M.R.; et al. Coronavirus disease 2019 infection and placental histopathology in women delivering at term. *Am. J. Obstet. Gynecol.* **2021**, *224*, e1–e382. [CrossRef]
77. Shanes, E.D.; Mithal, L.B.; Otero, S.; Azad, H.A.; Miller, E.S.; Goldstein, J.A. Placental Pathology in COVID-19. *Am. J. Clin. Pathol.* **2020**, *154*, 23–32. [CrossRef]
78. Lista, G.; Castoldi, F.M.L.R.; Compagnoni, G.; Maggioni, C.; Cornélissen, G.; Halberg, F. Neonatal and maternal concentrations of hydroxil radical and total antioxidant system: Protective role of placenta against fetal oxidative stress. *Neuro Endocrinol Lett.* **2010**, *31*, 319–324.
79. Sharps, M.C.; Hayes, D.J.L.; Lee, S.; Zou, Z.; Brady, C.A.; Almoghrabi, Y.; Kerby, A.; Tamber, K.K.; Jones, C.J.; Waldorf, K.M.A.; et al. A structured review of placental morphology and histopathological lesions associated with SARS-CoV-2 infection. *Placenta* **2020**, *101*, 13–29. [CrossRef] [PubMed]
80. Chisholm, K.M.; Heerema-McKenney, A. Fetal Thrombotic Vasculopathy. *Am. J. Surg. Pathol.* **2015**, *39*, 274–280. [CrossRef] [PubMed]
81. Redline, R.W. Clinical and pathological umbilical cord abnormalities in fetal thrombotic vasculopathy. *Hum. Pathol.* **2004**, *35*, 1494–1498. [CrossRef]
82. Redline, R.W.; Ariel, I.; Baergen, R.N.; Desa, D.J.; Kraus, F.T.; Roberts, D.J.; Sander, C.M. Fetal Vascular Obstructive Lesions: Nosology and Reproducibility of Placental Reaction Patterns. *Pediatr. Dev. Pathol.* **2004**, *7*, 443–452. [CrossRef] [PubMed]
83. Roberts, D.J.; Post, M.D. The placenta in pre-eclampsia and intrauterine growth restriction. *J. Clin. Pathol.* **2008**, *61*, 1254–1260. [CrossRef] [PubMed]
84. Ernst, L.M. Maternal vascular malperfusion of the placental bed. *APMIS* **2018**, *126*, 551–560. [CrossRef] [PubMed]
85. Hsu, A.L.; Guan, M.; Johannesen, E.; Stephens, A.J.; Khaleel, N.; Kagan, N.; Tuhlei, B.C.; Wan, X.-F. Placental SARS-CoV-2 in a pregnant woman with mild COVID-19 disease. *J. Med. Virol.* **2021**, *93*, 1038–1044. [CrossRef]
86. Suhren, J.-T.; Meinardus, A.; Hussein, K.; Schaumann, N. Meta-analysis on COVID-19-pregnancy-related placental pathologies shows no specific pattern. *Placenta* **2021**, *117*, 72–77. [CrossRef] [PubMed]
87. Levitan, D.; London, V.; McLaren, R.A.; Mann, J.D.; Cheng, K.; Silver, M.; Balhotra, K.S.; McCalla, S.; Loukeris, K. Histologic and Immunohistochemical Evaluation of 65 Placentas From Women With Polymerase Chain Reaction–Proven Severe Acute Respiratory Syndrome Coronavirus 2 (SARS-CoV-2) Infection. *Arch. Pathol. Lab. Med.* **2021**, *145*, 648–656. [CrossRef] [PubMed]
88. Al-Rawaf, S.A.; Mousa, E.T.; Kareem, N.M. Correlation between Pregnancy Outcome and Placental Pathology in COVID-19 Pregnant Women. *Infect. Dis. Obstet. Gynecol.* **2022**, *2022*, 1–5. [CrossRef] [PubMed]
89. Nascimento, A.C.M.; Avvad-Portari, E.; Meuser-Batista, M.; Conde, T.C.; de Sá, R.A.M.; Salomao, N.; Rabelo, K.; Ciasca, E.S.; Brendolin, M.d.O.; Vasconcelos, Z.; et al. Histopathological and clinical analysis of COVID-19-infected placentas. *Surg. Exp. Pathol.* **2024**, *7*, 1–9. [CrossRef]
90. Baergen, R.N.; Heller, D.S. Placental Pathology in COVID-19 Positive Mothers: Preliminary Findings. *Pediatr. Dev. Pathol.* **2020**, *23*, 177–180. [CrossRef] [PubMed]
91. Hosier, H.; Farhadian, S.F.; Morotti, R.A.; Deshmukh, U.; Lu-Culligan, A.; Campbell, K.H.; Yasumoto, Y.; Vogels, C.B.; Casanovas-Massana, A.; Vijayakumar, P.; et al. SARS–CoV-2 infection of the placenta. *J. Clin. Investig.* **2020**, *130*, 4947–4953. [CrossRef]
92. Smithgall, M.C.; Liu-Jarin, X.; Hamele-Bena, D.; Cimic, A.; Mourad, M.; Debelenko, L.; Chen, X. Third-trimester placentas of severe acute respiratory syndrome coronavirus 2 (SARS-CoV-2)-positive women: Histomorphology, including viral immunohistochemistry and in-situ hybridization. *Histopathology* **2020**, *77*, 994–999. [CrossRef]
93. Corbetta-Rastelli, C.M.; Altendahl, M.; Gasper, C.; Goldstein, J.D.; Afshar, Y.; Gaw, S.L. Analysis of placental pathology after COVID-19 by timing and severity of infection. *Am. J. Obstet. Gynecol. MFM* **2023**, *5*, 100981. [CrossRef] [PubMed]
94. Schaumann, N.; Suhren, J.-T. An Update on COVID-19-Associated Placental Pathologies. *Z. Fur Geburtshilfe Und Neonatol.* **2024**, *228*, 42–48. [CrossRef] [PubMed]
95. Gulersen, M.; Prasannan, L.; Tam, H.T.; Metz, C.N.; Rochelson, B.; Meirowitz, N.; Shan, W.; Edelman, M.; Millington, K.A. Histopathologic evaluation of placentas after diagnosis of maternal severe acute respiratory syndrome coronavirus 2 infection. *Am. J. Obstet. Gynecol. MFM* **2020**, *2*, 100211. [CrossRef] [PubMed]
96. Belay, G. Article Review on Histopathologic Features of Placenta and Adverse Outcome in Pregnant Women with COVID-19 Positive. *Pathol. Lab. Med.* **2023**, *7*, 4–11. [CrossRef]
97. Arts, N.; Schiffer, V.; Severens-Rijvers, C.; Bons, J.; Spaanderman, M.; Al-Nasiry, S. Cumulative effect of maternal vascular malperfusion types in the placenta on adverse pregnancy outcomes. *Placenta* **2022**, *129*, 43–50. [CrossRef]
98. Wright, E.; Audette, M.C.; Ye, X.Y.; Keating, S.; Hoffman, B.; Lye, S.J.; Shah, P.S.; Kingdom, J.C. Maternal Vascular Malperfusion and Adverse Perinatal Outcomes in Low-Risk Nulliparous Women. *Obstet. Gynecol.* **2017**, *130*, 1112–1120. [CrossRef] [PubMed]
99. Parks, W.T.; Catov, J.M. The Placenta as a Window to Maternal Vascular Health. *Obstet. Gynecol. Clin. N. Am.* **2020**, *47*, 17–28. [CrossRef] [PubMed]

100. Zur, R.L.; Kingdom, J.C.; Parks, W.T.; Hobson, S.R. The Placental Basis of Fetal Growth Restriction. *Obstet. Gynecol. Clin. N. Am.* **2019**, *47*, 81–98. [CrossRef] [PubMed]
101. Gordijn, S.J.; Beune, I.M.; Thilaganathan, B.; Papageorghiou, A.; Baschat, A.A.; Baker, P.N.; Silver, R.M.; Wynia, K.; Ganzevoort, W. Consensus definition of fetal growth restriction: A Delphi procedure. *Ultrasound Obstet. Gynecol.* **2016**, *48*, 333–339. [CrossRef] [PubMed]
102. Heider, A. Fetal Vascular Malperfusion. *Arch. Pathol. Lab. Med.* **2017**, *141*, 1484–1489. [CrossRef] [PubMed]
103. Gullo, G.; Scaglione, M.; Cucinella, G.; Chiantera, V.; Perino, A.; Greco, M.E.; Laganà, A.S.; Marinelli, E.; Basile, G.; Zaami, S. Neonatal Outcomes and Long-Term Follow-Up of Children Born from Frozen Embryo, a Narrative Review of Latest Research Findings. *Medicina* **2022**, *58*, 1218. [CrossRef]
104. Roescher, A.M.; Timmer, A.; Erwich, J.J.H.M.; Bos, A.F. Placental Pathology, Perinatal Death, Neonatal Outcome, and Neurological Development: A Systematic Review. *PLoS ONE* **2014**, *9*, e89419. [CrossRef] [PubMed]
105. Fajardo-Martinez, V.; Ferreira, F.; Fuller, T.; Cambou, M.C.; Kerin, T.; Paiola, S.; Mok, T.; Rao, R.; Mohole, J.; Paravastu, R.; et al. Neurodevelopmental delay in children exposed to maternal SARS-CoV-2 in-utero. *Sci Rep.* **2024**, *14*, 11851. [CrossRef]
106. Gullo, G.; Scaglione, M.; Buzzaccarini, G.; Laganà, A.S.; Basile, G.; Chiantera, V.; Cucinella, G.; Zaami, S. Cell-Free Fetal DNA and Non-Invasive Prenatal Diagnosis of Chromosomopathies and Pediatric Monogenic Diseases: A Critical Appraisal and Medicolegal Remarks. *J. Pers. Med.* **2022**, *13*, 1. [CrossRef] [PubMed]
107. Ministarstvo zdravlja Republike Srbije. Stručno-metodološko uputstvo za sprovođenje vanredne preporučene imunizacije protiv COVID-19 u Republici Srbiji vakcinama: Pfizer-BioNTech COVID-19 Vaccine (Comirnaty), Gam-COVID-Vak, SARS-CoV-2 Vaccine (Vero Cell), Inactivated, ChAdOx1 nCoV-19 Corona Virus Vaccine (Recombinant) COV-ISHIELD/AstraZeneca, Spikevax. [Online]. Available online: https://www.batut.org.rs/download/smuZaVanrednuPreporucenuImunizacijuProtivCOVID19.poslednji (accessed on 16 September 2024).
108. Maranto, M.; Gullo, G.; Bruno, A.; Minutolo, G.; Cucinella, G.; Maiorana, A.; Casuccio, A.; Restivo, V. Factors Associated with Anti-SARS-CoV-2 Vaccine Acceptance among Pregnant Women: Data from Outpatient Women Experiencing High-Risk Pregnancy. *Vaccines* **2023**, *11*, 454. [CrossRef]
109. Incognito, G.G.; Distefano, R.E.C.; Campo, G.; Gulino, F.A.; Gulisano, C.; Gullotta, C.; Gullo, G.; Cucinella, G.; Tuscano, A.; Bruno, M.T.; et al. Comparison of Maternal and Neonatal Outcomes between SARS-CoV-2 Variants: A Retrospective, Monocentric Study. *J. Clin. Med.* **2023**, *12*, 6329. [CrossRef] [PubMed]
110. Burgio, S.; Polizzi, C.; Alesi, M.; Perino, A.; Cucinella, G.; Kotlik, Y.; Lopez, A.; Vassiliadis, A.; Gullo, G. Personality Traits and Depression in Infertile Couples during the COVID-19. *J. Clin. Med.* **2024**, *13*, 4827. [CrossRef] [PubMed]
111. Burgio, S.; Cucinella, G.; Perino, A.; Baglio, G.; Crifasi, L.; Krysiak, R.; Kowalcze, K.; Gullo, G. Effectiveness of Psychological Counseling Intervention in High-Risk Pregnancies in Italy. *J. Pers. Med.* **2024**, *14*, 976. [CrossRef] [PubMed]

Journal of
Clinical Medicine

MDPI

Article

# Impact of COVID-19 on Pregnancy Outcomes: A Phase-Based Analysis from a Spanish Tertiary Hospital (2020–2023)

María-Asunción Quijada-Cazorla [1,2,3,*], María-Virgilia Simó-Rodríguez [3], Ana-María Palacios-Marqués [1,2,3], María Peláez-García [1] and José-Manuel Ramos-Rincón [2,4,5]

1 Department of Obstetrics and Gynecology, Dr. Balmis General University Hospital, 03010 Alicante, Spain; apalacios@umh.es (A.-M.P.-M.)
2 Alicante Institute for Health and Biomedical Research (ISABIAL), 03010 Alicante, Spain; jose.ramosr@umh.es
3 Department of Public Health, History of Science and Gynecology, Miguel Hernández University, 03550 San Juan de Alicante, Spain
4 Department of Internal Medicine, Dr. Balmis General University Hospital, 03010 Alicante, Spain
5 Department of Clinical Medicine, Miguel Hernández University, 03550 San Juan de Alicante, Spain
* Correspondence: mquijada@umh.es

## Abstract

**Background/Objectives:** Pregnancy has been considered a risk factor for severe SARS-CoV-2 infection, as well as for adverse maternal and neonatal outcomes. This study aimed to assess the clinical impact of COVID-19 on pregnant women managed at a Spanish tertiary care hospital across different phases of the pandemic. **Methods:** A retrospective observational study was conducted at Dr. Balmis General University Hospital (Alicante, Spain) between March 2020 and May 2023. All pregnant women who received hospital care with confirmed SARS-CoV-2 infection were included. Maternal and neonatal outcomes were analyzed and compared with the 6120 total births recorded during the same period. **Results:** A total of 249 pregnant women with COVID-19 were included, with 30.8%, 25.0%, and 7.9% hospitalized during each respective pandemic phase. The overall incidence of infection was 41 cases per 1000 births. Hospitalized pregnant women showed significantly higher rates of preterm birth, labor induction (70.4% vs. 47.0%; OR: 2.67; 95% CI: 1.12–6.43), and cesarean delivery (46.9% vs. 24.9%, OR: 2.60; 95% CI: 1.27–5.50). Neonatal outcomes included lower Apgar scores, increased admission to the neonatal unit (25.8% vs. 8.2%, $p = 0.007$), and a higher rate of neonatal complications (23.3% vs. 7.7%, $p = 0.015$). Maternal obesity and non-Spanish nationality were associated with more severe maternal disease. Vaccination against SARS-CoV-2 significantly reduced the risk of hospitalization due to the infection (OR: 0.30; 95% CI: 0.13–0.69). **Conclusions:** Pregnant women admitted with COVID-19 had increased risks of adverse obstetric and neonatal outcomes, underscoring the importance of preventive strategies, such as vaccination.

**Keywords:** COVID-19; SARS-CoV-2; pregnancy; cesarean delivery; maternal outcomes; neonatal outcomes; risk factors; vaccination

## 1. Introduction

Since the World Health Organization (WHO) declared COVID-19 a global pandemic on 11 March 2020, its impact on pregnancy has become a significant clinical concern due to its potential maternal and perinatal consequences. Pregnancy has been recognized as a risk factor for more severe SARS-CoV-2 infection as well as for adverse obstetric and neonatal outcomes [1]. Although most pregnant women presented with mild symptoms, with 73–86% remaining asymptomatic [2], approximately 16% progressed to severe disease [3].

Throughout the pandemic, the literature has reported variable effects of this coronavirus on maternal and neonatal health. Multiple studies have shown that SARS-CoV-2 infection during pregnancy is associated with higher maternal mortality [4], an increased risk of intensive care unit (ICU) admission compared to nonpregnant women, and up to a 3.5-fold increase in hospitalization rates [5–7]. Advanced maternal age, elevated body mass index (BMI), non-White ethnicity, and preexisting comorbidities have been associated with a worse prognosis [5].

The impact of SARS-CoV-2 on pregnancy-related outcomes has also been extensively discussed. Several studies have reported increased cesarean delivery rates [6,8] and higher risks of pregnancy-associated complications, including gestational diabetes, hypertensive disorders, and preterm labor [8,9]. In contrast, no significant differences have been observed in the incidence of other obstetric complications, such as postpartum hemorrhage [10].

Importantly, across the different phases of the pandemic, each SARS-CoV-2 variant has been associated with distinct clinical implications. The original Wuhan wild-type strain was initially considered the most virulent, with potentially more severe clinical outcomes involving the highest rate of cesarean deliveries [11]. The Delta variant demonstrated approximately 60% greater transmissibility than its predecessor and was linked to a significantly higher incidence of adverse clinical events [11,12]. In contrast, the Omicron variant, although more transmissible, was generally associated with milder clinical manifestations compared to earlier variants [11,13]. Despite these findings, few studies have explored the evolving impact of COVID-19 across the different pandemic phases, variant waves, and their specific implications for pregnancy.

In summary, the COVID-19 pandemic has presented a significant challenge to maternal and perinatal health, with an impact that remains incompletely characterized. Although the acute phase of the pandemic has passed, limited evidence is available regarding the progression of its clinical effects across successive viral variants, the role of vaccination, and its overall consequences for pregnancy. To address these gaps, we conducted a study to evaluate the clinical outcomes of SARS-CoV-2 infection during pregnancy, as well as its evolution throughout the different phases of the pandemic.

This study aims to provide real-world evidence of the temporal progression of the COVID-19 pandemic and its impact on maternal and perinatal outcomes at a Spanish tertiary care hospital from 2020 to 2023.

## 2. Materials and Methods

### 2.1. Study Design and Type

A retrospective cohort study was conducted, including all pregnant women diagnosed with COVID-19 during pregnancy who received care for this reason at Dr. Balmis General University Hospital (DBGUH) in Alicante, Spain, between 11 March 2020 and 5 May 2023. DBGUH is a tertiary-level referral center equipped with a neonatal intensive care unit (NICU) and serving a healthcare area of approximately 290,000 inhabitants. In addition to providing routine obstetric care, the hospital manages high-risk pregnancies, particularly those in which neonatal complications are anticipated and NICU admission is expected.

### 2.2. Study Population

Inclusion criteria: Those considered eligible for participation in this study fit the following criteria: pregnant women who received care at DBGUH and were diagnosed with SARS-CoV-2 infection using reverse transcription polymerase chain reaction (RT-PCR) during pregnancy between 11 March 2020 and 5 May 2023, and who subsequently gave birth at the same hospital. Therefore, moderate-to-severe cases of pregnant women with confirmed SARS-CoV-2 infection and COVID-19-related symptoms who attended the hospital emergency department for this reason were included.

All COVID-19 diagnoses included in the study were confirmed through reverse transcription polymerase chain reaction (RT-PCR) performed by medical professionals at the hospital. Home-based self-tests were not included, as the study was based on hospital medical records and laboratory-confirmed cases.

Exclusion criteria: The following cases were excluded: (1) patients incorrectly coded with COVID-19 who were not pregnant at the time of infection, and (2) pregnant women in whom SARS-CoV-2 infection was ruled out or could not be microbiologically confirmed.

The study group was compared in terms of obstetric outcomes with a control group. The inclusion criteria for the control group consisted of pregnant women without a confirmed SARS-CoV-2 infection (either a negative COVID-19 PCR test or no available test results) who gave birth at the same tertiary hospital during the study period, and who were not treated in the emergency department for COVID-19 infection during pregnancy.

### 2.3. Study Periods and Phase Definitions

Three study periods were defined based on the predominant circulating SARS-CoV-2 variants and the progression of the national COVID-19 vaccination campaign in Spain, according to epidemiological surveillance data:

- Period 1 (11 March 2020–28 February 2021): Characterized by the original Wuhan strain and a non-vaccinated population. 28 February 2021 was selected as the cutoff point because it marked the beginning of sustained circulation of the Alpha variant in Spain and the initial rollout of COVID-19 vaccination in pregnant women.
- Period 2 (1 March 2021–31 December 2021): Defined by the predominance of the Delta variant and a partially vaccinated population. During this phase, vaccination coverage among pregnant women began to progressively increase.
- Period 3 (1 January 2022–5 May 2023): Corresponding to the predominance of the Omicron variant and widespread vaccination coverage. This period was associated with high vaccination rates and reduced COVID-19 severity, in line with the evolving behavior of circulating variants and the national public health response.

These cutoff dates were selected to reflect key epidemiological and clinical transitions throughout the pandemic that may have influenced maternal and neonatal outcomes.

The results for each study period were compared with those recorded for a cohort of pregnant women without COVID-19 who delivered at the same hospital during the corresponding timeframe.

### 2.4. Data Collection and Definitions

Clinical data were obtained from electronic medical records and systematically recorded in an anonymized data collection form.

The following variables were collected:

- Maternal history: Maternal age, gestational age at the time of infection, country of birth, height, weight, body mass index (BMI), pregestational comorbidities (e.g., chronic respiratory disease, chronic hypertension, pregestational diabetes), COVID-19 vaccination status, parity, and history of previous spontaneous abortion.
- COVID-19-related variables: Symptoms (fever, cough, sore throat, dyspnea, myalgia, anosmia), emergency department visits, hospitalization, length of hospital stay, ICU admission and length of stay, treatments received (low molecular weight heparin, corticosteroids, oxygen therapy), and complications (bilateral pneumonia, thromboembolic events, maternal death, use of invasive or non-invasive mechanical ventilation).

- Pregnancy-related variables: Pregnancy outcome (miscarriage, preterm delivery, or term delivery), gestational complications (gestational diabetes, hypertensive disorders, threatened preterm labor), and fetal conditions (intrauterine growth restriction (IUGR)/small for gestational age (SGA), congenital anomalies, or other fetal complications).
- Delivery and perinatal outcomes: Date of delivery, gestational age at delivery, onset of labor (spontaneous or induced), and mode of delivery (vaginal or cesarean).
- Maternal postpartum complications: Postpartum hemorrhage, need for maternal blood transfusion, postpartum fever, ICU admission, and other maternal complications.
- Neonatal outcomes: Birth weight, Apgar scores, arterial and venous umbilical cord pH, NICU admission, perinatal complications, and neonatal death.

The two primary outcomes of the study focused on pregnant women with confirmed SARS-CoV-2 infection. The first outcome was the need for hospital admission after emergency department evaluation. The second outcome was the development of severe maternal COVID-19, defined as ICU admission, the use of invasive or non-invasive mechanical ventilation (IMV/NIMV), and/or maternal death.

### 2.5. Statistical Analysis

Statistical analyses were performed using IBM SPSS Statistics for Windows, version 25.0 (IBM Corp., Armonk, NY, USA). All variables were subjected to descriptive analysis. The distribution of quantitative variables was assessed using the Kolmogorov–Smirnov test. Variables with a normal distribution were reported as mean and standard deviation (SD), while non-normally distributed variables were expressed as the median and interquartile range (IQR). Categorical variables were summarized as absolute frequencies and percentages.

To compare quantitative variables between groups, Student's *t*-test was used for normally distributed variables and the Mann–Whitney U test was applied for non-normally distributed ones. For categorical variables, comparisons were performed using the chi-square test or Fisher's exact test, as appropriate. The strength of association was quantified using odds ratios (ORs) with 95% confidence intervals (95% CI). A $p$-value < 0.05 was considered statistically significant.

A complete case analysis was conducted for each variable. Due to the retrospective nature of the study and the variability in the completeness of clinical records, the number of available observations (N) differed slightly between variables.

### 2.6. Ethical Approach

The study was conducted following the ethical principles of the Declaration of Helsinki. The protocol was approved by the Ethics Committee of the Alicante Health Department-General Hospital, with project identification code CEIm PI2024-036/ISABIAL 2024-0049, on 7 March 2024. All data were collected in an anonymized form, and patient confidentiality was rigorously maintained throughout the study.

## 3. Results

### 3.1. COVID-19 in Pregnant Women

A total of 319 pregnant women diagnosed with SARS-CoV-2 infection during pregnancy and evaluated in the emergency department were initially identified.

After applying the exclusion criteria, 70 women were excluded, resulting in a final study population of 249 pregnant women for analysis. The included and excluded patients are presented in Figure 1. Figure 1 illustrates the selection process of the study cohort:

A total of 319 pregnant women were initially identified with a diagnosis of COVID-19 during pregnancy. Of these, 70 were excluded due to not meeting the inclusion criteria (e.g., incomplete data, delivery outside the hospital), and 9 experienced a miscarriage before 22 weeks of gestation. Therefore, the final study cohort—meeting all inclusion and exclusion criteria—consisted of 240 pregnant women with confirmed SARS-CoV-2 infection whose pregnancies progressed beyond 22 weeks and who delivered at the hospital.

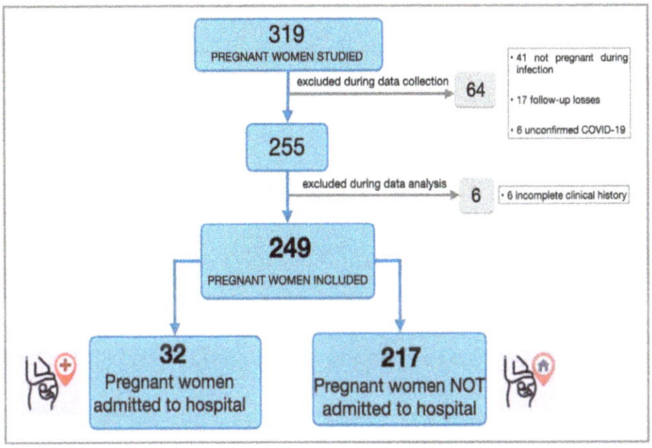


**Figure 1.** Flowchart of the inclusion and exclusion process for pregnant women with confirmed. SARS-CoV-2 infection during the study period. This figure represents the selection of the COVID-19 cohort only.

Between 11 March 2020, and 28 February 2021 (Period 1), 39 women (15.7%) were managed. Between March 1 2021 and 31 December 2021 (Period 2), 20 women (8.0%) were included. Most cases occurred between 1 January 2022 and 5 May 2023 (Period 3), involving 190 women (76.3%). Overall, 12.9% of the pregnant women evaluated in the emergency department required hospitalization. The hospital admission rates were 30.8% in Period 1, 25.0% in Period 2, and 7.9% in Period 3. These trends are shown in Figure 2.

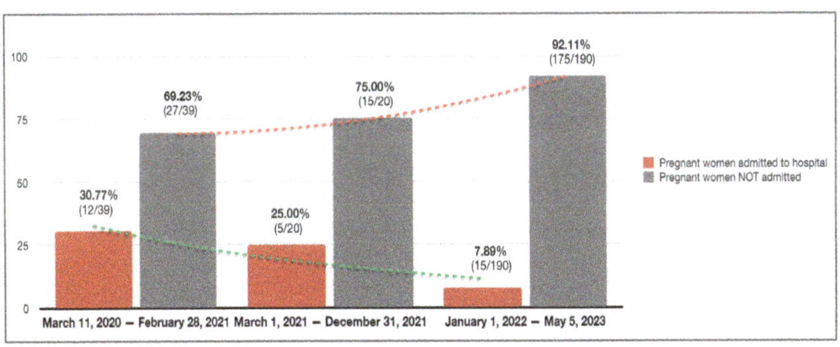


**Figure 2.** Number and percentage of pregnant women with confirmed COVID-19 and hospital admission rates across the different phases of the pandemic.

### *3.2. Obstetric Outcomes: COVID-19 vs. Non-COVID-19 Pregnancies*

During the study period, a total of 6120 deliveries occurred at the hospital. Of these, 5880 involved pregnant women without COVID-19, whose deliveries took place at the hospital but who did not meet the inclusion criteria for the study cohort. The remaining 240 deliveries involved pregnant women with confirmed SARS-CoV-2 infection during pregnancy, all of whom were evaluated and managed at the hospital's obstetric emergency department, and whose deliveries also occurred at the same institution. This corresponds to an incidence of 4.1%, or 41 cases per 1000 deliveries.

Of the initial 249 COVID-19 cases managed at the hospital (Figure 1), 9 pregnancies ended in miscarriage before 22 weeks of gestation and were excluded from the analysis. The final study cohort included 240 pregnant women who met all the eligibility criteria.

Pregnant women with COVID-19 showed a significantly higher rate of preterm birth compared to the non-COVID-19 group (18.3% vs. 8.7%, $p < 0.001$). Comparative results between both groups, stratified by gestational age and study period, are presented in Table 1.

**Table 1.** (**a**) Gestational age at delivery in pregnant women with and without COVID-19, stratified by gestational age and study period. (**b**) Obstetric outcomes across different phases of the study period.

**(a)**

| | | Gestational Age at Birth<br><28 Weeks<br>28–37 Weeks<br>≥37 Weeks | | |
|---|---|---|---|---|
| **Period of Study** | **Overall<br>% (n/N) [a]** | **COVID-19<br>% (n/N¹)** | **Non-COVID-19<br>% (n/N²)** | ***p*-Value** |
| 4 March 2020–28 February 2021 | 1.11 (21/1894)<br>8.08 (153/1894)<br>90.81 (1720/1894) | 5.56 (2/36)<br>36.11 (13/36)<br>58.33 (21/36) | 1.02 (19/1858)<br>7.53 (140/1858)<br>91.44 (1699/1858) | **<0.001** |
| 1 March 2021–31 December 2021 | 0.74 (12/1630)<br>8.83 (144/1630)<br>90.43 (1474/1630) | 0 (0/18)<br>22.22 (4/18)<br>77.78 (14/18) | 0.74 (12/1612)<br>8.68 (140/1612)<br>90.57 (1460/1612) | 0.125 |
| 1 January 2022–5 May 2023 | 0.96 (25/2596)<br>7.82 (203/2596)<br>91.22 (2368/2596) | 0 (0/186)<br>13.44 (25/186)<br>86.56 (161/186) | 1.04 (25/2410)<br>7.39 (178/2410)<br>91.58 (2207/2410) | **0.005** |
| Overall | 0.95 (58/6120)<br>8.17 (500/6120)<br>90.88 (5562/6120) | 0.83 (2/240)<br>17.5 (42/240)<br>81.67 (196/240) | 0.95 (56/5880)<br>7.79 (458/5880)<br>91.26 (5366/5880) | **<0.001** |

**(b)**

| | Cesarean Section | | | Induced Labor | | |
|---|---|---|---|---|---|---|
| **Period of study** | **COVID-19<br>% (n/N¹)** | **No COVID-19<br>% (n/N²)** | ***p*-value** | **COVID-19<br>% (n/N¹)** | **No COVID-19<br>% (n/N²)** | ***p*-value** |
| 4 March 2020–28 February 2021 | 36.1 (13/36) | 23.3 (433/1858) | 0.072 | 47.2 (17/36) | 40.3 (749/1858) | 0.441 |
| 1 March 2021–31 December 2021 | 33.3 (6/18) | 23.8 (384/1612) | 0.181 | 66.7 (12/18) | 41.1 (662/1612) | **0.028** |
| 1 January 2022–5 May 2023 | 27.4 (51/186) | 24.1 (582/2410) | 0.321 | 41.4 (77/186) | 34.9 (842/2410) | 0.075 |
| Overall | 29.2 (70/240) | 23.8 (1399/5880) | 0.052 | 44.2 (106/240) | 38.3 (2253/5880) | 0.521 |

[a] Data are presented as percentages (%), number of events (n), and total number of cases (N). $N^1$: total number of deliveries in women with COVID-19; $N^2$: total number of deliveries in women without COVID-19. In bold: $p < 0.05$.

Cesarean section rates were higher in COVID-19 pregnancies across all periods, although the differences were not statistically significant: 36.1% vs. 23.3% in Period 1 ($p = 0.072$); 33.3% vs. 23.8% in Period 2 ($p = 0.181$); and 27.4% vs. 24.1% in Period 3 ($p = 0.321$). The overall cesarean section rate approached statistical significance: 29.2% vs. 23.8% ($p = 0.052$).

The induction of labor was also more frequent among patients with COVID-19 across all periods: 47.2% vs. 40.3% in Period 1 ($p = 0.411$), 66.7% vs. 41.1% in Period 2 ($p = 0.028$), and 41.5% vs. 34.9% in Period 3 ($p = 0.075$). Table 1 presents detailed data on cesarean sections and labor inductions for each phase.

### 3.3. Epidemiological and Clinical Characteristics in Pregnant Women with COVID-19: Admitted vs. Non-Admitted

Of the 249 pregnant women included, 32 (12.9%) required hospitalization due to COVID-19. Table 2 summarizes the epidemiological characteristics, comorbidities, clinical symptoms, complications, and outcomes among the pregnant women with COVID-19 evaluated in the emergency department, comparing those who were admitted to those who were not. The proportion of admissions was higher during the first and second periods of the study (37.0% and 15.6% vs. 12.4% and 6.9%), whereas it was lower in the third period (46.9% vs. 80.6%; $p < 0.001$). A history of pulmonary disease was significantly more frequent among admitted pregnant women (15.6% vs. 5.1%, $p = 0.04$).

**Table 2.** Epidemiological characteristics, comorbidities, clinical symptoms, complications, and outcomes in pregnant women hospitalized with COVID-19.

| | **Overall (n = 249) % (n/N) [a]** | **Non-Admitted (n = 217) % (n/N) [a]** | **Admitted (n = 32) % (n/N) [a]** | ***p*-Value** |
|---|---|---|---|---|
| **Age**. Mdn (IQR) | 32 (26–36) | 31 (26–36) | 33 (27.5–36.5) | 0.251 |
| **Country of birth** | | | | |
| Spain | 62.7 (156/249) | 64.5 (140/217) | 50 (16/32) | 0.113 |
| South America | 21.7 (54/249) | 20.7 (45/217) | 28.1 (9/32) | |
| Africa | 12.4 (31/249) | 11.1 (24/217) | 21.9 (7/32) | |
| Europe | 2.8 (7/249) | 3.2 (7/217) | 0 (0/32) | |
| **Period of study** | | | | **<0.001** |
| 4 March 2020–28 February 2021 | 15.7 (39/249) | 12.4 (27/217) | 37.5 (12/32) | |
| 1 March 2021–31 December 2021 | 8.0 (20/249) | 6.9 (15/217) | 15.6 (5/32) | |
| 1 January 2022–5 May 2023 | 76.3 (190/249) | 80.6 (175/217) | 46.9 (15/32) | |
| **Comorbidities** | | | | |
| Obesity * | 20.6 (50/243) | 20.9 (44/211) | 19.4 (6/31) | 0.847 |
| Pulmonary disease | 6.4 (16/249) | 5.1 (11/217) | 15.6 (5/32) | **0.040** |
| Other comorbidities ** | 26.9 (67/249) | 25.8 (56/217) | 34.4 (11/32) | 0.308 |
| **Clinical symptoms** | | | | |
| Fever | 40.5 (94/232) | 36.5 (73/200) | 65.6 (21/32) | **<0.001** |
| Cough | 32 (74/231) | 27 (54/200) | 64.5 (20/31) | **<0.001** |
| Myalgia | 19.8 (46/232 | 17.5 (35/200) | 34.4 (11/32) | **0.026** |
| Odynophagia | 18.1 (42/232) | 14.5 (29/200) | 40.6 (13/32) | **<0.001** |
| Dyspnea | 12 (28/233) | 4.5 (9/201) | 59.4 (19/32) | **<0.001** |
| Anosmia | 3.4 (8/233) | 2 (4/201) | 12.5 (4/32) | **0.014** |
| **Clinical complications** | | | | |
| Bilateral pneumonia | 10.0 (25/249) | 0 (0/217) | 25 (8/32) | **<0.001** |
| Thromboembolism | 0.4 (1/249) | 0.5 (1/217) | 0 (0/32) | 1.000 |
| **Outcomes** | | | | |
| Admission ICU | 1.2 (3/248) | 0 (0/217) | 9.7 (3/31) | **0.002** |
| NIMV | 0.8 (2/248) | 0 (0/217) | 6.4 (2/31) | **0.015** |
| Death | 0.4 (1/248) | 0 (0/217) | 3.2 (1/31) | 0.120 |

[a] Data are presented as percentages (%), number of events (n), and total number of events (N). Continuous variables are shown as median (Mdn) and interquartile range (IQR) * BMI $\geq$ 30. ** Other comorbidities: chronic hypertension, pregestational diabetes, or history of previous spontaneous abortion. Abbreviations: Mdn, median; IQR, interquartile range; NIMV, non-invasive mechanical ventilation; ICU, intensive care unit. In bold: $p < 0.05$.

COVID-19-related symptoms (such as fever, cough, myalgia, odynophagia, dyspnea, and anosmia) were more commonly reported in hospitalized women. Notably, pneumonia was diagnosed in 25% of admitted patients, whereas none of the non-admitted patients developed pneumonia ($p < 0.001$).

### 3.4. Obstetric Outcomes in Pregnant Women with COVID-19: Admitted vs. Non-Admitted

Obstetric outcomes according to hospitalization status are detailed in Table 3. Hospitalized pregnant women were more frequently at earlier gestational ages (<24 and 24–34 weeks) and less commonly at ≥ 35 weeks compared to non-hospitalized women ($p = 0.037$).

**Table 3.** Comparative analysis of obstetric outcomes according to hospital admission.

| | **Overall (n = 249) % (n/N) [a]** | **Non-Admitted (n = 217) % (n/N) [a]** | **Admitted (n = 32) % (n/N) [a]** | ***p*-Value** |
|---|---|---|---|---|
| **Gestational age at the time of infection** | | | | |
| Mdn (IQR) | 32 (22–38) | 32 (21–38) | 29.50 (23.75–34.5) | 0.160 |
| <24 weeks | 27.6 (68/246) | 28 (60/214) | 25 (8/32) | **0.037** |
| 24–34 weeks | 30.9 (76/246) | 28 (60/214) | 50 (16/32) | |
| ≥35 weeks | 41.5 (102/246) | 43.9 (94/214) | 25 (8/32) | |
| **Obstetric history** | | | | |
| Number of pregnancies, Mdn (IQR) | 2 (1–3) | 2 (1–3) | 2 (1–3.75) | 0.657 |
| Number of previous miscarriages | 30.1 (75/249) | 30.9 (67/217) | 25 (8/32) | 0.499 |
| Previous vaginal deliveries | 38.2 (95/249) | 38.7 (84/217) | 34.4 (11/32) | 0.637 |
| Previous cesarean sections | 15.8 (39/247) | 15.3 (33/216) | 19.4 (6/31) | 0.598 |
| **Pregnancy complications** | | | | |
| Gestational diabetes | 11.2 (28/249) | 11.5 (25/217) | 9.4 (3/32) | 1.000 |
| Hypertensive disorders | 9.2 (23/249) | 8.8 (19/217) | 12.5 (4/32) | 0.520 |
| Threatened of preterm labor | 5.4 (13/217) | 5.7 (12/210) | 3.2 (1/31) | 1.000 |
| Fetal pathology * | 5 (12/242) | 4.8 (10/210) | 6.3 (2/32) | 0.663 |
| **Delivery outcomes** | | | | |
| Gestational age at birth, weeks. Mdn. (IQR) | 39 (26–38) | 39 (37–40) | 38 (37–39) | 0.251 |
| <34 weeks | 4.6 (11/240) | 3.8 (8/208) | 9.4 (3/32) | 0.121 |
| ≥34 weeks | 95.4 (229/240) | 96.2 (200/208) | 90.6 (29/32) | 0.168 |
| Term delivery | 86.7 (216/249) | 87.1 (189/217) | 84.4 (27/32) | 0.437 |
| Induced labor | 42.2 (105/249) | 39.6 (86/217) | 59.4 (19/32) | **0.023** |
| Unsatisfactory intrapartum fetal cardiotocography | 11.3 (26/230) | 10.6 (21/199) | 16.1 (5/31) | 0.363 |
| Cesarean section | 27.7 (69/249) | 24.9 (54/217) | 46.9 (15/32) | **0.009** |
| Postpartum hemorrhage | 4.9 (11/224) | 5.1 (10/195) | 3.4 (1/29) | 1.000 |
| **Maternal complications** | | | | |
| Maternal blood transfusion | 0.4 (1/239) | 0.5 (1/207) | 0 (0/32) | 1.000 |
| Maternal admission to ICU | 1.3 (3/238) | 0 (0/207) | 9.7 (3/31) | **0.002** |
| Postpartum fever | 2.5 (6/239) | 2.9 (6/207) | 0 (0/32) | 1.000 |

[a] Data are presented as percentages (%), number of events (n), and total number of events (N). Continuous variables are shown as median (Mdn) and interquartile range (IQR). * Fetal pathology: includes congenital malformations and/or fetal growth abnormalities. Abbreviations: Mdn: median; IQR: interquartile range; ICU: intensive care unit. In bold: $p < 0.05$.

The obstetric history and pregnancy-related complications were similar in both groups. However, the rates of induced labor (59.4% vs. 39.6%, $p = 0.023$) and cesarean section (46.9% vs. 24.9%, $p = 0.009$) were significantly higher in hospitalized patients. Maternal admission to the intensive care unit (ICU) due to pregnancy-related complications from COVID-19 occurred exclusively in admitted women (9.7% vs. 0%, $p < 0.002$). Full results are provided in Table 3.

### 3.5. Neonatal Outcomes in Pregnant Women with COVID-19: Admitted vs. Non-Admitted

Birth weight did not differ significantly between groups. However, neonates born to hospitalized mothers had significantly lower Apgar scores at 1 min (18.7% vs. 2.9%, $p < 0.001$), higher NICU admission (25.8% vs. 8.2%, $p = 0.007$), and more neonatal complications (23.3% vs. 7.7%, $p = 0.015$). Detailed findings are shown in Table 4.

**Table 4.** Characteristics of newborns of pregnant women with COVID-19 according to hospital admission.

| | **Overall % (n/N) [a]** | **Non-Admitted % (n/N) [a]** | **Admitted % (n/N) [a]** | ***p*-Value** |
|---|---|---|---|---|
| Birth weight; g | | | | |
| Mdn (IQR) | 3168 (2920–3501) | 3248 (2937–3542) | 3.090 (2837–3535) | 0.132 |
| <2500 g | 6.3 (15/223) | 5.8 (12/194) | 9.4 (3/29) | 0.433 |
| Apgar 1 score (1st min) | | | | **<0.001** |
| <7 | 5.0 (12/240) | 2.9 (6/208) | 18.7 (6/32) | |
| ≥7 | 95.0 (228/240) | 97.1 (202/208) | 81.3 (26/32) | |
| Apgar score (5th min) | | | | **0.133** |
| <7 | 0.4 (1/240) | 0 | 3.1 (1/32) | |
| ≥7 | 99.6 (239/240) | 100 (208/208) | 96.9 (31/32) | |
| Newborn admitted in NICU | 10.5 (25/238) | 8.2 (17/207) | 25.8 (8/31) | **0.007** |
| Neonatal complications * | 9.7 (23/237) | 7.7 (16/207) | 23.3 (7/30) | **0.015** |
| Umbilical arterial pH | 7.25 (7.24–7.27) | 7.25 (7.24–7.28) | 7.25 (7.23–7.29) | 0.921 |
| Umbilical venous pH | 7.33 (7.27–7.37) | 7.33 (7.28–7.36) | 7.32 (7.28–7.34) | 0.585 |

[a] Data are presented as percentages (%), number of events (n), and total number of events (N). Continuous variables are shown as median (Mdn) and interquartile range (IQR). * Neonatal complications include respiratory distress syndrome, necrotizing enterocolitis, neonatal sepsis, and hypoxic–ischemic encephalopathy. Abbreviations: Mdn: median; IQR: interquartile range; NICU: neonatal intensive care unit. In bold: $p < 0.05$.

### 3.6. Risk Factors for Severe COVID-19 Among Pregnant Women Admitted

Of the 32 pregnant women who were hospitalized, clinical data were unavailable for one patient. Therefore, the analysis included 31 women, of whom 5 (16.1%) experienced a severe episode, defined as ICU admission (n = 3), requirement for invasive or non-invasive mechanical ventilation (IMV/NIMV) (n = 5), and/or death (n = 1). The mean length of hospital stay for these patients was 15.4 days (SD ± 22.6).

Risk factors significantly associated with severe COVID-19 included non-Spanish nationality (100% vs. 38.5%, $p = 0.018$) and obesity (60% vs. 12%, $p = 0.041$). Detailed data are presented in Table 5.

**Table 5.** Risk factors for severe COVID-19 in hospitalized pregnant women.

| | **Severe COVID-19 % (n/N) [a]** | **Non-Severe COVID-19 % (n/N) [a]** | **Crude OR** | ***p*-Value** |
|---|---|---|---|---|
| Age ≥ 35 years | 0 (0/5) | 38.5 (10/26) | NA | 0.147 |
| Gestational age at delivery, (weeks) | | | | 1.000 |
| <35 | 80.0 (4/5) | 74.1 (20/27) | 1 | |
| ≥35 | 20.0 (1/5) | 27.9 (7/26) | 0.71 (0.07–7.6) | |

**Table 5.** *Cont.*

| | Severe COVID-19 % (n/N) [a] | Non-Severe COVID-19 % (n/N) [a] | Crude OR | *p*-Value |
|---|---|---|---|---|
| Born in Spain | 0 (0/5) | 61.5 (16/26) | NA | **0.018** |
| **Comorbidities** | | | | |
| Obesity * | 60.0 (3/5) | 12.0 (3/25) | 11.0 (1.27–95) | **0.041** |
| Pulmonary diseases | 20.0 (1/5) | 11.5 (3/26) | 1.91 (0.15–23) | 0.525 |
| Hypertension | 0 | 15.4 (4/26) | NA | 1.000 |
| **Clinical presentation** | | | | |
| Fever | 100 (5/5) | 61.5 (16/26) | NA | 0.147 |
| Cough | 75.0 (3/4) | 65.4 (17/26) | 1.58 (0.14–17) | 1.000 |
| Odynophagia | 6.0 (3/5) | 38.5 (10/26) | 2.40 (0.33–17) | 0.625 |
| Anosmia | 0 (0/5) | 15.4 (4/26) | NA | 1.000 |
| Dyspnea | 100 (5/5) | 53.8 (14/26) | NA | 0.128 |
| Myalgia | 60 (3/5) | 30.8 (8/26) | 3.37 (0.46–24) | 0.317 |
| **Treatment** | | | | |
| LMWH | 80 (4/5) | 84.6 (22/26) | 0.77 (0.64–8.31) | 1.000 |
| Steroid | 100 (5/5) | 26.9 (7/26) | NA | **0.005** |
| **Complication/outcome** | | | | |
| Bilateral pneumonia | 100 (5/5) | 11.5 (3/26) | NA | **<0.001** |
| Thromboembolism | 0 | 3.8 (1/26) | NA | 1.000 |
| Death | 20 (1/5) | 0 | NA | 0.161 |

[a] Data are presented as percentages (%), number of events (n), and total number of events (N). Continuous variables are expressed as median (Mdn) and interquartile range (IQR). * BMI $\geq$ 30. Abbreviations: LMWH, low-molecular-weight heparin. In bold: $p < 0.05$.

### 3.7. *Effect of Vaccination on Hospital Admission in Pregnant Women*

Among the hospitalized pregnant women, 71.9% were unvaccinated, compared to 56.2% of those not admitted who had received at least one dose of a COVID-19 vaccine. This difference was statistically significant (OR = 0.30; 95% CI: 0.13–0.69), indicating a protective effect of vaccination against hospital admission. Detailed results are provided in Table 6.

**Table 6.** Comparative analysis of hospital admissions according to vaccination status.

| | Overall % (n/N) [a] | Non-Admitted % (n/N) [a] | Admitted % (n/N) [a] | *p*-Value |
|---|---|---|---|---|
| **Vaccination status** | | | | |
| Not vaccinated | 47.4 (118/249) | 43.8 (95/217) | 71.9 (23/32) | **0.003** |
| Vaccinated (1 or 2 doses) | 52.6 (131/249) | 56.2 (122/217) | 28.1 (9/32) | |

[a] Data are presented as percentages (%), number of events (n), and total number (N). In bold: $p < 0.05$.

## 4. Discussion

This study provides important insights into the clinical characteristics, obstetric outcomes, and neonatal complications associated with COVID-19 among pregnant women in Spain, a country that experienced a particularly high burden of infections and hospitalizations during the pandemic. Although the overall incidence of COVID-19 in our cohort remained relatively low, it increased markedly during the Omicron wave, likely due to the relaxation of public health measures and the higher transmissibility of this variant. Severe maternal infection was associated with complications such as preeclampsia, preterm birth, and cesarean delivery, emphasizing the importance of close maternal monitoring. Neonatal outcomes—particularly NICU admissions—were more frequent among neonates born to women with severe disease, consistent with previous studies [6].

Additionally, COVID-19 vaccination emerged as a protective factor against severe disease and hospitalization, underscoring the importance of immunization during pregnancy.

### *4.1. Prevalence and Incidence of COVID-19*

The incidence of COVID-19 among pregnant women during the study period (11 March 2020–5 May 2023), based on total deliveries, was 4.1%. However, this rate is lower than that reported in other studies. For instance, a meta-analysis [5] found an incidence of up to 10% among pregnant women who presented to or were admitted to hospitals during the early stages of the pandemic. Similarly, a large retrospective cohort study by Son et al. [13] reported an SARS-CoV-2 positivity rate of 6.9% in pregnant women between March and December 2020.

The lower incidence observed in our study may be explained by our inclusion criteria, which focused on pregnant women who received hospital care for COVID-19-related symptoms—representing more severe cases—rather than on all pregnant women with COVID-19. This likely excluded many asymptomatic or mildly symptomatic cases managed in outpatient settings.

By pandemic phase, incidence rates were 20.6 and 12.3 per 1000 deliveries during the first and second phases, respectively, closely aligning with Donati et al. [14], who reported rates of 23.5 and 16.6 per 1000 deliveries during the same periods. However, a substantial increase was observed during the third phase, with the incidence rate rising to 73.2 per 1000 deliveries. These findings are consistent with data from England, where a population-based study by Vousden et al. [15] confirmed increases in infection and disease severity during the Delta and Omicron waves compared to the wild-type and Alpha variants. This surge is likely attributable to the combination of relaxed public health measures and the greater transmissibility of the Omicron variant compared to previous strains.

In relation to SARS-CoV-2 variants, studies such as the Italian study by Incognito et al. [11] found that the Delta variant was linked to the most severe maternal and neonatal outcomes, including higher rates of ICU admission, preterm birth, and mortality. Alpha showed intermediate severity, while Omicron was associated with milder disease.

### *4.2. Obstetric Outcomes: COVID-19 vs. Non-COVID-19 Pregnancies*

Over the 3 years and 2 months of the COVID-19 pandemic covered by this study, we observed an increased incidence of preterm birth among pregnant women with SARS-CoV-2 infection. Although this rate declined across pandemic waves, it remained elevated during the third wave (13.44%), compared to the 8.43% observed among non-infected pregnant women. These results align with prior studies reporting an increased risk of preterm delivery associated with SARS-CoV-2 infection, particularly during the initial phases of the pandemic [9,14,16]. Our findings are also consistent with Seaton et al. [17], who reported a reduced preterm birth rate during the Omicron period compared to earlier waves. This reduction may be attributed to the lower virulence of the Omicron variant and the protective effect of COVID-19 vaccination, as highlighted by Hui et al. [18].

The relationship between COVID-19 and the mode of delivery has evolved over time. Early in the pandemic, some studies reported an increased rate of cesarean sections [11,17,19]. However, more recent evidence has not supported a significant association between SARS-CoV-2 infection and delivery mode [6,14,20]. The results of our study are consistent with the latter body of evidence, as we did not observe a statistically significant increase in cesarean deliveries among infected pregnant women.

The impact of SARS-CoV-2 infection on labor induction has been less extensively studied. In our cohort, a rising trend in induction rates was observed among infected pregnant women, reaching statistical significance exclusively during the second wave of the pandemic. Other authors have similarly reported increased rates of labor induction and planned cesarean sections among pregnant women with moderate-to-severe COVID-19 [21,22]. This trend probably indicates the need for closer monitoring and proactive obstetric management in infected patients.

### 4.3. Epidemiological Characteristics and Clinical Outcomes: Admitted vs. Non-Admitted Pregnant Women

In our cohort, 12.9% of pregnant women diagnosed with COVID-19 required hospitalization due to the infection. A significant variation in hospitalization rates was observed across different phases of the pandemic, with more admissions during the first and third waves.

A single case of maternal death was reported, corresponding to a maternal mortality rate of 0.4%, which is comparable to the 0.1% reported by Jering et al. [23]. However, the overall in-hospital mortality rate among pregnant women in our cohort was 3.1%, notably higher than the 1.1% reported by Pineles et al. [7]. This discrepancy may be attributable to the timing of infection, as most severe cases in our cohort occurred during the early phase of the pandemic, when clinical experience and evidence-based management strategies were still evolving [24].

All COVID–19-related symptoms—including fever, cough, sore throat, anosmia, dyspnea, and myalgia—were significantly more frequent among hospitalized patients. Bilateral pneumonia was diagnosed exclusively in this group, affecting 25% of those admitted. A history of preexisting respiratory disease was also identified as a risk factor for hospitalization. As expected, patients requiring admission had more severe clinical presentations and symptomatologies.

### 4.4. Obstetric Outcomes: Admitted vs. Non-Admitted Pregnant Women

In our study, 75% of hospitalized pregnant women had a gestational age of less than 35 weeks at the time of admission. In contrast to our findings, previous studies, such as those by Lassi et al. [3] and Donati et al. [14], have reported higher infection and hospitalization rates during the second and third trimesters.

Our data did not demonstrate a significantly higher frequency of obstetric complications among hospitalized pregnant women with COVID-19 compared to those who were not admitted. The preeclampsia rate in hospitalized patients was 12.5%, higher than the 8.8% observed in the non-hospitalized group, although this difference did not reach statistical significance. Several studies have established an association between SARS-CoV-2 infection and an increased risk of preeclampsia, particularly in severe cases, as shown in meta-analyses by Wei et al. [9] and Conde-Agudelo et al. [25]. The limited number of preeclampsia cases in our cohort may have reduced the ability to detect significant differences.

We found that pregnant women with COVID-19 who required hospitalization had a significantly higher rate of cesarean delivery and labor induction. These findings may indicate that deliveries were expedited due to maternal complications associated with infection. While most studies have not identified a consistent association between COVID-19 infection and mode of delivery [6,14,20], some evidence suggests that cesarean birth is more common in cases of moderate to higher disease severity [18], which is consistent with our results.

We also observed a higher incidence of preterm birth among hospitalized pregnant women (15.6% vs. 8.8%), although this difference did not reach statistical significance, likely due to the relatively small number of hospitalized patients. Nonetheless, the existing literature consistently reports increased odds of preterm birth in pregnancies complicated by SARS-CoV-2 infection, particularly in cases involving moderate-to-severe illness [9,

20,26]. A national study conducted in Slovakia analyzed SARS-CoV-2 positive cases throughout the entire pandemic period (March 2020–May 2023), also reporting an increased incidence of cesarean deliveries and preterm births among pregnant women infected [8].

As expected, the need for ICU admission was greater among hospitalized patients, further reflecting the more severe clinical course of the infection. The ICU admission rate in our cohort was 9.7%, slightly lower than the 12.8% reported by Metz et al. [20].

### *4.5. Neonatal Outcomes in Pregnant Women with COVID-19: Admitted vs. Non-Admitted Pregnancies*

Meta-analyses by Allotey et al. [5] and Smith et al. [12] have reported a significant increase in neonatal mortality among infants born to mothers with COVID-19. Specifically, Allotey et al. [5] documented a neonatal mortality rate of 0.5%. In our study, no neonatal deaths were recorded during the study period. However, neonates born to women hospitalized with COVID-19 exhibited a higher incidence of adverse outcomes, including lower 1 min Apgar scores, increased rates of NICU admission, and a greater frequency of neonatal complications. These findings are consistent with previous studies that have also documented elevated NICU admission rates among neonates born to women with SARS-CoV-2 infection, particularly in cases of severe maternal illness [5,6,20,26]. A meta-analysis by Deng et al. [27] further supports this, showing that neonates born during periods dominated by more transmissible variants—such as Delta and Omicron—had significantly higher risks of adverse outcomes, including NICU admission and respiratory complications, compared to those born during the early (wild-type) phase of the pandemic.

In contrast to the findings of Berumen-Lechuga et al. [26], who reported significantly lower neonatal birth weights in pregnancies complicated by severe COVID-19, our study did not identify any statistically significant differences in birth weight between neonates born to hospitalized and non-hospitalized mothers.

Our findings are consistent with reports from other European countries, where the pandemic has been shown to negatively affect not only obstetric and neonatal outcomes but also the psychological well-being of pregnant individuals (e.g., increased anxiety, stress, and depressive symptoms) [28–30]. These studies support the need for comprehensive perinatal care that addresses both medical and psychological aspects during pandemics.

### *4.6. Severity of COVID-19 in Hospitalized Pregnant Women*

The rate of severe COVID-19 in our study—defined as ICU admission, mechanical ventilation, and/or maternal death—was 16.1%, slightly higher than the rates reported by Boettcher et al. [6] (5.4–12%) and Schell et al. [31] (10%). Other authors, such as Jering et al. [23], have described lower rates (3.3%) among women admitted for delivery.

In our cohort, obesity (BMI $\geq$ 30) and non-Spanish nationality were significantly associated with severe cases of COVID-19. Obesity has also been identified as a risk factor for severe disease in pregnant populations, as documented in multiple studies [5,12,32]. Our findings also align with those of Donati et al. [14] and Engjom et al. [32], who identified that foreign nationality—particularly among migrant women—was associated with an increased risk of adverse maternal outcomes. Nevertheless, it must be taken into account that, while nationality was associated with an increased risk of severe maternal COVID-19 in our study, it likely serves as a proxy for unmeasured structural and social factors, such as socioeconomic disadvantage, migrant status, language or cultural barriers, and access to healthcare. It should not be interpreted as a biological or ethnic determinant, and future research should incorporate more nuanced indicators of social and ethnic vulnerability to better understand these disparities.

Additionally, a study conducted in the United States in 2023 [6] identified several pregestational comorbidities, including diabetes, hypertension, and cardiovascular disease, as significant risk factors for maternal mortality, which were included within the definition of severe COVID-19 in our study. However, in our cohort, these comorbidities did not reach statistical significance, possibly due to the limited number of severe cases in our study.

### *4.7. Vaccination*

Vaccination against SARS-CoV-2 was identified as a protective factor against COVID-19-related hospitalization in our cohort. A significantly higher proportion of hospitalized pregnant women were unvaccinated. This finding is consistent with previous studies that have recognized unvaccinated status as a significant risk factor for the development of severe COVID-19 during pregnancy [26,32].

In our study, 62.2% of pregnant women had received at least one dose of a COVID-19 vaccine. By the end of the second wave of the pandemic, vaccination coverage among pregnant women varied widely across Europe, ranging from 20% in Lombardy, Italy, to 80% in Norway [32,33]. These differences in vaccination uptake highlight the need for consistent international guidance. In its 2024 interim guidance, the World Health Organization reaffirmed that COVID-19 vaccination during pregnancy is both safe and strongly recommended, particularly for women at high risk of severe disease [34].

These findings reinforce the importance of promoting COVID-19 vaccination among pregnant women, particularly in light of ongoing viral mutations and potential future waves. Recent evidence also supports the safety and effectiveness of booster doses during pregnancy. In a recent multicenter study, Barros et al. [35] reported that newborns of booster-vaccinated mothers had a significantly lower risk of SARS-CoV-2 infection, as well as reduced rates of preterm birth, neonatal respiratory distress, and NICU stay.

Lastly, it is important to note that although our results suggest a protective effect of COVID-19 vaccination during pregnancy, detailed data regarding the number of doses received, type of vaccine administered, and gestational timing were not consistently available due to limitations in retrospective documentation. This limits the depth of our analysis and should be considered when interpreting the findings.

### *4.8. Strengths and Limitations*

A major strength of this study is its focus on the epidemiological and clinical impact of COVID-19 in pregnant women in Spain, a country that experienced one of the highest burdens of infection, hospitalization, and mortality during the pandemic. While extensive data exist regarding the general population, obstetric outcomes related to COVID-19 in Spain have remained underexplored. This study helps fill that gap by providing valuable longitudinal data on maternal and neonatal outcomes across multiple phases of the pandemic, contributing to a more comprehensive understanding of the obstetric implications of SARS-CoV-2 infection in a high-risk setting.

However, several limitations must be acknowledged. First, this was a single-center (monocentric) study conducted at a tertiary-care hospital, which may limit the generalizability of the findings to other settings or healthcare systems. Second, due to its retrospective nature, data collection relied on the accuracy and completeness of medical records, which may have resulted in missing, inconsistent, or erroneous information. Third, selection bias is possible, as case identification depended on available documentation and coding, which may have led to missed or misclassified cases. For all the reasons mentioned above, and although we acknowledge the importance of adjusted models for controlling potential confusion, multivariable logistic regression was not performed due to limitations in data completeness and the small number of events for certain outcomes, which could have compromised the reliability of the estimates. This represents an inherent limitation of our retrospective design and should be taken into account when interpreting the findings.

Lastly, given that the study was conducted at a single tertiary referral center specializing in high-risk pregnancies, the study population may disproportionately represent moderate-to-severe cases of COVID-19. As a result, mild or asymptomatic cases—particularly those managed in outpatient settings—may be underrepresented, potentially limiting the generalizability of the findings.

Another important point to consider is that some comparisons—particularly those involving subgroups such as hospitalized patients—may have lacked sufficient statistical power to detect significant differences due to limited sample sizes. This limitation should be taken into account when interpreting nonsignificant results, as a type II error cannot be ruled out. This aspect has been addressed throughout the Section 4. Moreover, it is important to acknowledge that this study spans a four-year period, during which significant changes were introduced in the clinical management of COVID-19, including the availability of vaccination and updates in treatment protocols. These evolving healthcare strategies may have influenced the observed obstetric and neonatal outcomes across different phases of the pandemic. This limitation should be taken into account when interpreting the results, as the heterogeneity in clinical practices over time may have introduced confounding factors.

Additional limitations include the lack of genomic confirmation for SARS-CoV-2 variant classification, which was based on prevailing epidemiological phases, given that routine genomic sequencing was not available for individual cases during the study period; the absence of long-term follow-up data on neonatal outcomes; and the potential for case misclassification due to reliance on retrospective clinical coding. Moreover, maternal mental health data were not systematically collected, limiting our ability to evaluate the psychological dimension of COVID-19 during pregnancy, which has been associated with adverse outcomes, such as preterm birth, low birth weight, and increased NICU admission. These limitations should be considered when interpreting the findings and their generalizability.

Further multicenter studies with broader geographic representation and prospective designs are warranted to confirm these findings and guide global obstetric management in future pandemics or SARS-CoV-2 resurgence scenarios.

## 5. Conclusions

This study demonstrates that hospital admission due to COVID-19 during pregnancy is associated with an increased risk of adverse obstetric and neonatal outcomes. Specifically, higher rates of preterm birth, labor induction, and cesarean delivery were observed among hospitalized women. Moreover, neonates born to these patients experienced more complications, including lower 1 min Apgar scores and increased NICU admission rates. These findings underscore the need for vigilant monitoring, early intervention, and the promotion of COVID-19 vaccination during pregnancy to mitigate risks for both mothers and newborns.

**Author Contributions:** Conceptualization, investigation, formal analysis, and project administration, M.-A.Q.-C. and J.-M.R.-R.; investigation and data curation, M.-V.S.-R. and M.P.-G.; writing—original draft preparation, M.-A.Q.-C.; methodology, visualization, and writing—review and editing, M.-A.Q.-C., A.-M.P.-M., and J.-M.R.-R.; supervision, A.-M.P.-M. and J.-M.R.-R. All authors have read and agreed to the published version of the manuscript.

**Funding:** This manuscript was supported by funding from the Alicante Institute for Health and Biomedical Research (ISABIAL) for its publication.

**Institutional Review Board Statement:** This study was conducted in accordance with the Declaration of Helsinki of 1975, which was revised in 2013. The study protocol was approved by the Ethics Committee of Alicante Health Department-General Hospital, with project identification code CEIm PI2024-036/ISABIAL 2024-0049, and date of approval 7 March 2024.

**Informed Consent Statement:** Patient consent was waived due to the nature of the research: a retrospective, observational study with a large sample size and wide temporal range, which made it impossible to obtain consent from all study participants. The Ethics Committee of the Health Department of Alicante-General Hospital approved the exemption from informed consent according to the protocol presented, given the characteristics of the study.

**Data Availability Statement:** The original contributions presented in this study are included in the article. Further inquiries can be directed to the corresponding author.

**Conflicts of Interest:** The authors declare no conflicts of interest.

## Abbreviations

The following abbreviations are used in this manuscript:

| | |
|---|---|
| BMI | Body mass index |
| CI | Confidence interval |
| DBGUH | Doctor Balmis General University Hospital |
| ICU | Intensive care unit |
| IMV | Invasive mechanical ventilation |
| IQR | Interquartile range |
| IUGR | Intrauterine growth restriction |
| LMWH | Low-molecular-weight heparin |
| Mdn | Median |
| NICU | Neonatal intensive care unit |
| NIMV | Non-invasive mechanical ventilation |
| OR | Odds ratio |
| RT-PCR | Reverse transcription polymerase chain reaction |
| SD | Standard deviation |
| SGA | Small for gestational age |
| WHO | World Health Organization |

## References


1. Ellington, S.; Strid, P.; Tong, V.T.; Woodworth, K.; Galang, R.R.; Zambrano, L.D.; Nahabedian, J.; Anderson, K.; Gilboa, S.M. Characteristics of Women of Reproductive Age with Laboratory-Confirmed SARS-CoV-2 Infection by Pregnancy Status—United States, January 22–June 7, 2020. *MMWR Morb. Mortal. Wkly. Rep.* **2020**, *69*, 769–775. [CrossRef] [PubMed]
2. Royal College of Obstetricians and Gynaecologists. *Coronavirus (COVID-19) Infection in Pregnancy. Information for healthcare professionals*; Version 16; RCOG: London, UK, 2022.
3. Lassi, Z.S.; Ana, A.; Das, J.K.; Salam, R.A.; Padhani, Z.A.; Irfan, O.; Bhutta, Z.A. A systematic review and meta-analysis of data on pregnant women with confirmed COVID-19: Clinical presentation, and pregnancy and perinatal outcomes based on COVID-19 severity. *J. Glob. Health.* **2021**, *11*, 05018. [CrossRef] [PubMed]
4. Molina, R.L.; Tsai, T.C.; Dai, D.; Soto, M.; Rosenthal, N.; Orav, E.J.; Figueroa, J.F. Comparison of Pregnancy and Birth Outcomes Before vs During the COVID-19 Pandemic. *JAMA Netw. Open.* **2022**, *5*, e2226531. [CrossRef] [PubMed]
5. Allotey, J.; Stallings, E.; Bonet, M.; Yap, M.; Chatterjee, S.; Kew, T.; Debenham, L.; Llavall, A.C.; Dixit, A.; Zhou, D.; et al. Clinical manifestations, risk factors, and maternal and perinatal outcomes of coronavirus disease 2019 in pregnancy: Living systematic review and meta-analysis. *BMJ* **2020**, *370*, m3320. [CrossRef] [PubMed]
6. Boettcher, L.B.; Metz, T.D. Maternal and neonatal outcomes following SARS-CoV-2 infection. *Semin. Fetal Neonatal Med.* **2023**, *28*, 101428. [CrossRef] [PubMed]
7. Pineles, B.L.; Goodman, K.E.; Pineles, L.; O'HAra, L.M.; Nadimpalli, G.; Magder, L.S.; Baghdadi, J.D.; Parchem, J.G.; Harris, A.D. Pregnancy and the Risk of In-Hospital Coronavirus Disease 2019 (COVID-19) Mortality. *Obstet. Gynecol.* **2022**, *139*, 846–854. [CrossRef] [PubMed]

8. Goldbergerová, A.; Kováč, L.; Marcišová, C.; Borovský, M.; Kotríková, D.; Izáková, Ľ.; Mikas, J.; Námešná, J.; Krištúfková, Z.; Krištúfková, A. Assessing the Impact of COVID-19 on Pregnancy and Maternal Outcomes: A Slovak National Study. *Reprod. Med.* **2024**, *5*, 319–334. [CrossRef]
9. Wei, S.Q.; Bilodeau-Bertrand, M.; Liu, S.; Auger, N. The impact of COVID-19 on pregnancy outcomes: A systematic review and meta-analysis. *Can. Med Assoc. J.* **2021**, *193*, E540–E548. [CrossRef] [PubMed]
10. Mullins, E.; Perry, A.; Banerjee, J.; Townson, J.; Grozeva, D.; Milton, R.; Kirby, N.; Playle, R.; Bourne, T.; Lees, C.; et al. Pregnancy and neonatal outcomes of COVID-19: The PAN_COVID study. *Eur. J. Obstet. Gynecol. Reprod. Biol.* **2022**, *276*, 161–167. [CrossRef] [PubMed]
11. Incognito, G.; Distefano, R.E.; Campo, G.; Gulino, F.A.; Gulisano, C.; Gullotta, C.; Gullo, G.; Cucinella, G.; Tuscano, A.; Bruno, M.T.; et al. Comparison of Maternal and Neonatal Outcomes between SARS-CoV-2 Variants: A Retrospective, Monocentric Study. *J. Clin. Med.* **2023**, *12*, 6329. [CrossRef] [PubMed]
12. Smith, E.R.; Oakley, E.; Grandner, G.W.; Rukundo, G.; Farooq, F.; Ferguson, K.; Baumann, S.; Waldorf, K.M.A.; Afshar, Y.; Ahlberg, M.; et al. Clinical risk factors of adverse outcomes among women with COVID-19 in the pregnancy and postpartum period: A sequential, prospective meta-analysis. *Am. J. Obstet. Gynecol.* **2023**, *228*, 161–177. [CrossRef] [PubMed]
13. Son, M.; Gallagher, K.; Lo, J.Y.; Lindgren, E.J.; Burris, H.H.; Dysart, K.; Greenspan, J.; Culhane, J.F.; Handley, S.C.M. Coronavirus Disease 2019 (COVID-19) pandemic and pregnancy outcomes in a U. *S. population. Obstet. Gynecol.* **2021**, *138*, 542–551. [CrossRef] [PubMed]
14. Donati, S.; Corsi, E.; Maraschini, A.; Salvatore, M.A.; the ItOSS-COVID-19 Working Group. SARS-CoV-2 infection among hospitalised pregnant women and impact of different viral strains on COVID-19 severity in Italy: a national prospective population-based cohort study. *BJOG* **2022**, *129*, 221–231. [CrossRef] [PubMed]
15. Vousden, N.; Ramakrishnan, R.; Bunch, K.; Morris, E.; Simpson, N.; Gale, C.; O'Brien, P.; Quigley, M.; Brocklehurst, P.; Kurinczuk, J.J.; et al. Impact of different SARS-CoV-2 variants on maternal and perinatal outcomes: A population-based study in England. *BMJ* **2023**, *381*, e074259. [CrossRef]
16. Chmielewska, B.; Barratt, I.; Townsend, R.; Kalafat, E.; van der Meulen, J.; Gurol-Urganci, I.; O'Brien, P.; Morris, E.; Draycott, T.; Thangaratinam, S.; et al. Effects of the COVID-19 pandemic on maternal and perinatal outcomes: A systematic review and meta-analysis. *Lancet Glob. Health.* **2021**, *9*, e759–e772. [CrossRef] [PubMed]
17. Seaton, C.L.; Cohen, A.; Henninger, E.M.; Gendlina, I.; Hou, W.; Bernstein, P.S.; Duong, T.Q. Coronavirus disease 2019 (COVID-19) perinatal outcomes across the pandemic at an academic medical center in New York City. *Obstet. Gynecol.* **2023**, *141*, 144–151. [CrossRef] [PubMed]
18. Hui, L.; Marzan, M.B.; Rolnik, D.L.; Potenza, S.; Pritchard, N.; Said, J.M.; Palmer, K.R.; Whitehead, C.L.; Sheehan, P.M.; Ford, J.; et al. Reductions on stillbirths and preterm birth in COVID-19 vaccinated women: A multicenter cohort study of vaccination uptake and perinatal outcomes. *Am. J. Obstet. Gynecol.* **2023**, *228*, e1–e585.e16. [CrossRef] [PubMed]
19. Parazzini, F.; Bartolus, R.; Mauri, P.A.; Favilli, A.; Gerli, S.; Ferrazzi, E. Delivery in pregnant women infected with SARS-CoV-2: A fast review. *Int. J. Gynaecol. Obstet.* **2020**, *150*, 41–46. [CrossRef] [PubMed]
20. Metz, T.D.; Clifton, R.G.; Hughes, B.L.; Sandoval, G.J.; Grobman, W.A.; Saade, G.R.; Manuck, T.A.; Longo, M.; Sowles, A.; Clark, K.; et al. Association of SARS-Cov-2 infection with serious maternal morbidity and mortality from obstetric complications. *JAMA* **2022**, *327*, 748–759. [CrossRef] [PubMed]
21. Morán Antolín, E.; Broullón Molanes, J.R.; de la Cruz Conty, M.L.; Pardilla, M.B.E.; Martín, M.d.P.G.; Bueno, J.A.S.; Acebal, L.F.; Recarte, P.P.; Bartolomé, A.Á.; Cendán, J.P.M.; et al. SARS-CoV-2 infection and C-section: A prospective observational study. *Virus* **2021**, *13*, 2330. [CrossRef] [PubMed]
22. Trinh, L.T.T.; Achat, H.M.; Pesce, A. Caesarean sections before and during the COVID-19 pandemic in western Sydney, Australia. *J. Obstet. Gynaecol.* **2023**, *43*, 2265668. [CrossRef] [PubMed]
23. Jering, K.S.; Claggett, B.L.; Cunningham, J.W.; Rosenthal, N.; Vardeny, O.; Greene, M.F.; Solomon, S.D. Clinical characteristics and outcomes of hospitalized women giving birth with and without COVID-19. *JAMA Intern. Med.* **2021**, *181*, 714–717. [CrossRef] [PubMed]
24. Pinargote-Celorio, H.; Moreno-Pérez, Ó.; González-De-La-Aleja, P.; Llenas-García, J.; Pérez-Crespo, P.M.M.; Rodríguez-Díaz, J.-C.; Martínez-López, B.; Gutiérrez, N.M.; Ramos-Rincón, J.-M.; Merino, E. Real-world effectiveness of early anti-SARS therapy in severely immunocompromised COVID-19 outpatients during the SARS-CoV-2 omicron variant era: A propensity score-adjusted retrospective cohort study. *J. Antimicrob. Chemother.* **2024**, *79*, 3248–3253. [CrossRef] [PubMed]
25. Conde-Agudelo, A.; Romero, R. SARS-CoV-2 infection during pregnancy and risk of preeclampsia: A systematic review and meta-analysis. *Am. J. Obstet. Gynecol.* **2022**, *226*, 68–89.e3. [CrossRef] [PubMed]
26. Berumen-Lechuga, M.G.; Leaños-Miranda, A.; Molina-Pérez, C.J.; García-Cortés, L.R.; Palomo-Piñón, S. Risk factors for severe-critical COVID-19 in pregnant women. *J. Clin. Med.* **2023**, *12*, 5812. [CrossRef] [PubMed]

27. Deng, J.; Ma, Y.; Liu, Q.; Du, M.; Liu, M.; Liu, J. Association of infection with different SARS-CoV-2 variants during pregnancy with maternal and perinatal outcomes: A systematic review and meta-analysis. *Int. J. Environ. Res. Public Health* **2022**, *19*, 15932. [CrossRef] [PubMed]
28. La Rosa, V.L.; Oddo-Sommerfeld, S.; Schermelleh-Engel, K.; Commodari, E. From lockdown to cradle: Navigating the psychological challenges of childbirth during the COVID-19 pandemic in Italy–Evidence from a 3-year analysis. *Curr. Psychol.* **2024**, *43*, 35616–35629. [CrossRef]
29. Giesbrecht, G.F.; Rojas, L.; Patel, S.; Kuret, V.; MacKinnon, A.L.; Tomfohr-Madsen, L.; Lebel, C. Fear of COVID-19, mental health, and pregnancy outcomes in the pregnancy during the COVID-19 pandemic study: Fear of COVID-19 and pregnancy outcomes. *J. Affect. Disord.* **2022**, *299*, 483–491. [CrossRef] [PubMed]
30. Tauqeer, F.; Ceulemans, M.; Gerbier, E.; Passier, A.; Oliver, A.; Foulon, V.; Panchaud, A.; Lupattelli, A.; Nordeng, H. Mental health of pregnant and postpartum women during the third wave of the COVID-19 pandemic: A European cross-sectional study. *BMJ Open* **2023**, *13*, e063391. [CrossRef] [PubMed]
31. Schell, R.C.; Macias, D.A.; Garner, W.H.; White, A.M.; McIntire, D.D.; Pruszynski, J.; Adhikari, E.H. Examining the impact of trimester of diagnosis on COVID-19 disease progression in pregnancy. *Am. J. Obstet. Gynecol. MFM.* **2022**, *4*, 100728. [CrossRef] [PubMed]
32. Engjom, H.; Aabakke, A.J.M.; Klungsoyr, K.; Svanvik, T.; Äyräs, O.; Jonasdottir, E.; Thurn, L.; Jones, E.; Pettersson, K.; Nyfløt, L.T.; et al. COVID-19 in pregnancy-characteristics and outcomes of pregnant women admitted to hospital because of SARS-CoV-2 infection in the Nordic countries. *Acta Obstet. Gynecol. Scand.* **2021**, *100*, 1611–1619. [CrossRef] [PubMed]
33. Carbone, L.; Trinchillo, M.G.; Di Girolamo, R.; Raffone, A.; Saccone, G.; Iorio, G.G.; Gabrielli, O.; Maruotti, G.M. COVID-19 vaccine and pregnancy outcomes: A systematic review and meta-analysis. *Int. J. Gynaecol. Obstet.* **2022**, *159*, 651–661. [CrossRef] [PubMed]
34. World Health Organization (WHO). Interim Recommendations for the Use of COVID-19 Vaccines in Pregnant and Lactating Women—March 2024. Available online: https://www.who.int (accessed on 1 November 2024).
35. Barros, F.C.; Gunier, R.B.; Rego, A.; Sentilhes, L.; Rauch, S.; Gandino, S.; Teji, J.S.; Thornton, J.G.; Kachikis, A.B.; Nieto, R.; et al. Maternal vaccination against COVID-19 and neonatal outcomes during Omicron: INTERCOVID-2022 study. *Am. J. Obstet. Gynecol.* **2024**, *231*, 460.e1–460.e17. [CrossRef] [PubMed]

Journal of
Clinical Medicine

MDPI

*Review*

# Neurodevelopmental Outcomes in Children Born to Mothers Infected with SARS-CoV-2 During Pregnancy: A Narrative Review

**Daniela Păcurar [1,2], Alexandru Dinulescu [1,2,*], Ana Prejmereanu [1,2], Alexandru Cosmin Palcău [1,3], Irina Dijmărescu [1,2] and Mirela-Luminița Pavelescu [1,2]**

1 Faculty of Medicine, "Carol Davila" University of Medicine and Pharmacy, 050474 Bucharest, Romania; daniela.pacurar@umfcd.ro (D.P.); ana.prejmereanu@rez.umfcd.ro (A.P.); alexandru-cosmin.palcau@drd.umfcd.ro (A.C.P.); irina.dijmarescu@umfcd.ro (I.D.); mirela.pavelescu@umfcd.ro (M.-L.P.)
2 Department of Pediatrics, Emergency Hospital for Children "Grigore Alexandrescu", 011743 Bucharest, Romania
3 Department of General Surgery, University Emergency Hospital of Bucharest, 050098 Bucharest, Romania
* Correspondence: alexandru.dinulescu@drd.umfcd.ro; Tel.: +40-720-548-233

**Abstract**

**Background**: The potential impact of maternal SARS-CoV-2 infection during pregnancy on the neurodevelopment of offspring has raised considerable concern. Emerging studies have evaluated various developmental domains in exposed infants, yet findings remain inconsistent. **Objective**: To synthesize current evidence regarding neurodevelopmental outcomes in infants born to mothers with confirmed SARS-CoV-2 infection during pregnancy. Methods: We conducted a narrative review following PRISMA guidelines. A literature search was performed in PubMed, Cochrane, and ScienceDirect using keywords including "COVID-19", "pregnancy", "neurodevelopment", and "SARS-CoV-2". Nineteen studies were included. Data were extracted regarding study design, sample size, timing of exposure, age at assessment, developmental tools used, and key findings. Study quality was assessed using the Newcastle–Ottawa Scale. **Results**: Among 19 included studies, 12 reported at least some neurodevelopmental delays, particularly in motor and language domains. However, these delays were generally mild, domain-specific, and often not statistically significant. Seven studies, most of which were high-quality and low-risk, reported no significant differences between exposed and unexposed groups. Assessment tools and follow-up durations varied widely, limiting comparability. **Conclusions**: Current evidence does not support a consistent association between in utero SARS-CoV-2 exposure and an unfavorable neurodevelopmental outcome up to 24 months. However, heterogeneity in methods and short-term follow-up warrant further high-quality longitudinal research.

**Keywords:** SARS-CoV-2; COVID-19; pregnancy; neurodevelopment; infants; maternal infection; developmental delay; prenatal exposure

## 1. Introduction

The intrauterine environment plays a pivotal role in fetal development, including the processes of brain growth and maturation [1–3]. Maternal infections during pregnancy are well-documented contributors to negative neurodevelopmental outcomes in offspring, as pathogens or the maternal immune response can disrupt fetal brain development at critical stages [1,4–8]. Among the diverse etiologies that may impair fetal and early neurodevelopment—including metabolic, genetic, endocrine, and structural disorders, congenital infections represent a significant and potentially preventable cause of adverse outcomes [9–14]. Numerous viral infections, such as cytomegalovirus (CMV), Epstein–Barr virus (EBV), Zika virus (ZIKV), and influenza, have been associated with a spectrum of neurodevelopmental sequelae, including sensorineural hearing loss, intellectual disability, motor dysfunction, and autism spectrum disorders (ASD) [15–21]. CMV, for instance, is the most common congenital viral infection and a leading cause of neurodevelopmental disability, while prenatal exposure to maternal influenza has been linked to increased risks of schizophrenia and neurocognitive impairments in later life, although this statement needs more reliable data [20,22–24].

In this context, the emergence of SARS-CoV-2 as a novel coronavirus with global reach has raised concerns about its potential impact on children's neurodevelopment [25–27]. Although vertical transmission of SARS-CoV-2 appears to be rare, the maternal immune activation (MIA) associated with COVID-19, characterized by systemic inflammation, cytokine release, and placental pathology, may represent a mechanism by which SARS-CoV-2 prenatal exposure could affect the developing fetal brain [26,28–32]. Furthermore, the pandemic has brought additional stressors such as altered prenatal care, maternal mental health issues, and social isolation, all of which may compound neurodevelopmental risks [33–35].

COVID-19 infection in pregnancy is a known factor for preterm birth, especially if the infection occurs in the third trimester or is a severe one [36–38]. There were also other complications described in COVID-19 pregnancy, such as an increased risk of hypertensive disorders of pregnancy, gestational diabetes, or an increased rate of neonatal intensive care unit (NICU) admission [39–42]. One important aspect is that the mRNA COVID-19 vaccine administered before pregnancy was not associated with an increased risk of any of those complications [43,44].

While initial concerns focused on obstetric complications such as preterm birth and vertical transmission, attention has increasingly turned to potential long-term consequences for offspring, particularly in the domain of neurodevelopment [43–45]. Recent reviews have begun to explore the early neurodevelopmental trajectories of children born to mothers infected with SARS-CoV-2 during pregnancy, with some reports suggesting subtle delays in motor, language, or social-emotional development during infancy [26,46]. It remains critical to disentangle the direct effects of the virus from indirect influences such as maternal emotional dysregulation and psychosocial stress during the pandemic, including social isolation and healthcare disruption, which may have further contributed to altered mother–infant interactions and long-term neurodevelopmental impact [47–49]. However, findings remain inconclusive, and methodological heterogeneity, regarding timing of maternal infection, severity of disease, gestational age at exposure, and follow-up duration, limits the generalizability of available evidence.

This review aims to synthesize current evidence on neurodevelopmental outcomes in children with in utero exposure to SARS-CoV-2. By exploring current epidemiologic findings, we seek to highlight both the knowns and unknowns in this evolving field and underscore the need for long-term, high-quality follow-up studies to fully understand the impact of COVID-19 on the next generation.

## 2. Materials and Methods

This study was conducted as a narrative review, with elements of systematic methodology applied to ensure rigor and transparency. A comprehensive literature search was performed in databases such as PubMed and Cochrane using predefined keywords. The selection process followed PRISMA principles, and study quality was assessed using the Newcastle–Ottawa Scale (NOS).

### 2.1. Inclusion Criteria

- Peer-reviewed observational studies (cohort or case–control).
- Neurodevelopment assessed via standardized tools (e.g., ASQ 3, Bayley scales) or clinical examination during infancy or early childhood (≤24 months), standardized parent-reported questionnaires (e.g., Ages and Stages Questionnaire), or direct neurological clinical examination during infancy or early childhood (≤24 months).

### 2.2. Exclusion Criteria

- Narrative reviews, animal studies (except mechanistic discussion), case reports without neurodevelopmental follow-up.
- Studies reporting exclusively biological outcomes (e.g., cytokine profiles, epigenetic changes) without separate reporting of standardized neurodevelopmental assessments.

### 2.3. Search Strategy, Selection and Data Extraction

A comprehensive literature search was conducted using PubMed, Cochrane Library, and ScienceDirect databases up to July 2025. The following keywords were used: ("SARS-CoV-2" OR "COVID-19") AND ("pregnancy" OR "maternal infection") AND ("neurodevelopment" OR "neurodevelopmental outcomes" OR "infant development"). Data extraction included sample size, neurodevelopmental tools used, follow-up age, and key outcomes. The search yielded 1083 articles. After removing duplicates and screening titles and abstracts, the full texts of potentially relevant studies were reviewed. Borderline-eligible studies were excluded if they did not report standardized neurodevelopmental outcomes separately, if they focused exclusively on biological outcomes without clinical correlation, or if they involved animal models. A total of 21 studies met the final inclusion criteria and were included in the review (Figure 1).

**Data extraction**

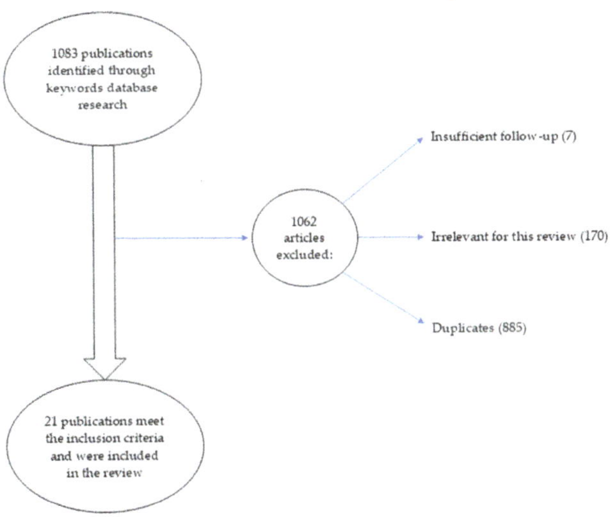


**Figure 1.** Data extraction.

### 2.4. Data Synthesis

Due to substantial heterogeneity across the included studies in terms of neurodevelopmental assessment tools, follow-up duration, outcome domains, and reporting formats, a meta-analysis was not feasible. Instead, a narrative synthesis was performed. Results were organized thematically according to developmental domains (e.g., motor, language, cognitive, and social-emotional) and by the type and timing of maternal SARS-CoV-2 exposure. Consistencies and discrepancies across studies were qualitatively assessed, with attention to study quality, sample size, and methodological rigor as evaluated by the Newcastle–Ottawa Scale, interpreted as low risk of bias: 7–9; moderate risk of bias: 4–6 and high risk of bias: 0–3 (Table 1) [50].

**Table 1.** Risk of Bias Assessment (Newcastle–Ottawa Scale).

| Number | Study | Selection (Max 4) | Comparability (Max 2) | Outcome (Max 3) | Total Score | Risk Level |
|---|---|---|---|---|---|---|
| 1 | Shuffrey et al., 2021 [51] | 4 | 2 | 3 | 9 | Low |
| 2 | Roffman et al., 2021 [52] | 3 | 1 | 2 | 6 | Moderate |
| 3 | Cheng et al., 2021 [53] | 3 | 1 | 1 | 5 | Moderate |
| 4 | Wu et al., 2021 [54] | 3 | 1 | 2 | 6 | Moderate |
| 5 | Schuh et al., 2021 [55] | 2 | 1 | 1 | 4 | Moderate |
| 6 | Edlow et al., 2022 [56] | 4 | 2 | 2 | 8 | Low |
| 7 | Ayed et al., 2022 [57] | 3 | 2 | 2 | 7 | Low |
| 8 | Buonsenso et al., 2022 [58] | 3 | 1 | 1 | 5 | Moderate |
| 9 | Aldrete-Cortez et al., 2022 [59] | 3 | 1 | 2 | 6 | Moderate |
| 10 | Liu et al., 2022 [60] | 3 | 1 | 2 | 6 | Moderate |
| 11 | Martenot et al., 2022 [61] | 3 | 1 | 1 | 5 | Moderate |
| 12 | Martinez et al., 2023 [62] | 4 | 1 | 2 | 7 | Low |
| 13 | Silva et al., 2023 [63] | 3 | 1 | 2 | 6 | Moderate |
| 14 | Ayesa-Arriola et al., 2023 [64] | 2 | 1 | 2 | 5 | Moderate |
| 15 | Rood et al., 2023 [65] | 2 | 0 | 1 | 3 | High |
| 16 | Vrantsidis et al., 2024 [66] | 4 | 2 | 3 | 9 | Low |
| 17 | Jaswa et al., 2024 [67] | 4 | 2 | 3 | 9 | Low |
| 18 | Hill et al., 2024 [68] | 4 | 2 | 2 | 8 | Low |
| 19 | Silva et al., 2025 [69] | 3 | 1 | 2 | 6 | Moderate |
| 20 | Kehdi et al., 2025 [70] | 4 | 2 | 3 | 9 | Low |
| 21 | Berg et al., 2025 [71] | 4 | 2 | 3 | 9 | Low |

Note: Risk levels were defined as Low (7–9), Moderate (4–6), or High (0–3).

Among the 21 included studies, 9 were rated as low risk of bias, 11 as moderate, and 1 as high risk. Studies with high total scores (e.g., Jaswa et al., Vrantsidis et al., Shuffrey et al.) were typically large, prospective cohorts with appropriate comparators and robust outcome assessment [51,66,67]. Studies rated as moderate risk tended to have smaller sample sizes, limited follow-up durations, or used less validated assessment tools.

## 3. Results

A total of 21 studies met the inclusion criteria for this narrative review, evaluating neurodevelopmental outcomes in infants born to mothers infected with SARS-CoV-2 during pregnancy. The sample sizes of the exposed groups ranged from 9 to 555, and neurodevelopmental assessments were performed at ages ranging from 6 weeks to 24 months postpartum. The most frequently used assessment tool was the Ages and Stages Questionnaire (ASQ-3). Other instruments used were the Denver Developmental Screening Test, General Movement Assessment (GMA), Motor Optimality Scores Revised (MOS-R), Neonatal Behavioral Assessment Scale (NBAS), Age and Stage Questionnaire Social-Emotional (ASQ:SE-2), Van Wiechen Scheme, International Statistical Classification of Diseases and Related Health Problems, Tenth Revision (ICD-10), Survey of Well-Being of

Young Children (SWYC), Baby Pediatric Symptom Checklist (BPSC), and various clinical or parent-report measures.

Based on Table 2, 13 out of 21 studies (62%) reported at least some neurodevelopmental delays among SARS-CoV-2-exposed infants. These delays were most frequently observed in motor, language, and socioemotional domains, though the clinical significance and persistence of these delays varied considerably across studies.

**Table 2.** Consolidated characteristics of included studies.

| Study | Design/N (Exposed) | Maternal Infection Timing (Trimester) | Maternal Disease Severity | Neurodevelopment Tool | Follow-Up Age | Key Findings | Adjustment for Confounders |
|---|---|---|---|---|---|---|---|
| Shuffrey et al., 2021 [51] | Cohort/$N$ = 317 (114 exposed) | 1st: $n$ = 42, 2nd: $n$ = 90, 3rd: $n$ = 67;) | 34% asymptomatic, 62% mild/moderate, 4% severe | ASQ-3 | 6 months | No major neurodevelopmental differences in infants born during the pandemic (exposed vs. non-exposed), but those born during the pandemic had significantly lower scores on gross motor, fine motor, and personal-social subdomains when compared to a cohort born prior to the onset of the pandemic. | Yes—adjusted for maternal education, race/ethnicity, infant sex, GA, mode of delivery, NICU admission |
| Roffman et al., 2021 [52] | Cohort/$N$ = 34 (19 exposed) | Not reported (NR) | NR | ASQ-3, BPSC | 12 months | Gross motor delay and high irritability ($p$ = 0.015). | NR |
| Cheng et al., 2021 [53] | Cohort/$N$ = 18 (9 exposed) | All in the 3rd trimester | 100% mild/moderate | ASQ-3 | 8–10 months | The infants from SARS-CoV-2-exposed mothers had lower scores in communication, gross movement, fine movement, problem solving, and personal-social domains, but only fine motor movement was significantly lower ($p$ = 0.03). | NR |
| Wu et al., 2021 [54] | Cohort/$N$ = 135 (57 exposed) | 1st: $n$ = 0, 2nd: $n$ = 4, 3rd: $n$ = 53 | 86% mild/moderate, 14% severe | ASQ-3, ASQ:SE-2 | 3 months | No significant neurodevelopmental differences between exposed and unexposed groups. | Yes—adjusted for mother–infant separation, low birth weight (LBW), infant sex, preterm birth, NICU admission, breastfeeding at 3 months |
| Schuh et al., 2021 [55] | Cohort/$N$ = 15 (15 exposed) | NR | 100% severe | ASQ-3 | 6 months | All of them were reported as normal development. | NR |
| Edlow et al., 2022 [56] | Cohort/$N$ = 7772 (222 exposed) | 1st: $n$ = 1, 2nd: $n$ = 61, 3rd: $n$ = 160 | NR | ICD-10 codes | 12 months | Maternal SARS-CoV-2 positivity during pregnancy was associated with a greater rate of neurodevelopmental diagnoses (Odds ratio (OR) = 1.86, $p$ = 0.04). | Yes—adjusted for maternal age, race/ethnicity, insurance status, gestational age (GA), birthweight, infant sex, |
| Ayed et al., 2022 [57] | Cohort/$N$ = 298 (298 exposed) | 1st: $n$ = 5, 2nd: $n$ = 20, 3rd: $n$ = 273 | 39.5% asymptomatic, 53.6% mild/moderate, 6.9% severe | ASQ-3 | 10–12 months | The rate of development delays was 10%. The risk of developmental delays was higher with first-trimester (OR: 8.2, $p$ = 0.039) and second-trimester maternal SARS-CoV-2 infections (OR: 8.1, $p$ = 0.001) than with third-trimester. | Yes—adjusted for maternal age, maternal infection timing, GA, birthweight, infant sex, parental education and type of feeding in the first 6 months |
| Buonsenso et al., 2022 [58] | Cohort/$N$ = 199 (199 exposed) | 1st: $n$ = 6, 2nd: $n$ = 6, 3rd: $n$ = 187 | 57.6% asymptomatic, 36.9% mild/moderate, 5.5% severe | Clinical exam | 3-6-9-12 months | All of them were reported as normal neurological development. | NR |

**Table 2.** *Cont.*

| Study | Design/N (Exposed) | Maternal Infection Timing (Trimester) | Maternal Disease Severity | Neurodevelopment Tool | Follow-Up Age | Key Findings | Adjustment for Confounders |
|---|---|---|---|---|---|---|---|
| Aldrete-Cortez et al., 2022 [59] | Cohort/$N = 56$ (28 exposed) | All in 3rd trimester | 100% mild/moderate | GMA | 3–5 months | The exposed group had a significantly reduced total MOS-R; the median was lower in the exposed group (21 vs. 25, $p = 0.002$). | Yes—adjusted for maternal/infant characteristics differing between groups: maternal age, marital status, education level, preeclampsia, hypothyroidism, gestational diabetes, GA, infant sex, type of delivery, Hyper-bilirubinemia, APGAR score, days of hospitalization, birthweight, length at birth, birth head circumference |
| Liu et al., 2022 [60] | Cohort/$N = 98$ (31 exposed) | All in the 3rd trimester | 100% mild/moderate | Denver II | 9 months | Fine motor abnormalities higher in the exposed group (15.2% vs. 2.1%; $p = 0.02$). | Yes—adjusted using for age, sex, infection status |
| Martenot et al., 2022 [61] | Cohort/$N = 24$ (24 exposed) | All in the 3rd trimester | 4% asymptomatic, 96% symptomatic (severity NR) | ASQ-2 | 10 months | All of them were reported as normal neurological development. | NR |
| Martinez et al., 2023 [62] | Cohort/$N = 239$ (124 exposed) | 1st: $n = 17$, 2nd: $n = 37$, 3rd: $n = 70$ | 14.5% asymptomatic, 67.7% mild/moderate, 17.7% severe | GMA, MOS-R, clinical exam | 3–8 months | Suboptimal neuromotor development in exposed infants. The median of MOS-R was lower in the exposed group (23 vs. 25, $p < 0.001$), and 16 exposed infants had MOS-R scores <20 vs. 0 controls ($p < 0.001$). At 6–8 months clinical exam, 13 exposed vs. 0 controls had developmental delay. | Yes—adjusted for COVID-19 severity, trimester of infection, neonatal and maternal comorbidities, fetal sex, maternal age, maternal fever during COVID-19 and preterm birth |
| Silva et al., 2023 [63] | Cross-sectional study, $N = 54$ (27 exposed); | NR | NR | SWYC | From 1 to 12 months | Motor developmental delay in COVID-19-exposed infants (OR = 6.3, $p = 0.01$); socioemotional developmental delay (OR = 4.0; $p = 0.02$); Inflexibility (OR = 14.0; $p = 0.02$); Parental concerns about behavior, learning, or development of the infant (OR = 9.7; $p = 0.01$). | Yes—adjusted for sex, GA and family context. |
| Ayesa-Arriola et al., 2023 [64] | Cohort/$N = 42$ (21 exposed) | 1st: $n = 3$, 2nd: $n = 8$, 3rd: $n = 10$ | 95.2% mild/moderate, 4.8% severe | NBAS (0–3 mo) | 6 weeks | Lower affectionate response in the exposed group ($p = 0.009$), especially those exposed in the third trimester ($p = 0.043$). | Yes—for maternal age, GA, trimester of infection, infant age at assessment and infant sex |
| Rood et al., 2023 [65] | Cohort/$N = 13$ (13 exposed) | All in 3rd trimester | 46% mild/moderate, 54% severe | Van Wiechen Scheme | 3 months | Follow-up similar to children born to COVID-19-negative mothers, mild neurodevelopmental delay in 2 (15.3%). | NR |
| Vrantsidis et al., 2024 [66] | Cohort/$N = 896$ (96 exposed) | 1st: $n = 21$, 2nd: $n = 45$, 3rd: $n = 30$ | 1% asymptomatic, 74% mild/moderate, 25% severe | ASQ-3 | 6–24 months | No significant neurodevelopmental differences between the exposed and unexposed groups | Yes—for maternal comorbidities and household socioeconomic status |

**Table 2.** *Cont.*

| Study | Design/N (Exposed) | Maternal Infection Timing (Trimester) | Maternal Disease Severity | Neurodevelopment Tool | Follow-Up Age | Key Findings | Adjustment for Confounders |
|---|---|---|---|---|---|---|---|
| Jaswa et al., 2024 [67] | Cohort/$N$ = 2003 (217 exposed) | 1st: $n$ = 122, 2nd: $n$ = 42, 3rd: $n$ = 53 | NR | ASQ-3 | 12–24 months | No significant neurodevelopmental differences between exposed and unexposed groups, or by the trimester of infection in the exposed group. | Yes—for maternal age, race, education level, income, maternal generalized anxiety and depression symptoms at baseline. |
| Hill et al., 2024 [68] | Cohort/$N$= 30 (16 expoed) | 1st: $n$ = 0, 2nd: $n$ = 4, 3rd: $n$ = 12 | 100% severe | ASQ-3 | 12 months | Lower ASQ-3 scores in children exposed to severe SARS-CoV-2 maternal infection in communication, problem solving and personal-social domains ($p < 0.005$); correlations with cytokine profiles and epigenetic markers. | NR |
| Silva et al., 2025 [69] | Cohort/$N$ = 41 (41 exposed) | 1st: $n$ = 5, 2nd: $n$ = 9, 3rd: $n$ = 27 | NR | ASQ-3 | 18 months | 22 (53%) children performed below the cutoff value in communication and 19 (46%) in gross motor coordination. | Yes—for maternal age, GA, type of delivery, sex, Apgar score, birth weight, the child's need for prolonged hospitalization after birth, and trimester infection |
| Kehdi et al., 2025 [70] | Cohort/$N$ = 41 (18 exposed) | All in 3rd trimester | 55% mild/moderate, 55% severe | Bayley-III | 6–24 months | At 6 and 24 months, up to 36% cognitive, 64% communication, and 57% motor delays were observed. Specific cord blood cytokines correlated with respective domain delays. | No adjustment for confounders; BSID-III scores corrected for gestational age |
| Berg et al., 2025 [71] | Cohort/$N$ = 1446 (555 exposed) | 1st: $n$ = 63, 2nd: $n$ = 278, 3rd: $n$ = 214 | 95.5% mild/asymptomatic, 4.5% severe | ASQ-3 | 4 months | There was no group difference in ASQ total mean scores, but those exposed to severe maternal COVID-19 had an increased risk of total ASQ scores below the cutoff (exposed: 16.0% vs. unexposed: 6.1%; OR 3.57; 95% CI, 1.14–11.24). | Yes—for mother BMI, education, country of origin, maternal age, pre-pregnancy comorbidity, GA, APGAR, type of delivery, birthweight, type of feeding |

### *3.1. Motor Development Findings*

Motor development was the most commonly affected domain, with 11 studies reporting motor-related concerns. Shuffrey et al. (2021) found that both exposed and unexposed infants born during the pandemic had significantly lower scores in gross motor and fine motor domains compared to pre-pandemic cohorts, suggesting broader pandemic-related effects beyond direct viral exposure [51]. Several studies specifically identified fine motor delays: Cheng et al. (2021) reported significantly lower fine motor scores ($p$ = 0.03) in exposed infants at 8–10 months, while Liu et al. (2022) found higher rates of fine motor abnormalities in exposed versus unexposed groups (15.2% vs. 2.1%; $p$ = 0.02) [53,60]. Studies utilizing more sensitive motor assessment tools detected subtle neuromotor differences. Martinez et al. (2023) and Aldrete-Cortez et al. (2022), both using the Motor Optimality Score-Revised (MOS-R), found significantly lower median scores in exposed infants (23 vs. 25, $p < 0.001$; and 21 vs. 25, $p$ = 0.002, respectively) [59,62]. Martinez et al. additionally reported that 16 exposed infants had MOS-R scores < 20 versus 0 controls ($p < 0.001$), and 13 exposed versus 0 controls showed developmental delays at 6–8 months clinical examination [62]. Kehdi et al. (2025) observed that 40% had motor delays at 6 months, this percentage increasing to 64.3% at 24 months, with specific cord blood cytokines correlating with motor delays (IL-6, IL-8, IL-17, and IL-1β) [70].

### 3.2. Communication and Language Development Findings

Communication delays were reported in several studies, with varying degrees of severity. Silva et al. (2025) found that 22 of 41 exposed children (53%) performed below the cutoff value in communication domains at 18 months [69]. Hill et al. (2024) reported lower ASQ-3 scores in communication domains among children exposed to severe maternal SARS-CoV-2 infection ($p < 0.005$), with findings correlating with specific cytokine profiles and epigenetic markers [68]. Berg et al. (2025), in one of the largest cohorts ($N = 1446$, 555 exposed), found no group differences in total ASQ scores, but noted increased risk of scores below cutoff among those exposed to severe maternal COVID-19 (16.0% vs. 6.1%; OR 3.57; 95% CI, 1.14–11.24) [71]. Finally, the only study rated as high risk of bias, Rood et al. (2023), suggested a mild delay but lacked a control group and included only 14 infants, limiting its reliability [65].

### 3.3. Socioemotional and Behavioral Outcomes

Several studies examined socioemotional development with mixed findings. Silva et al. (2023) reported increased odds of socioemotional developmental delay (OR = 4.0; $p = 0.02$) and inflexibility (OR = 14.0; $p = 0.02$) in exposed infants [63]. Ayesa-Arriola et al. (2023) found lower affectionate response scores in exposed groups ($p = 0.009$), particularly among those exposed in the third trimester ($p = 0.043$) [64]. Roffman et al. (2021) noted high irritability in exposed infants ($p = 0.015$) [52].

### 3.4. Timing of Maternal Infection

The trimester of maternal infection showed variable associations with outcomes. Ayed et al. (2022) found a higher risk of developmental delays with first-trimester (OR: 8.2, $p = 0.039$) and second-trimester (OR: 8.1, $p = 0.001$) infections compared to third-trimester exposure, but Ayesa-Arriola et al. (2023) reported more pronounced effects in third-trimester exposures, particularly for affectionate response measures ($p = 0.043$) [57,64]. It should be noted that more than a quarter (6/21) of the studies included had subjects only from the 3rd trimester infection, and three studies did not report this variable.

### 3.5. Disease Severity

Disease severity appeared to influence outcomes in some studies. Berg et al. (2025) specifically found increased risk only among infants exposed to severe maternal COVID-19 [71]. Hill et al. (2024) focused exclusively on severe maternal infections and reported significant developmental impacts with biological correlates [68].

### 3.6. Studies Reporting No Significant Differences

Seven studies reported no significant neurodevelopmental differences between exposed and unexposed groups. These included some of the largest and highest-quality studies: Jaswa et al. (2024) with 2003 participants (217 exposed) followed to 12–24 months, Vrantsidis et al. (2024) with 896 participants (96 exposed) followed to 6–24 months, and Wu et al. (2021) with 135 participants (57 exposed) assessed at 3 months [54,66,67]. These studies were notable for their larger sample sizes, appropriate control groups, and adjustment for multiple confounders, including maternal comorbidities, socioeconomic status, gestational age, and infant characteristics.

### 3.7. Adjustment for Confounders

Adjustment for confounders varied substantially across studies. Higher-quality studies typically adjusted for key variables, including gestational age, birthweight, maternal age, education, socioeconomic status, and infection characteristics. Studies with limited or no confounder adjustment showed more pronounced associations, raising questions about residual confounding.

## 4. Discussion

This narrative review synthesizes current evidence regarding neurodevelopment in infants born to mothers infected with SARS-CoV-2 during pregnancy, incorporating quality assessment using the Newcastle–Ottawa Scale to contextualize findings. While methodological heterogeneity presents interpretive challenges, emerging patterns regarding gestational timing, infection severity, and biological mechanisms warrant deeper clinical and scientific consideration alongside careful evaluation of study design limitations.

### 4.1. Overall Pattern of Findings and Study Quality Considerations

While 67% of studies reported some neurodevelopmental concerns, this proportion requires careful interpretation within the context of study quality and design. The highest-quality studies with low risk of bias (Jaswa et al., Vrantsidis et al., Shuffrey et al.) consistently reported no major developmental differences between exposed and unexposed groups [51,66,67]. This pattern suggests that apparent associations in lower-quality studies may reflect methodological limitations rather than true causal relationships.

The domains most frequently affected, motor development, communication, and socioemotional function, align with areas particularly vulnerable to early disruption and most readily assessed in infancy. However, the transient and mild nature of most reported delays, combined with their absence in well-controlled studies, suggests these findings may not represent clinically significant or persistent developmental alterations in the majority of exposed infants.

Overall, this review supports the statement that SARS-CoV-2 infection during pregnancy is not consistently associated with clinically significant neurodevelopmental delays in early infancy, but it remains essential to distinguish between the effects of being born during the pandemic and direct intrauterine exposure to SARS-CoV-2. Some delays may reflect broader societal disruptions rather than biological effects of the virus.

### 4.2. Gestational Timing of SARS-CoV2 Infection

The timing of maternal SARS-CoV-2 infection during pregnancy emerges as a critical determinant of neurodevelopmental risk, with evidence suggesting trimester-specific vulnerabilities that align with established principles of fetal brain development.

First-trimester exposure shows the strongest association with developmental delays, consistent with this period's critical role in neural tube closure, neurulation, and establishment of basic brain architecture [72,73]. Ayed et al. (2022) provided compelling evidence for this vulnerability window, reporting dramatically increased odds ratios for developmental delays with first-trimester exposure (OR: 8.2, $p = 0.039$) [57]. During the first trimester, the blood–brain barrier is still developing, potentially allowing greater cytokine penetration into fetal neural tissue [74]. Established literature describes that first-trimester maternal immune activation affects fundamental neurodevelopmental processes, including neurogenesis, neuronal migration, and synaptic pruning [75,76]. The motor and reflex deficits specifically associated with first-trimester exposure may reflect disruption of brainstem and spinal cord development, which occurs primarily during weeks 4–8 of gestation.

These structures are particularly vulnerable to inflammatory insults during their critical formation periods [77].

Second-trimester findings present complex findings, with Ayed et al. similarly reporting elevated risk (OR: 8.1, $p = 0.001$), while other studies suggest more subtle effects [57]. This period (weeks 13–26) encompasses peak cortical neurogenesis and the establishment of fundamental cortical architecture [78]. The apparent inconsistency in second-trimester findings across studies may reflect the diverse nature of developmental processes occurring during this extended period.

Third-trimester exposure presents the most intriguing findings, with studies reporting both protective and adverse effects. Ayesa-Arriola et al. (2023) found reduced affectionate response specifically in third-trimester exposed infants ($p = 0.043$), while several studies focusing exclusively on third-trimester exposure reported relatively preserved outcomes [64]. This apparent paradox may reflect the dual nature of late pregnancy immune activation. While the fetal brain is more mature and potentially more resistant to inflammatory disruption, this period encompasses critical synaptogenesis, circuit refinement, and the establishment of neurotransmitter systems crucial for social-emotional development [79].

### 4.3. Infection Severity

Studies focusing on mild to moderate maternal infections generally report reassuring outcomes. Berg et al. (2025), in their large cohort study ($N = 1446$), found no group differences in overall ASQ scores when analyzing the full spectrum of infection severity [71]. This suggests that the typical maternal inflammatory response to mild SARS-CoV-2 infection may be insufficient to significantly disrupt fetal neurodevelopment. The predominance of mild infections in many cohorts (often 80–95% of cases) likely contributes to the generally reassuring overall findings.

Neurodevelopmental effects are more consistently reported in studies examining severe maternal infections. Berg et al. specifically identified increased risk of developmental concerns only among infants exposed to severe maternal COVID-19 (16.0% vs. 6.1%; OR 3.57; 95% CI, 1.14–11.24) [71]. This finding suggests a dose–response relationship between maternal inflammatory burden and fetal neurodevelopmental risk. Hill et al. (2024) provided crucial mechanistic insights by focusing exclusively on severe maternal infections and demonstrating correlations between infant DNA methylation patterns and neurodevelopmental outcomes with specific cytokine profiles. Their finding of lower ASQ-3 scores in multiple domains (communication, problem solving, and personal-social; $p < 0.005$) coupled with epigenetic evidence provides the strongest support for biologically mediated effects [68].

### 4.4. Maternal Immune Activation

The concept of MIA provides a unifying framework for understanding SARS-CoV-2 effects on fetal neurodevelopment. Rather than requiring direct viral invasion of fetal neural tissue, MIA suggests that the maternal inflammatory response itself, can disrupt fetal brain development through shared inflammatory pathways [80]. This mechanism has been demonstrated across diverse maternal infections, from influenza to bacterial infections, suggesting common downstream effects despite different initial triggers [18,81]. The MIA model explains why SARS-CoV-2 effects on neurodevelopment show similarities to those observed with other prenatal infections, despite the virus's unique characteristics. The key mediators are pro-inflammatory cytokines (such as IL-6, TNF-$\alpha$, and IL-1$\beta$) that can cross the placenta and blood–brain barrier, triggering neuroinflammation in the developing fetal brain [31]. This neuroinflammation can then disrupt critical developmental processes, including neurogenesis, neuronal migration, synaptic formation, and myelination, regardless of whether the original pathogen directly infected neural tissue [76].

Kehdi et al. (2025) provided direct evidence of cytokine-mediated mechanisms, demonstrating that specific cord blood cytokines (IFN-$\gamma$, TNF-$\alpha$, IL-6, IL-8, IL-17, IL-1$\beta$, CXCL10) correlated with domain-specific developmental delays [70]. The specificity of these correlations suggests that different cytokine profiles may preferentially affect distinct neurodevelopmental domains. Pro-inflammatory cytokines like TNF-$\alpha$ and IL-6 have established roles in disrupting neurogenesis and synaptic development, while chemokines like CXCL10 may affect microglial activation and neuroinflammation [82–85].

Beyond direct cytokine effects, SARS-CoV-2 infection can cause placental pathology, including thrombosis, infarction, and chronic villitis [86]. Liu et al. (2022) specifically linked fine motor abnormalities in exposed infants to placental hypoxia and ischemia, suggesting that vascular-mediated effects may be as important as direct inflammatory mechanisms [60].

Hill et al. (2024) provided groundbreaking evidence of epigenetic changes in infants exposed to severe maternal SARS-CoV-2 infection [68]. These DNA methylation alterations correlated with specific neurodevelopmental deficits, suggesting that maternal immune activation may program persistent changes in gene expression that influence long-term neurodevelopmental trajectories [87–89].

### *4.5. Specific Areas of Development Affected*

Motor delays represent the most frequently reported and consistent finding across studies, appearing in 11 of 21 included studies. This consistency may reflect both the early emergence and relatively straightforward assessment of motor skills, but also suggests genuine vulnerability of motor systems to prenatal inflammatory insults. The progression from gross motor delays detected by standard screening tools to fine motor deficits identified by more sensitive instruments (MOS-R, GMA) indicates that motor effects may be subtle but persistent. Martinez et al. (2023) and Aldrete-Cortez et al. (2022) both demonstrated that specialized motor assessment tools could detect deficits missed by standard screening instruments, with significantly lower median MOS-R scores in exposed groups (23 vs. 25, $p < 0.001$; and 21 vs. 25, $p = 0.002$, respectively) [59,62]. The basal ganglia and cerebellar systems, vulnerable to prenatal inflammatory insults, are integral to both motor control and higher-order cognitive functions, potentially predicting later learning difficulties and attention problems [90,91].

Communication delays, while less consistently reported across all studies, may represent more clinically significant long-term effects when present. Silva et al. (2025) found that 53% of exposed children performed below cutoff values in communication domains at 18 months, a proportion that substantially exceeds the typical population prevalence of language delays (10–15%) [69]. The correlation between communication delays and specific cytokine profiles (Kehdi et al., 2025) suggests that neuroinflammation may particularly affect perisylvian cortical regions critical for language development [70,92].

Social-emotional findings are reported in fewer studies. Ayesa-Arriola et al. (2023) documented reduced affectionate response, while Silva et al. (2023) reported increased inflexibility (OR = 14.0; $p = 0.02$) and socioemotional developmental delays (OR = 4.0; $p = 0.02$) [63,64]. These findings align with established research linking prenatal immune activation to autism spectrum disorders, social anxiety, and other social-emotional difficulties [93–95].

## *4.6. Methodological Heterogeneity Impact on Interpretation*

### 4.6.1. Assessment Tools and Their Clinical Implications

The choice of neurodevelopmental assessment tool significantly influenced findings and their clinical interpretation. Parent-reported questionnaires such as the ASQ-3, while cost-effective and widely used, may be influenced by recall bias, parental stress, and pandemic-related anxiety [96]. These tools have known limitations in sensitivity for mild to moderate delays, and maternal education level significantly influences their accuracy [97]. The high prevalence of ASQ-3 use across studies (12 of 21) may contribute to apparent consistency of findings while actually reflecting shared methodological limitations rather than true developmental effects.

In contrast, studies using more sensitive, clinician-administered tools like the Motor Optimality Score-Revised (MOS-R) or General Movement Assessment (GMA) detected subtle neuromotor differences that may have greater clinical significance. However, these tools require specialized training and are resource-intensive, limiting their use to smaller cohorts and potentially introducing selection bias [98–100].

Direct neurological examination, while valuable for detecting overt abnormalities, may miss subtle cognitive or socioemotional delays that become apparent only with standardized developmental assessments [101]. This methodological diversity substantially contributes to the heterogeneity of findings and complicates direct comparison of results across studies.

### 4.6.2. Follow-Up Duration and Developmental Windows

The variation in follow-up duration (6 weeks to 24 months) represents another critical limitation with important clinical implications. Most studies focused on early infancy, when many neurodevelopmental domains are still emerging and may not yet manifest subtle deficits. Domains such as executive function, attention regulation, and complex social behaviors typically become measurable only in later childhood, meaning that current evidence may not capture the full spectrum of potential effects.

Furthermore, the timing of assessment relative to critical developmental windows varies across studies, making it difficult to determine whether observed differences represent persistent delays, transient perturbations, or normal developmental variation. This limitation is particularly important given that some prenatal exposures may have effects that only become apparent during school age or adolescence.

### 4.6.3. Distinguishing Viral Effects from Pandemic Context

A particularly important finding emerges from studies that attempted to distinguish direct viral effects from broader pandemic-related impacts. Shuffrey et al. (2021) [51] provided crucial insight by comparing three groups: pre-pandemic infants, pandemic-born unexposed infants, and pandemic-born exposed infants. Their finding that both pandemic-born groups showed lower developmental scores compared to pre-pandemic cohorts, regardless of maternal infection status, highlights the challenge of attributing developmental differences specifically to SARS-CoV-2 exposure [51]. This observation suggests that many reported developmental concerns may reflect broader pandemic-related disruptions, including altered prenatal care, maternal mental health impacts, reduced social stimulation, and disrupted healthcare access rather than direct viral effects [102,103]. The failure of many studies to account for these contextual factors represents a significant limitation in interpreting current literature.

#### 4.6.4. Confounding and Study Quality Considerations

The inconsistent approach to confounder adjustment across studies represents a major limitation affecting interpretation. Key confounders, including preterm birth, small for gestational age status, maternal mental health, socioeconomic factors, and healthcare access disruption, were variably addressed. Large registry-based studies and well-funded cohorts generally provided more comprehensive adjustment, while smaller studies often presented unadjusted comparisons.

Where adjustment was limited or absent, observed associations, particularly modest developmental score differences, should be interpreted cautiously, given the potential for residual confounding. The observation that studies with more comprehensive confounder adjustment were less likely to report significant associations supports this concern.

Among the 21 included studies, the 9 studies rated as low risk of bias using the Newcastle–Ottawa Scale were predominantly large, prospective cohorts with appropriate control groups and robust outcome assessments. Notably, most studies rated as low risk (6 of 9) reported no significant neurodevelopmental differences, while studies reporting delays were more frequently rated as moderate or high risk due to limitations in sample size, control group quality, follow-up duration, or assessment methodology. The only study rated as high risk of bias, Rood et al. (2023), suggested a mild delay but lacked a control group and included only 14 infants, limiting its reliability [65].

### 4.7. Similar Studies

Our finding is in concordance with other studies: a meta-analysis comparing infants born during compared to those born before the pandemic published by Hessami et al. (2022) found no overall rise in neurodevelopmental impairment, except for communication delay regardless of maternal infection and among infants with confirmed prenatal SARS-CoV-2, only fine motor performance showed a notable increase in risk (OR $\approx$ 3.5) [104]. A systematic review conducted by Veloso et al. (2024) focusing on the first postnatal year reported that while most SARS-CoV-2-exposed infants achieved age-appropriate development, mild deficits emerged, particularly in gross and fine motor domains and early on, and language/social domains, especially by parental report tools such as ASQ 3, NBAS, and BPSC [105]. Another meta-analysis published by Jackson et al. (2024), which included four studies up to 11 months postpartum, found no statistically significant increased risk of delay in communication, motor, problem-solving, or social domains among term infants [106].

### 4.8. Limitations

This review has several limitations. First, there is a substantial heterogeneity among included studies regarding neurodevelopmental assessment tools, timing of evaluations, and definitions of delay. Second, most studies had short-term follow-up, typically ending before 24 months, precluding evaluation of later-emerging deficits in domains such as executive function, attention, and social behavior. Third, while some studies used standardized clinical assessments, many relied on parent-report tools, which may be subject to re-reporting bias.

Additionally, confounding factors such as maternal stress, preterm birth, or pandemic-related changes in healthcare access were variably controlled. Only one study distinguished between direct viral effects and indirect environmental consequences of the pandemic, by comparing 3 groups: pre-pandemic group and 2 pandemic groups exposed and non-exposed [51].

### 4.9. Future Directions

Future research should focus on large-scale, longitudinal cohort studies that follow children with in utero SARS-CoV-2 exposure into later childhood and adolescence, allowing for the assessment of cognitive, behavioral, and emotional outcomes beyond the early developmental window. Standardized neurodevelopmental assessment tools, consistent follow-up intervals, and appropriate control groups (including both pandemic-born but unexposed children and pre-pandemic cohorts) are essential to improving comparability across studies. Investigations should also explore potential modifiers such as the timing of maternal infection during pregnancy, maternal mental health, preterm birth, and infant sex.

## 5. Conclusions

Based on the Newcastle–Ottawa Scale analysis, current evidence does not indicate consistent neurodevelopmental harm from prenatal SARS-CoV-2 exposure. Most well-designed studies support normal developmental trajectories up to 24 months; however, emerging evidence suggests that specific subgroups, particularly those exposed to severe maternal illness or during vulnerable gestational periods, may be at increased risk for subtle developmental effects. Nonetheless, further high-quality longitudinal research is needed to track potential late-emerging outcomes, especially in cognitive, emotional, and behavioral domains during school age. While reassuring trends emerge from high-quality studies, the nuanced nature of prenatal exposures, direct viral effects versus indirect psychosocial or immunological impacts, underscores the complexity of this topic. Thus, continued surveillance and rigorous, harmonized research protocols remain essential.

**Author Contributions:** Conceptualization, D.P., A.D. and M.-L.P.; methodology, D.P., A.D. and M.-L.P.; software, A.D.; validation, D.P., I.D. and M.-L.P.; data curation, A.D., A.C.P. and A.P.; writing—original draft preparation, A.D., A.C.P. and A.P.; writing—review and editing, D.P., I.D. and M.-L.P.; visualization, A.D. and A.P.; supervision, D.P., I.D. and M.-L.P.; All authors have read and agreed to the published version of the manuscript.

**Funding:** This research received no external funding.

**Data Availability Statement:** Data are contained within the article.

**Acknowledgments:** Publication of this paper was supported by the University of Medicine and Pharmacy Carol Davila through the institutional program Publish not Perish.

**Conflicts of Interest:** The authors declare no conflicts of interest.

## Abbreviations

The following abbreviations are used in this manuscript:

| | |
|---|---|
| COVID 19 | Coronavirus disease 2019 |
| SARS-CoV-2 | Severe acute respiratory syndrome coronavirus 2 |
| PRISMA | Preferred Reporting Items for Systematic reviews and Meta-Analyses |
| ASD | Autism spectrum disorders |
| CMV | Cytomegalovirus |
| EBV | Epstein–Barr virus |
| NOS | Newcastle–Ottawa Scale |
| OR | Odds ratio |
| ASQ-3 | Ages and Stages Questionnaire |
| BPSC | Baby Pediatric Symptom Checklist |
| GMA | General Movement Assessment |
| MOS-R | Motor Optimality Scores Revised |
| NBAS | Neonatal Behavioral Assessment Scale |

| | |
|---|---|
| ICD-10 | International Statistical Classification of Diseases and Related Health Problems, Tenth Revision |
| SWYC | Survey of Well-Being of Young Children |
| ASQ:SE-2 | Age and Stage Questionnaire Social-Emotional |
| MIA | Maternal Immune Activation |
| LBW | Low birth weight |
| GA | Gestational age |
| OR | Odds ratio |

## References


1. Fitzgerald, E.; Hor, K.; Drake, A.J. Maternal Influences on Fetal Brain Development: The Role of Nutrition, Infection and Stress, and the Potential for Intergenerational Consequences. *Early Hum. Dev.* **2020**, *150*, 105190. [CrossRef]
2. Buss, C.; Entringer, S.; Wadhwa, P.D. Fetal Programming of Brain Development: Intrauterine Stress and Susceptibility to Psychopathology. A Presentation from the European Society for Paediatric Endocrinology (ESPE) New Inroads to Child Health (NICHe) Conference on Stress Response and Child Health in Heraklion, Crete, Greece, 18–20 May 2012. *Sci. Signal* **2012**, *5*, pt7. [CrossRef]
3. Leibovitz, Z.; Lerman-Sagie, T.; Haddad, L. Fetal Brain Development: Regulating Processes and Related Malformations. *Life* **2022**, *12*, 809. [CrossRef]
4. Kwon, H.-K.; Choi, G.B.; Huh, J.R. Maternal Inflammation and Its Ramifications on Fetal Neurodevelopment. *Trends Immunol.* **2022**, *43*, 230–244. [CrossRef]
5. Goeden, N.; Velasquez, J.; Arnold, K.A.; Chan, Y.; Lund, B.T.; Anderson, G.M.; Bonnin, A. Maternal Inflammation Disrupts Fetal Neurodevelopment via Increased Placental Output of Serotonin to the Fetal Brain. *J. Neurosci.* **2016**, *36*, 6041–6049. [CrossRef] [PubMed]
6. Sokou, R.; Lianou, A.; Lampridou, M.; Panagiotounakou, P.; Kafalidis, G.; Paliatsiou, S.; Volaki, P.; Tsantes, A.G.; Boutsikou, T.; Iliodromiti, Z.; et al. Neonates at Risk: Understanding the Impact of High-Risk Pregnancies on Neonatal Health. *Medicina* **2025**, *61*, 1077. [CrossRef] [PubMed]
7. Lubrano, C.; Parisi, F.; Cetin, I. Impact of Maternal Environment and Inflammation on Fetal Neurodevelopment. *Antioxidants* **2024**, *13*, 453. [CrossRef]
8. Lungu, N.; Popescu, D.-E.; Jura, A.M.C.; Zaharie, M.; Jura, M.-A.; Roșca, I.; Boia, M. Enhancing Early Detection of Sepsis in Neonates through Multimodal Biosignal Integration: A Study of Pulse Oximetry, Near-Infrared Spectroscopy (NIRS), and Skin Temperature Monitoring. *Bioengineering* **2024**, *11*, 681. [CrossRef]
9. Sood, E.; Newburger, J.W.; Anixt, J.S.; Cassidy, A.R.; Jackson, J.L.; Jonas, R.A.; Lisanti, A.J.; Lopez, K.N.; Peyvandi, S.; Marino, B.S. Neurodevelopmental Outcomes for Individuals with Congenital Heart Disease: Updates in Neuroprotection, Risk-Stratification, Evaluation, and Management: A Scientific Statement From the American Heart Association. *Circulation* **2024**, *149*, e997–e1022. [CrossRef]
10. Doi, M.; Usui, N.; Shimada, S. Prenatal Environment and Neurodevelopmental Disorders. *Front. Endocrinol.* **2022**, *13*, 860110. [CrossRef]
11. De Felice, A.; Ricceri, L.; Venerosi, A.; Chiarotti, F.; Calamandrei, G. Multifactorial Origin of Neurodevelopmental Disorders: Approaches to Understanding Complex Etiologies. *Toxics* **2015**, *3*, 89–129. [CrossRef]
12. Năstase, L.; Cristea, O.; Diaconu, A.; Stoicescu, S.-M.; Mohora, R.; Pascu, B.M.; Tala, S.T.; Roșca, I. Two Cases of Congenital Hypothyroidism Revealing Thyroid Agenesis. *Medicina* **2023**, *59*, 1887. [CrossRef]
13. Rosca, I.; Turenschi, A.; Nicolescu, A.; Constantin, A.T.; Canciu, A.M.; Dica, A.D.; Bratila, E.; Coroleuca, C.A.; Nastase, L. Endocrine Disorders in a Newborn with Heterozygous Galactosemia, Down Syndrome and Complex Cardiac Malformation: Case Report. *Medicina* **2023**, *59*, 856. [CrossRef]
14. Bratan, C.A.; Gheorghe, M.; Ispas, I.; Franti, E.; Dascalu, M.; Stoicescu, S.M.; Rosca, I.; Gherghiceanu, F.; Dumitrache, D.; Nastase, L. Dunstan Baby Language Classification with CNN. In Proceedings of the 2021 International Conference on Speech Technology and Human-Computer Dialogue (SpeD), Bucharest, Romania, 13–15 October 2021; IEEE: New York, NY, USA; pp. 167–171.
15. Pesch, M.H.; Leung, J.; Lanzieri, T.M.; Tinker, S.C.; Rose, C.E.; Danielson, M.L.; Yeargin-Allsopp, M.; Grosse, S.D. Autism Spectrum Disorder Diagnoses and Congenital Cytomegalovirus. *Pediatrics* **2024**, *153*, e2023064081. [CrossRef]
16. Wang, J.; Li, Y.; Geng, X.; Zhang, X.; Xiao, Y.; Wang, W. Associations of Epstein-Barr Virus Infection with Attention Deficit Hyperactivity Disorder, Learning Disability, and Special Education in U.S. Children. *Int. J. Gen. Med.* **2021**, *15*, 2187–2195. [CrossRef] [PubMed]
17. Egorova, M.; Egorov, V.; Zabrodskaya, Y. Maternal Influenza and Offspring Neurodevelopment. *Curr. Issues Mol. Biol.* **2024**, *46*, 355–366. [CrossRef] [PubMed]

18. Otero, A.M.; Connolly, M.G.; Gonzalez-Ricon, R.J.; Wang, S.S.; Allen, J.M.; Antonson, A.M. Influenza A Virus During Pregnancy Disrupts Maternal Intestinal Immunity and Fetal Cortical Development in a Dose- and Time-Dependent Manner. *Mol. Psychiatry* **2025**, *30*, 13–28. [CrossRef] [PubMed]
19. Guardado, K.; Varela-Cardoso, M.; Pérez-Roa, V.O.; Morales-Romero, J.; Zenteno-Cuevas, R.; Ramos-Ligonio, Á.; Guzmán-Martínez, O.; Sampieri, C.L.; Ortiz-Chacha, C.S.; Pérez-Varela, R.; et al. Evaluation of Anomalies and Neurodevelopment in Children Exposed to ZIKV During Pregnancy. *Children* **2022**, *9*, 1216. [CrossRef]
20. Pesch, M.H.; Lauer, C.S.; Weinberg, J.B. Neurodevelopmental Outcomes of Children with Congenital Cytomegalovirus: A Systematic Scoping Review. *Pediatr. Res.* **2024**, *95*, 418–435. [CrossRef]
21. Seblany, H.T.; Dinu, I.S.; Safer, M.; Plesca, D.A. FACTORS THAT HAVE A NEGATIVE IMPACT ON QUALITY OF LIFE IN CHILDREN WITH ADHD. *Farmacia* **2014**, *62*, 350–357.
22. Fung, S.G.; Fakhraei, R.; Condran, G.; Regan, A.K.; Dimanlig-Cruz, S.; Ricci, C.; Foo, D.; Sarna, M.; Török, E.; Fell, D.B. Neuropsychiatric Outcomes in Offspring after Fetal Exposure to Maternal Influenza Infection During Pregnancy: A Systematic Review. *Reprod. Toxicol.* **2022**, *113*, 155–169. [CrossRef]
23. Moreno, J.L.; Kurita, M.; Holloway, T.; López, J.; Cadagan, R.; Martínez-Sobrido, L.; García-Sastre, A.; González-Maeso, J. Maternal Influenza Viral Infection Causes Schizophrenia-Like Alterations of 5-$HT_{2A}$ and $MGlu_2$ Receptors in the Adult Offspring. *J. Neurosci.* **2011**, *31*, 1863–1872. [CrossRef] [PubMed]
24. Selten, J.-P.; Termorshuizen, F. The Serological Evidence for Maternal Influenza as Risk Factor for Psychosis in Offspring Is Insufficient: Critical Review and Meta-Analysis. *Schizophr. Res.* **2017**, *183*, 2–9. [CrossRef] [PubMed]
25. Shook, L.L.; Sullivan, E.L.; Lo, J.O.; Perlis, R.H.; Edlow, A.G. COVID-19 in Pregnancy: Implications for Fetal Brain Development. *Trends Mol. Med.* **2022**, *28*, 319–330. [CrossRef] [PubMed]
26. Dubey, H.; Sharma, R.K.; Krishnan, S.; Knickmeyer, R. SARS-CoV-2 (COVID-19) as a Possible Risk Factor for Neurodevelopmental Disorders. *Front. Neurosci.* **2022**, *16*, 1021721. [CrossRef]
27. Popescu, D.-E.; Cerbu, S.; Rosca, I.; Lungu, N.; Trușculescu, A.A.; Belengeanu, V.; Manea, A.M.; Dima, M.A.; Gorun, F.; Popa, Z.L.; et al. Comparative Analysis of Hematological and Biochemical Changes in Neonates among Women with and Without COVID-19 Infection During Pregnancy. *Children* **2023**, *10*, 1370. [CrossRef]
28. De Luca, D.; Vauloup-Fellous, C.; Benachi, A.; Vivanti, A. Transmission of SARS-CoV-2 from Mother to Fetus or Neonate: What to Know and What to Do? *Semin. Fetal Neonatal Med.* **2023**, *28*, 101429. [CrossRef]
29. Jeganathan, K.; Paul, A.B. Vertical Transmission of SARS-CoV-2: A Systematic Review. *Obs. Med.* **2022**, *15*, 91–98. [CrossRef]
30. Lins, B. Maternal Immune Activation as a Risk Factor for Psychiatric Illness in the Context of the SARS-CoV-2 Pandemic. *Brain Behav. Immun. Health* **2021**, *16*, 100297. [CrossRef]
31. Hofsink, N.; Groenink, L.; Plösch, T. The Fetal Programming Effect of Maternal Immune Activation (MIA) on the Offspring's Immune System. *Semin. Immunopathol.* **2024**, *46*, 14. [CrossRef]
32. Popescu, D.E.; Roșca, I.; Jura, A.M.C.; Cioca, A.; Pop, O.; Lungu, N.; Popa, Z.-L.; Rațiu, A.; Boia, M. Prompt Placental Histopathological and Immunohistochemical Assessment after SARS-CoV-2 Infection During Pregnancy—Our Perspective of a Small Group. *Int. J. Mol. Sci.* **2024**, *25*, 1836. [CrossRef]
33. Kasaven, L.S.; Raynaud, I.; Jalmbrant, M.; Joash, K.; Jones, B.P. The Impact of the COVID-19 Pandemic on Perinatal Services and Maternal Mental Health in the UK. *BJPsych Open* **2023**, *9*, e13. [CrossRef] [PubMed]
34. Kotlar, B.; Gerson, E.M.; Petrillo, S.; Langer, A.; Tiemeier, H. The Impact of the COVID-19 Pandemic on Maternal and Perinatal Health: A Scoping Review. *Reprod. Health* **2021**, *18*, 10. [CrossRef] [PubMed]
35. Zhu, P.; Sun, M.; Hao, J.; Chen, Y.; Jiang, X.; Tao, R.; Huang, K.; Tao, F. Does Prenatal Maternal Stress Impair Cognitive Development and Alter Temperament Characteristics in Toddlers with Healthy Birth Outcomes? *Dev. Med. Child. Neurol.* **2014**, *56*, 283–289. [CrossRef] [PubMed]
36. Perelli, F.; Vidiri, A.; Palomba, G.; Franco, R.; Gallitelli, V.; Parasiliti, M.; Bisanti, M.; Spanò, A.; Silvagni, A.; Lopez, A.; et al. Preterm Birth and SARS-CoV-2: Does a Correlation Exist? *Biomedicines* **2025**, *13*, 282. [CrossRef]
37. Smith, L.H.; Dollinger, C.Y.; VanderWeele, T.J.; Wyszynski, D.F.; Hernández-Díaz, S. Timing and Severity of COVID-19 During Pregnancy and Risk of Preterm Birth in the International Registry of Coronavirus Exposure in Pregnancy. *BMC Pregnancy Childbirth* **2022**, *22*, 775. [CrossRef]
38. Klein, A.Z.; Kunatharaju, S.; Golder, S.; Levine, L.D.; Figueiredo, J.C.; Gonzalez-Hernandez, G. Association Between COVID-19 During Pregnancy and Preterm Birth by Trimester of Infection: A Retrospective Cohort Study Using Longitudinal Social Media Data. *J. Med. Internet Res.* **2025**, *27*, e66097. [CrossRef]
39. Zamparini, J.; Saggers, R.; Buga, C.E. A Review of Coronavirus Disease 2019 in Pregnancy. *Semin. Respir. Crit. Care Med.* **2023**, *44*, 050–065. [CrossRef]
40. Metz, T.D.; Clifton, R.G.; Hughes, B.L.; Sandoval, G.J.; Grobman, W.A.; Saade, G.R.; Manuck, T.A.; Longo, M.; Sowles, A.; Clark, K.; et al. Association of SARS-CoV-2 Infection with Serious Maternal Morbidity and Mortality From Obstetric Complications. *JAMA* **2022**, *327*, 748. [CrossRef]

41. Zanardo, V.; Tortora, D.; Sandri, A.; Severino, L.; Mesirca, P.; Straface, G. COVID-19 Pandemic: Impact on Gestational Diabetes Mellitus Prevalence. *Diabetes Res. Clin. Pract.* **2022**, *183*, 109149. [CrossRef]
42. Murphy, C.A.; O'Reilly, D.P.; Edebiri, O.; Donnelly, J.C.; McCallion, N.; Drew, R.J.; Ferguson, W. The Effect of COVID-19 Infection During Pregnancy; Evaluating Neonatal Outcomes and the Impact of the B.1.1.7. Variant. *Pediatr. Infect. Dis. J.* **2021**, *40*, e475–e481. [CrossRef] [PubMed]
43. Pinheiro, G.S.M.A.; de Souza, R.C.; de Oliveira Azevedo, V.M.G.; Guimarães, N.S.; Pires, L.G.; Lemos, S.M.A.; Alves, C.R.L. Effects of Intrauterine Exposure to SARS-CoV-2 on Infants' Development: A Rapid Review and Meta-Analysis. *Eur. J. Pediatr.* **2023**, *182*, 2041–2055. [CrossRef] [PubMed]
44. Yao, Y.; Sun, L.; Luo, J.; Qi, W.; Zuo, X.; Yang, Z. The Effect of Long-Term COVID-19 Infection on Maternal and Fetal Complications: A Retrospective Cohort Study Conducted at a Single Center in China. *Sci. Rep.* **2024**, *14*, 17273. [CrossRef] [PubMed]
45. Goicea, L.; Buzoianu, E.; Davitoiu, A.M.; Chindris, S.; Zamfirescu, A.; Iancu, M.; Ghiorghiu, I.; Tincu, I.; Draganescu, A.; Dorobantu, A.; et al. Multisystemic Inflammatory Syndrome in Children Post-COVID-19: Clinical-Biological Characteristics of Patients in the First Year of the Pandemic. *J. Pediatr. Neonatal Individ. Med.* **2023**, *12*, e120210.
46. Dunn, A.; Malhotra, A. Neurodevelopmental Risks of SARS-CoV-2 Infection in Utero. *Pediatr. Res.* **2025**. [CrossRef]
47. Buechel, C.; Friedmann, A.; Eber, S.; Behrends, U.; Mall, V.; Nehring, I. The Change of Psychosocial Stress Factors in Families with Infants and Toddlers During the COVID-19 Pandemic. A Longitudinal Perspective on the CoronabaBY Study from Germany. *Front. Pediatr.* **2024**, *12*, 1354089. [CrossRef]
48. Nazzari, S.; Pili, M.P.; Günay, Y.; Provenzi, L. Pandemic Babies: A Systematic Review of the Association between Maternal Pandemic-Related Stress During Pregnancy and Infant Development. *Neurosci. Biobehav. Rev.* **2024**, *162*, 105723. [CrossRef]
49. Penna, A.L.; de Aquino, C.M.; Pinheiro, M.S.N.; do Nascimento, R.L.F.; Farias-Antúnez, S.; Araújo, D.A.B.S.; Mita, C.; Machado, M.M.T.; Castro, M.C. Impact of the COVID-19 Pandemic on Maternal Mental Health, Early Childhood Development, and Parental Practices: A Global Scoping Review. *BMC Public Health* **2023**, *23*, 388. [CrossRef]
50. Wells, G.; Shea, B.; Peterson, J.; Welch, V.; Losos, M.; Tugwell, P. The Newcastle-Ottawa Scale (NOS) for Assessing the Quality of Nonrandomised Studies in Meta-Analyses. Available online: https://www.ohri.ca/programs/clinical_epidemiology/oxford.asp (accessed on 24 June 2025).
51. Shuffrey, L.C.; Firestein, M.R.; Kyle, M.; Fields, A.; Alcántara, C.; Amso, D.; Austin, J.; Bain, J.M.; Barbosa, J.; Bence, M.; et al. Birth During the COVID-19 Pandemic, but Not Maternal SARS-CoV-2 Infection During Pregnancy, Is Associated with Lower Neurodevelopmental Scores at 6-Months. *medRxiv* **2021**. [CrossRef]
52. ACNP 60th Annual Meeting: Poster Abstracts P1–P275. *Neuropsychopharmacology* **2021**, *46*, 72–217. [CrossRef]
53. Cheng, Y.; Teng, H.; Xiao, Y.; Yao, M.; Yin, J.; Sun, G. Impact of SARS-CoV-2 Infection During Pregnancy on Infant Neurobehavioral Development: A Case-Control Study. *Front. Pediatr.* **2021**, *9*, 762684. [CrossRef]
54. Wu, T.; Chen, L.; Wang, Y.; Shi, H.; Niu, J.; Yin, X.; Li, M.; Tan, C.; Jiang, H.; Zheng, D.; et al. Effects of SARS-CoV-2 Infection During Late Pregnancy on Early Childhood Development: A Prospective Cohort Study. *Front. Pediatr.* **2021**, *9*, 750012. [CrossRef] [PubMed]
55. Schuh, T.L.; Mithal, L.B.; Naureckas, S.; Miller, E.S.; Garfield, C.F.; Shah, M.D. Outcomes from Birth to 6 Months of Publicly Insured Infants Born to Mothers with Severe Acute Respiratory Syndrome Coronavirus 2 Infection in the United States. *J. Perinat. Med.* **2022**, *50*, 334–342. [CrossRef] [PubMed]
56. Edlow, A.G.; Castro, V.M.; Shook, L.L.; Kaimal, A.J.; Perlis, R.H. Neurodevelopmental Outcomes at 1 Year in Infants of Mothers Who Tested Positive for SARS-CoV-2 During Pregnancy. *JAMA Netw. Open* **2022**, *5*, e2215787. [CrossRef] [PubMed]
57. Ayed, M.; Embaireeg, A.; Kartam, M.; More, K.; Alqallaf, M.; AlNafisi, A.; Alsaffar, Z.; Bahzad, Z.; Buhamad, Y.; Alsayegh, H.; et al. Neurodevelopmental Outcomes of Infants Born to Mothers with SARS-CoV-2 Infections During Pregnancy: A National Prospective Study in Kuwait. *BMC Pediatr.* **2022**, *22*, 319. [CrossRef]
58. Buonsenso, D.; Costa, S.; Giordano, L.; Priolo, F.; Colonna, A.T.; Morini, S.; Sbarbati, M.; Pata, D.; Acampora, A.; Conti, G.; et al. Short- and Mid-Term Multidisciplinary Outcomes of Newborns Exposed to SARS-CoV-2 in Utero or During the Perinatal Period: Preliminary Findings. *Eur. J. Pediatr.* **2022**, *181*, 1507–1520. [CrossRef]
59. Aldrete-Cortez, V.; Bobadilla, L.; Tafoya, S.A.; Gonzalez-Carpinteiro, A.; Nava, F.; Viñals, C.; Alvarado, E.; Mendizabal-Espinosa, R.; Gómez-López, M.E.; Ramirez-Garcia, L.A.; et al. Infants Prenatally Exposed to SARS-CoV-2 Show the Absence of Fidgety Movements and Are at Higher Risk for Neurological Disorders: A Comparative Study. *PLoS ONE* **2022**, *17*, e0267575. [CrossRef]
60. Liu, H.-Y.; Guo, J.; Zeng, C.; Cao, Y.; Ran, R.; Wu, T.; Yang, G.; Zhao, D.; Yang, P.; Yu, X.; et al. Transient Early Fine Motor Abnormalities in Infants Born to COVID-19 Mothers Are Associated with Placental Hypoxia and Ischemia. *Front. Pediatr.* **2022**, *9*, 793561. [CrossRef]
61. Martenot, A.; Labbassi, I.; Delfils-Stern, A.; Deruelle, P.; Kuhn, P. Medical and Neurodevelopmental Outcomes at 10 Months of Age in Infants Born at 34 Weeks plus to Mothers with COVID-19. *Acta Paediatr.* **2023**, *112*, 296–297. [CrossRef]

62. Fajardo Martinez, V.; Zhang, D.; Paiola, S.; Mok, T.; Cambou, M.C.; Kerin, T.; Rao, R.; Brasil, P.; Ferreira, F.; Fuller, T.; et al. Neuromotor Repertoires in Infants Exposed to Maternal COVID-19 During Pregnancy: A Cohort Study. *BMJ Open* **2023**, *13*, e069194. [CrossRef]
63. Silva, P.Y.F.; Lima da Cruz, M.C.; Guerra Azevedo, I.; Moreira, R.S.; Sousa, K.G.; Pereira, S.A. Risk of Global Developmental Delay in Infants Born from Mothers with COVID-19: A Cross-Sectional Study. *Int. J. Womens Health* **2023**, *15*, 467–474. [CrossRef] [PubMed]
64. Ayesa-Arriola, R.; Castro Quintas, Á.; Ortiz-García de la Foz, V.; Miguel Corredera, M.; San Martín González, N.; Murillo-García, N.; Neergaard, K.; Fañanás Saura, L.; de las Cuevas-Terán, I. Exploring the Impact of COVID-19 on Newborn Neurodevelopment: A Pilot Study. *Sci. Rep.* **2023**, *13*, 2983. [CrossRef]
65. Rood, M.; ten Kate, L.; Boeddha, N.P.; van't Kruys, K. Clinical Characteristics, Transmission Rate and Outcome of Neonates Born to COVID-19-Positive Mothers: A Prospective Case Series From a Resource-Limited Setting. *Pediatr. Infect. Dis. J.* **2023**, *42*, 35–42. [CrossRef] [PubMed]
66. Vrantsidis, D.M.; van de Wouw, M.; Hall, E.R.M.; Kuret, V.; Rioux, C.; Conrad, M.L.; Mesa, C.; Harris, A.; Lebel, C.; Tomfohr-Madsen, L.; et al. Neurodevelopment in the First 2 Years of Life Following Prenatal Exposure to Maternal SARS-CoV-2 Infection. *JAMA Netw. Open* **2024**, *7*, e2443697. [CrossRef] [PubMed]
67. Jaswa, E.G.; Huddleston, H.G.; Lindquist, K.J.; Wu, A.H.B.; Bishop, S.L.; Kim, Y.-S.; Kaing, A.; Prahl, M.; Gaw, S.L.; Corley, J.; et al. In Utero Exposure to Maternal COVID-19 and Offspring Neurodevelopment Through Age 24 Months. *JAMA Netw. Open* **2024**, *7*, e2439792. [CrossRef]
68. Hill, R.A.; Gibbons, A.; Suwakulsiri, W.; Taseska, A.; Darke, H.; Malhotra, A.; Yee, H.; Fahey, M.; Hunt, R.W.; Lim, I.; et al. Investigating the Impact of Severe Maternal SARS-CoV-2 Infection on Infant DNA Methylation and Neurodevelopment. *Mol. Psychiatry* **2025**, *30*, 1976–1984. [CrossRef]
69. Silva, L.M.; Melo, M.L.dO.; Alpes, M.F.; Santos, C.M.D. Risk of Neurodevelopmental Changes in 18-Month-Old Children Born to Mothers Infected with SARS-CoV-2. *Audiol. Commun. Res.* **2025**, *30*, e2963. [CrossRef]
70. Kehdi, R.C.; Silva, M.F.S.; Cavalcante, L.R.L.; Fiorenza, N.G.; Viana, M.; Leite, I.B.; dos Santos Silva, B.R.; de Assis, D.F.; Cortez, P.C.; Bezerra, D.L.; et al. Cord Blood Cytokines/Chemokines Linked to Delays in Toddlers Exposed to SARS-CoV-2 Prenatally. *Pediatr. Res.* **2025**. [CrossRef]
71. Berg, J.; Linden, K.; Zaigham, M.; Domellöf, M.; Ahlsson, F.; Elfvin, A.; Åden, U.; Abrahamsson, T.; Ohlin, A.; Berg, J.; et al. The Association between Antenatal SARS-CoV-2 Exposure and Infant Neurodevelopment at Four Months of Age: A Prospective Multicenter Cohort Survey within the COPE Study. *Int. J. Infect. Dis.* **2025**, *158*, 107973. [CrossRef]
72. Yamaguchi, Y.; Miyazawa, H.; Miura, M. Neural Tube Closure and Embryonic Metabolism. *Congenit. Anom.* **2017**, *57*, 134–137. [CrossRef]
73. Engelhardt, D.M.; Martyr, C.A.; Niswander, L. Pathogenesis of Neural Tube Defects: The Regulation and Disruption of Cellular Processes Underlying Neural Tube Closure. *WIREs Mech. Dis.* **2022**, *14*, e1559. [CrossRef] [PubMed]
74. Goasdoué, K.; Miller, S.M.; Colditz, P.B.; Björkman, S.T. Review: The Blood-Brain Barrier; Protecting the Developing Fetal Brain. *Placenta* **2017**, *54*, 111–116. [CrossRef] [PubMed]
75. Bergdolt, L.; Dunaevsky, A. Brain Changes in a Maternal Immune Activation Model of Neurodevelopmental Brain Disorders. *Prog. Neurobiol.* **2019**, *175*, 1–19. [CrossRef] [PubMed]
76. McEwan, F.; Glazier, J.D.; Hager, R. The Impact of Maternal Immune Activation on Embryonic Brain Development. *Front. Neurosci.* **2023**, *17*, 1146710. [CrossRef]
77. Chhetri, P.K.; Das, J.M. Neuroanatomy, Neural Tube Development and Stages. Available online: https://www.ncbi.nlm.nih.gov/books/NBK557414/ (accessed on 23 August 2025).
78. Kostović, I.; Judaš, M. Embryonic and Fetal Development of the Human Cerebral Cortex. In *Brain Mapping*; Elsevier: Amsterdam, The Netherlands, 2015; pp. 167–175.
79. National Research Council (US); Institute of Medicine (US). Committee on Integrating the Science of Early Childhood Development The Developing Brain. In *From Neurons to Neighborhoods: The Science of Early Childhood Development*; Shonkoff, J.P., Phillips, D.A., Eds.; National Academies Press (US): Washington, DC, USA, 2000.
80. Jackson, R.; Cornish, R.; Daskalopoulou, Z.; Gale, C.; Hurd, M.; Johnson, S.; Knight, M.; Kurinczuk, J.J.; Woodward, K.; Chakkarapani, E.; et al. Association of Antenatal or Neonatal SARS-CoV-2 Exposure with Developmental and Respiratory Outcomes, and Healthcare Usage in Early Childhood: A National Prospective Cohort Study. *EClinicalMedicine* **2024**, *72*, 102628. [CrossRef]
81. Hall, M.B.; Willis, D.E.; Rodriguez, E.L.; Schwarz, J.M. Maternal Immune Activation as an Epidemiological Risk Factor for Neurodevelopmental Disorders: Considerations of Timing, Severity, Individual Differences, and Sex in Human and Rodent Studies. *Front. Neurosci.* **2023**, *17*, 1135559. [CrossRef]

82. Groh, J.; Feng, R.; Yuan, X.; Liu, L.; Klein, D.; Hutahaean, G.; Butz, E.; Wang, Z.; Steinbrecher, L.; Neher, J.; et al. Microglia Activation Orchestrates CXCL10-Mediated CD8+ T Cell Recruitment to Promote Aging-Related White Matter Degeneration. *Nat. Neurosci.* **2025**, *28*, 1160–1173. [CrossRef]
83. Kummer, K.K.; Zeidler, M.; Kalpachidou, T.; Kress, M. Role of IL-6 in the Regulation of Neuronal Development, Survival and Function. *Cytokine* **2021**, *144*, 155582. [CrossRef]
84. Gonzalez Caldito, N. Role of Tumor Necrosis Factor-Alpha in the Central Nervous System: A Focus on Autoimmune Disorders. *Front. Immunol.* **2023**, *14*, 1213448. [CrossRef]
85. Zhang, W.; Xiao, D.; Mao, Q.; Xia, H. Role of Neuroinflammation in Neurodegeneration Development. *Signal Transduct. Target. Ther.* **2023**, *8*, 267. [CrossRef]
86. Bicanin Ilic, M.; Nikolic Turnic, T.; Ilic, I.; Nikolov, A.; Mujkovic, S.; Rakic, D.; Jovic, N.; Arsenijevic, N.; Mitrovic, S.; Spasojevic, M.; et al. SARS-CoV-2 Infection and Its Association with Maternal and Fetal Redox Status and Outcomes: A Prospective Clinical Study. *J. Clin. Med.* **2025**, *14*, 1555. [CrossRef]
87. LaSalle, J.M. DNA Methylation Biomarkers of Intellectual/Developmental Disability across the Lifespan. *J. Neurodev. Disord.* **2025**, *17*, 10. [CrossRef] [PubMed]
88. Neumann, A.; Walton, E.; Alemany, S.; Cecil, C.; González, J.R.; Jima, D.D.; Lahti, J.; Tuominen, S.T.; Barker, E.D.; Binder, E.; et al. Association between DNA Methylation and ADHD Symptoms from Birth to School Age: A Prospective Meta-Analysis. *Transl. Psychiatry* **2020**, *10*, 398. [CrossRef] [PubMed]
89. Trajkova, S.; Kerkhof, J.; Rossi Sebastiano, M.; Pavinato, L.; Ferrero, E.; Giovenino, C.; Carli, D.; Di Gregorio, E.; Marinoni, R.; Mandrile, G.; et al. DNA Methylation Analysis in Patients with Neurodevelopmental Disorders Improves Variant Interpretation and Reveals Complexity. *Hum. Genet. Genom. Adv.* **2024**, *5*, 100309. [CrossRef] [PubMed]
90. Hikosaka, M.; Parvez, M.S.A.; Yamawaki, Y.; Oe, S.; Liang, Y.; Wada, Y.; Hirahara, Y.; Koike, T.; Imai, H.; Oishi, N.; et al. Maternal Immune Activation Followed by Peripubertal Stress Combinedly Produce Reactive Microglia and Confine Cerebellar Cognition. *Commun. Biol.* **2025**, *8*, 296. [CrossRef]
91. Hagberg, H.; Mallard, C.; Ferriero, D.M.; Vannucci, S.J.; Levison, S.W.; Vexler, Z.S.; Gressens, P. The Role of Inflammation in Perinatal Brain Injury. *Nat. Rev. Neurol.* **2015**, *11*, 192–208. [CrossRef] [PubMed]
92. Henry, M.L.; Beeson, P.M.; Stark, A.J.; Rapcsak, S.Z. The Role of Left Perisylvian Cortical Regions in Spelling. *Brain Lang* **2007**, *100*, 44–52. [CrossRef]
93. Ellul, P.; Maruani, A.; Vantalon, V.; Humeau, E.; Amestoy, A.; Anchordoqui, A.; Atzori, P.; Baleyte, J.-M.; Benmansour, S.; Bonnot, O.; et al. Maternal Immune Activation During Pregnancy Is Associated with More Difficulties in Socio-Adaptive Behaviors in Autism Spectrum Disorder. *Sci. Rep.* **2023**, *13*, 17687. [CrossRef]
94. Quagliato, L.A.; de Matos, U.; Nardi, A.E. Maternal Immune Activation Generates Anxiety in Offspring: A Translational Meta-Analysis. *Transl. Psychiatry* **2021**, *11*, 245. [CrossRef]
95. Murlanova, K.; Begmatova, D.; Weber-Stadlbauer, U.; Meyer, U.; Pletnikov, M.; Pinhasov, A. Double Trouble: Prenatal Immune Activation in Stress Sensitive Offspring. *Brain Behav. Immun.* **2022**, *99*, 3–8. [CrossRef]
96. Duggan, C.; Irvine, A.D.; O'B Hourihane, J.; Kiely, M.E.; Murray, D.M. ASQ-3 and BSID-III's Concurrent Validity and Predictive Ability of Cognitive Outcome at 5 Years. *Pediatr. Res.* **2023**, *94*, 1465–1471. [CrossRef]
97. Lockhart, M.; Chaux, R.; Chevin, M.; Celle, M.; Raia-Barjat, T.; Patural, H.; Chabrier, S.; Giraud, A. Classification Performance of the Ages and Stages Questionnaire: Influence of Maternal Education Level. *Children* **2023**, *10*, 449. [CrossRef]
98. Crowle, C.; Jackman, M.; Webb, A.; Morgan, C. Use of the Motor Optimality Score-Revised (MOS-R) to Predict Neurodevelopmental Outcomes in Infants with Congenital Anomalies. *Early Hum. Dev.* **2023**, *187*, 105876. [CrossRef] [PubMed]
99. Einspieler, C.; Bos, A.F.; Spittle, A.J.; Bertoncelli, N.; Burger, M.; Peyton, C.; Toldo, M.; Utsch, F.; Zhang, D.; Marschik, P.B. The General Movement Optimality Score-Revised (GMOS-R) with Socioeconomically Stratified Percentile Ranks. *J. Clin. Med.* **2024**, *13*, 2260. [CrossRef] [PubMed]
100. Örtqvist, M.; Marschik, P.B.; Toldo, M.; Zhang, D.; Fajardo-Martinez, V.; Nielsen-Saines, K.; Ådén, U.; Einspieler, C. Reliability of the Motor Optimality Score-Revised: A Study of Infants at Elevated Likelihood for Adverse Neurological Outcomes. *Acta Paediatr.* **2023**, *112*, 1259–1265. [CrossRef] [PubMed]
101. Ossmy, O.; Donati, G.; Kaur, A.; Sotoodeh, M.S.; Forrester, G. Towards Automatic Assessment of Atypical Early Motor Development? *Brain Res. Bull.* **2025**, *224*, 111311. [CrossRef]
102. Kokkinaki, T.; Hatzidaki, E. COVID-19 Pandemic-Related Restrictions: Factors That May Affect Perinatal Maternal Mental Health and Implications for Infant Development. *Front. Pediatr.* **2022**, *10*, 846627. [CrossRef]
103. Firestein, M.R.; Dumitriu, D.; Marsh, R.; Monk, C. Maternal Mental Health and Infant Development During the COVID-19 Pandemic. *JAMA Psychiatry* **2022**, *79*, 1040. [CrossRef]
104. Hessami, K.; Norooznezhad, A.H.; Monteiro, S.; Barrozo, E.R.; Abdolmaleki, A.S.; Arian, S.E.; Zargarzadeh, N.; Shekerdemian, L.S.; Aagaard, K.M.; Shamshirsaz, A.A. COVID-19 Pandemic and Infant Neurodevelopmental Impairment. *JAMA Netw. Open* **2022**, *5*, e2238941. [CrossRef]

105. Veloso, A.H.N.; Barbosa, A.d.M.; Ribeiro, M.F.M.; Gervásio, F.M. Neurodevelopment in the First Year of Children Exposed to SARS-CoV-2 During Intrauterine Period: Systematic Review. *Rev. Gauch. Enferm.* **2024**, *45*, e20240020. [CrossRef]
106. Jackson, R.; Woodward, K.; Ireland, M.; Larkin, C.; Kurinczuk, J.J.; Knight, M.; Gale, C.; Johnson, S.; Cornish, R.; Chakkarapani, E. Antenatal and Neonatal Exposure to SARS-CoV-2 and Children's Development: A Systematic Review and Meta-Analysis. *Pediatr. Res.* **2024**, *96*, 40–50. [CrossRef]

Journal of
*Clinical Medicine*

MDPI

*Article*

# A Cohort Study Characterizing the Outcomes Following an Acute SARS-CoV-2 Infection in Pregnancy

**Clementine Adeyemi [1], Leticia Breuer [2], Raghad Kodvawala [2], Delia Miller [3] and Margaret V. Powers-Fletcher [4,*]**

1 Department of Internal Medicine, College of Medicine, University of Cincinnati, 3230 Eden Ave, Cincinnati, OH 45267, USA; adeyemce@mail.uc.edu
2 College of Medicine, University of Cincinnati, 3230 Eden Ave, Cincinnati, OH 45267, USA
3 Department of Environmental and Public Health Sciences, University of Cincinnati, 160 Panzeca Way, Cincinnati, OH 45267, USA; mille5dp@ucmail.uc.edu
4 College of Arts & Sciences, University of Cincinnati, 2700 Campus Way, Cincinnati, OH 45219, USA
* Correspondence: powersmg@ucmail.uc.edu

**Abstract**

**Background/Objectives:** Current estimates suggest that 6% of COVID-19 survivors develop a post-viral sequela known as Long COVID. Among those at risk for this sequela, pregnant individuals are a vulnerable patient population, but they are understudied as to the nature of their symptomology and potential adverse outcomes. **Methods:** This retrospective study evaluated a cohort of 150 pregnant individuals with a history of acute SARS-CoV-2 infection during pregnancy, observing for Long COVID symptoms and assessing for adverse outcomes. Of this cohort, 64% identified as Black and/or Latina, which provides a more diverse representation compared to previously published studies. **Results:** Within this cohort, 26.7% of individuals experienced at least one symptom of Long COVID; subcohorts, which were categorized based on presence or absence of Long COVID symptomology, presented with varying phenotypes. Pain, mental health dysfunction or psychological problems, and fatigue were the predominant symptoms documented for patients who averaged two Long COVID symptoms after at least 30 days following a COVID-19 diagnosis. Different adverse outcomes were higher in frequency among subcohorts, highlighting a need for continued study to explore the nuances of the impact of COVID-19 on this unique and vulnerable population. The most notable trends between subcohorts related to treatment patterns for acute COVID-19, vaccine status, and cesarean delivery rates. **Conclusions:** By providing a description of the documented health experience for a predominantly non-White cohort of individuals who were diagnosed with an acute SARS-CoV-2 during pregnancy, our study contributes to a foundation upon which future studies can build.

**Keywords:** COVID-19 and pregnancy; SARS-CoV-2 infection; maternal morbidity; pregnancy complication; management; maternal comorbidities; severe disease; prevention; diagnosis; treatment

## 1. Introduction

First described through social media by sufferers who characterized themselves as "long-haulers," the presence or continuation of symptoms for an extended period following acute COVID-19 is an accepted condition with various working definitions [1]. The 2022 definition by the Centers for Disease Control and Prevention (CDC) defined it as "a lack of return to normal health after a SARS-CoV-2 infection, specifically after at least four weeks," while the National Academies of Sciences, Engineering, and Medicine (NASEM) defines it as "an infection-associated chronic condition (IACC) that occurs after a SARS-CoV-2 infection and is present for at least 3 months as a continuous, relapsing and remitting, or progressive disease state that affects one or more organ systems" [2,3]. The phrase "Post-Acute Sequelae of SARS-CoV-2 infection," or PASC, is used by the National Institutes of Health (NIH) to refer to the worsening, continuation, reoccurrence of symptoms or the emergence of new symptoms 30 days or more after the initial manifestation of symptoms from a SARS-CoV-2 infection, while the World Health Organization (WHO) definition is specific to symptom continuation of three months or longer [4,5]. Using the WHO definition, at least 6% of the over 778 million cases with a history of COVID-19 globally are thought to have experienced Long COVID and, in the United States specifically, this condition afflicts an estimated ~43–45 million people [5–8]. Due to the variability in clinical definitions and challenges in diagnosis, however, this number is likely underestimated [9].

Not only does the variability within clinical definitions of Long COVID have an impact on epidemiology estimates, but it also has a negative impact on potential sufferers, delaying them from seeking care due to the lack of knowledge on the comprehensive or differential symptoms; this is amplified by healthcare access challenges such as frequently fragmented, siloed care across various clinical specialties [10,11]. This is particularly concerning for vulnerable patient populations who may be at higher risk for adverse outcomes. Researchers are working to better characterize Long COVID in such vulnerable groups [12–15], but there are still critical gaps in knowledge.

Pregnant individuals are within the group of particularly vulnerable patients for whom a better understanding of Long COVID is required. Adverse effects of acute COVID-19 have been documented during pregnancy, including higher risk of pre-eclampsia and increased incidence of neurodevelopmental disorders in offspring [16–18]. Moreover, because of safety concerns for the fetus, clinical trials and subsequently approved therapies for acute COVID-19 in pregnant individuals are limited [19–21]. Overall, there is a higher risk of respiratory-infection-associated maternal and fetal morbidity and mortality in pregnant individuals, including associated conditions such as influenza [22–24]. The exact nature of Long COVID in pregnant or recently pregnant individuals, however, is still poorly understood and is possibly unique from that of non-pregnant individuals. Pregnant individuals are known to have physiologically altered immune states during pregnancy and post-partum compared to non-pregnant individuals, among other physiological differences [25]. As a result, variation in susceptibility to and presentation of disease is not surprising [26]. Other diseases have been documented as presenting with distinct characteristics in pregnant individuals compared to non-pregnant individuals, including diabetes and hypertension [27–29]. Long COVID in the pregnant and post-partum population is still poorly understood, with the few published studies reporting conflicting conclusions [14,30–32]. Thus, to add to the emerging body of research and literature, this study aims to describe the health status of a cohort of individuals who experienced acute SARS-CoV-2 infection during pregnancy. This cohort was selected from those seeking care at an academic health center in an urban setting, which serves both rural and suburban areas. As a result, this study, with its comparatively diverse patient population, offers a distinct perspective from existing studies on Long COVID during pregnancy [14,15].

## 2. Methods

This study was a retrospective cohort study conducted in May through December of 2024 involving the chart review and unstructured data analysis of the electronic health records (EHRs) of pregnant individuals seen within a singular large academic healthcare system that consists of two regional hospitals and multiple clinical sites (Figure 1).

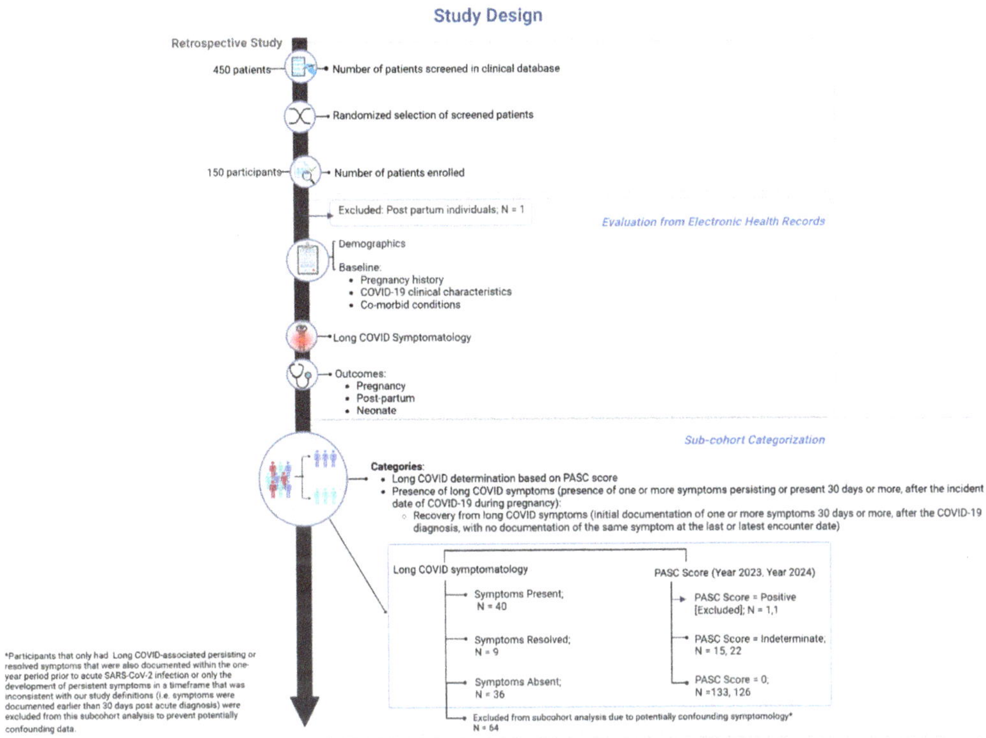


**Figure 1.** Study Design. In this descriptive study, electronic health records were retrospectively reviewed for 149 pregnant individuals with a history of acute SARS-CoV-2 infection during pregnancy, observing for Long COVID symptoms and assessing for adverse outcomes. Participants were classified according to two different classification systems, either based on overall Long COVID symptomatology or a PASC score derived from the NIH RECOVER protocol. Figure created using the web-based application, BioRender. Adeyemi, C. (2025) https://BioRender.com/g0xjvir (accessed on 30 September 2025).

### 2.1. Human Subjects Protection

This study was conducted with the review and approval of the University of Cincinnati Institutional Review Board (protocol # 2020-0313).

### 2.2. Cohort Selection and Definitions

A cohort of 150 participants, aged 15 years and above, was randomly selected from a pre-existing list of 450 patients that was generated by network providers to track pregnancy-related encounters, particularly labor and delivery, for patients with documented SARS-CoV-2 infections at any point during pregnancy. Pregnancy was noted by a clinician's observation of any gestational age for the patient and an indicator of pregnancy such as a prenatal visit, ultrasound visit, a delivery summary note or, a post-partum encounter detailing the date of delivery. Infection was documented by the clinician within patient's EHR based on either an in-house laboratory-confirmed positive SARS-CoV-2 PCR or antigen test or an at-home test result noted by the patient. The acute phase of a SARS-CoV-2 infection was defined as from the date of reported symptom onset up to 21 days. Upon EHR review, a single patient was identified who had a post-partum COVID-19 diagnosis date and was thus excluded from the study, resulting in a total of 149 participants.

### 2.3. Study Period

Participants records were reviewed from a year prior to their pregnancy-related COVID-19 diagnosis date until 31 December 2024.

### 2.4. EHR Review

Data collection was performed manually by a team of four researchers (C.A, R.K, L.B and D.M) using a data abstraction tool that was informed by expertise from a panel of individuals with maternal–fetal medicine, Long COVID, and/or EHR informatics expertise. Each investigator was trained using a protocol detailing search terms to use for each question on the two instruments used for this study (Supplemental Figure S1). These instruments evaluating symptomology and pregnancy were adapted for EHR data extraction from the NIH RECOVER instruments for the prospective study conducted on pregnant adults (Table 1). This adapted instrument included select symptomology associated with PASC along with variables associated with pregnancy history and outcomes.

**Table 1.** List of Symptoms Evaluated through Retrospective EHR Chart Review.

| Symptom List/Description |
|---|
| Poor appetite or overeating |
| Fatigue (being very tired) |
| Post-exertional malaise (Symptoms worse after even minor physical or mental effort) |
| Swelling of legs, Weakness in arms or legs, muscle cramps in legs and/or feet |
| Fever, chills, sweats or flushing |
| Loss of or change in smell or taste |
| Pain in any part of your body |
| Shortness of breath |
| Cough |
| Palpitations, racing heart, arrhythmia, skipped beats |
| Gastrointestinal (belly) symptoms (feeling full or vomiting after eating, diarrhea, constipation, cramping or colicky abdominal pain) |
| Bladder problems (incontinence, trouble passing urine or emptying bladder) |
| Nerve problems (tremor, shaking, abnormal movements, numbness, tingling, burning, cannot move part of body, new seizures) |
| Problems with anxiety, depression, stress, or trauma-related symptoms like nightmares or grief |
| Problems with sleep |
| Problems thinking or concentrating ("brain fog"), Feeling faint, dizzy, "goofy"; difficulty thinking soon after standing up from a sitting or lying position |
| Color changes in your skin, such as red, white or purple |
| Skin rash, sores |
| Excessively dry mouth, eyes |
| Excessive thirst |
| Vision problems (blurry, light sensitivity, difficulty reading or focusing, floaters, flashing lights, "snow") |
| Problems with hearing (hearing loss, ringing in ears) |

Table 1. *Cont.*

| Symptom List/Description |
| --- |
| Hair loss |
| Problems with teeth |
| Changes to menstrual cycle, reports of heavy periods |
| Changes in fertility or difficulty getting pregnant |
| Any other symptoms that were attributed to COVID-19 in EHR documentation |

### 2.5. Data Collection Variables

From the manual EHR review, clinical chart documentation of 26 selected symptoms that have previously been associated with Long COVID was recorded as outlined in Table 1. During the period of review, several time points were specifically assessed for symptom documentation, including the following windows relative to the COVID-19 diagnosis index date during pregnancy: a year before, 22 days after, 30 days after, and the final encounter at the time of record review. Participant demographic data included age (at the time of expected delivery date), race, and ethnicity, as well as SARS-CoV-2 vaccine status. In addition to symptom documentation, data was collected related to health during pregnancy and delivery outcomes. Included in the outcomes evaluated was COVID-19 severity indicated by a documentation of the need for ventilation or hospitalization due to acute COVID-19. Participants with missing data were retained for analysis to avoid a significant loss of information and a reduction in sample size.

### 2.6. Cohort Classification

For analysis of symptoms following COVID-19 diagnosis during pregnancy, participants were classified using two different approaches: (1) by overall symptom presence, recovery, or absence and (2) based on PASC score derived from the NIH RECOVER protocol (Figure 1).

#### 2.6.1. Overall Symptom Presence

Long COVID symptomology was classified as "Symptoms Present," "Symptoms Resolved," or "Symptoms Absent." For those classified as Symptoms Present, our study design required that the symptom be present at both 30 days or more following the acute COVID-19 and remain documented at the final encounter in the study period; if the symptom was no longer documented at the final encounter, the participant was classified as Symptoms Resolved. Participants who did not clearly meet the criteria for one of these three classifications were excluded from analysis as outlined in Figure 1. Additionally, Supplemental Table S1 lists each participant record by their subcohort classification group.

#### 2.6.2. PASC Score

The NIH RECOVER group developed an index scoring model for the description of patients suspected of or at-risk for PASC [4]. Briefly, the scoring was informed by the most distinct frequent symptoms experienced by their Long COVID participants compared to those who did not have Long COVID and those who did not have a positive case of SARS-CoV-2 infection. The cohort was an adult population of predominantly non-pregnant individuals. The initial index was published in 2023 with an updated 2024 index informed by the evolving knowledge of the Long COVID experience informed by their participants [33]. The categories are "PASC Zero", "PASC Indeterminate." or "PASC Positive." PASC Positive participants have a score of 12 or more in 2023 and 11 in 2024 with these scores determined from the aggregate score of the select symptoms reported or observed in participants.

For the purpose of our study, participants were classified as "PASC Positive" if they had documented persistence or presence of one or more PASC-specific symptoms, culminating in an aggregate score of 11 or 12, depending on the version of the PASC scoring system used that year. Participants were considered "PASC Indeterminate" if they had documented persistence or presence of one or more PASC symptoms with an aggregate score of less than 11 or 12, depending on the PASC score version used. Finally, participants were considered "PASC Zero" if they either: (1) only had a documented presence of one or more symptoms that were also present at some point during the year before the incident date of their COVID-19 diagnosis during pregnancy; (2) only had a documented presence of one or more symptoms persisting or present 30 days or more after their incident date of COVID-19 during pregnancy but a final PASC score of zero; (3) only had a documented presence of one or more symptoms present 30 days or more after their incident date of COVID-19 diagnosis during pregnancy but no longer had documentation of that symptom in their latest encounter at the time of chart review; or (4) had no documentation of any of the PASC score symptoms in their EHR.

### 2.7. Statistical Analysis

The sample size was determined to balance the intensive effort required for comprehensive manual review of each participant's electronic health record with the goal of assembling a preliminary yet informative cohort representative of this understudied population. Because the study was exploratory and descriptive, it was not designed for hypothesis testing or formal power analysis. Descriptive statistics are presented as frequencies, proportions and means, as appropriate. For categorical variables highlighted within the text and figures, we reported both observed proportions and corresponding 95% confidence intervals to convey the precision of the estimates. Given the relatively small subgroup sizes (approximately 20–40 participants), exact (Clopper–Pearson) binomial confidence intervals were used rather than large-sample approximations.

## 3. Results

### 3.1. Subcohorts Based on Overall Symptom Presence and PASC Score Classification

#### 3.1.1. Overall Symptom Presence

There were 36 (24%), 40 (27%), and 9 (6%) of the total participants that were classified as Symptoms Absent, Symptoms Present, and Symptoms Resolved, respectively (Figure 1 and Table 2). The remaining 43% of participants could not clearly be classified into one of these three groups because of either the presence of Long COVID-associated symptoms prior to acute SARS-CoV-2 infection or the development of persistent symptoms in a timeframe that was inconsistent with our study definitions (Figure 1 and Supplemental Table S1); they were excluded from analysis, rather than included in one of the three classifications, so as to prevent potentially confounding data. Demographic data for subcohorts are listed in Table 2. For each subcohort, the majority of participants were in their third trimester at the time of acute COVID-19 diagnosis (Symptoms Absent 69%, Symptoms Present 55% and Symptoms Resolved 78%). Only 30% of participants in the Symptoms Absent subcohort had documentation of either declined SARS-CoV-2 vaccination or vaccination occurring after their acute COVID-19 diagnosis during pregnancy, compared to 67.5% in the Symptoms Present and 55% in the Symptoms Resolved subcohorts (Table 2 and Figure 2).

**Table 2.** Subcohorts Based on Overall Symptoms and PASC Score.

| | | Symptoms Absent | Symptoms Present | Symptoms Resolved | PASC Zero 2023 | PASC Indeterminate 2023 | PASC Zero 2024 | PASC Indeterminate 2024 |
|---|---|---|---|---|---|---|---|---|
| Number of participants | | 36 | 40 | 9 | 133 | 15 | 126 | 22 |
| Proportion of participant pool | | 24.20% | 26.90% | 6.04% | 89.30% | 10.10% | 84.60% | 14.80% |
| Age (years) | Range | 16–41 | 20–44 | 17–36 | 15–41 | 20–39 | 16–41 | 15–39 |
| | Mean | 26.6 | 32.4 | 26.7 | 27.7 | 28.9 | 28.1 | 27.1 |
| Race/Ethnicity | Black | 31% | 47.50% | 22% | 43% | 47% | 44% | 36% |
| | White | 32% | 30% | 22% | 30% | 33% | 29% | 41% |
| | Latina | 32% | 17.50% | 56% | 22% | 13% | 22% | 14% |
| | Asian | 0% | 5% | 0% | 2% | 7% | 2% | 5% |
| | Native American or Alaska Native | 0% | 0% | 0% | 1% | 0% | 0% | 5% |
| | Native Hawaiian or Pacific Islander | 0% | 0% | 0% | 0% | 0% | 0% | 5% |
| | Multiracial | 5% | 0% | 0% | 2% | 0% | 2% | 0% |
| Vaccination Status | Before COVID-19 diagnosis | 17% | 15% | 11% | 21% | 7% | 21% | 9% |
| | After COVID-19 diagnosis | 19% | 27.50% | 33% | 20% | 40% | 21% | 32% |
| | Not documented | 53% | 17.50% | 33% | 33% | 13% | 33% | 18% |
| | Patient declined | 11% | 40% | 22% | 26% | 40% | 25% | 41% |
| Trimester on date of COVID-19 Diagnosis | 1st | 3% | 12.50% | 0% | 5% | 20% | 5% | 14% |
| | 2nd | 28% | 32.50% | 22% | 32% | 47% | 35% | 50% |
| | 3rd | 69% | 55% | 78% | 62% | 33% | 60% | 36% |
| Gestational Age (weeks) | Mean | 31.9 | 28 | 33.6 | 29 | 25.7 | 29.5 | 25.6 |
| Trimester | Mean | 3rd | 3rd | 3rd | 3rd | 2nd | 3rd | 2nd |

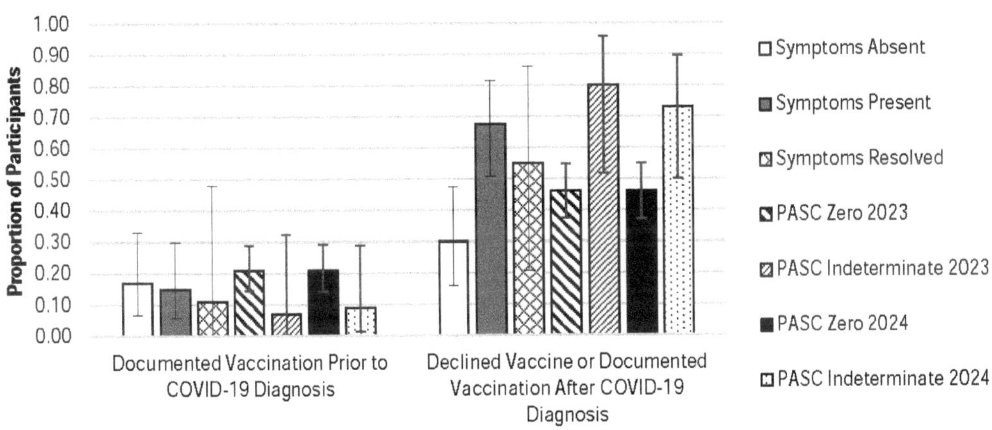


**Figure 2.** Observed Proportions of Vaccination History. For each subgroup, the observed proportions of participants for whom (1) COVID-19 vaccination was documented prior to the acute COVID-19 infection during pregnancy or (2) COVID-19 vaccination was either documented as declined by the participant or only documented after the acute COVID-19 diagnosis are reported. Corresponding 95% confidence intervals are shown to convey the precision of the estimates. The order of the chart legend entries (listed vertically) corresponds to the order of data categories shown in the graph (left to right).

#### 3.1.2. PASC Score

The PASC Score classification was completed using models derived from those published in 2023 and 2024 [4,33], and thus subcohorts are labeled as such. Using the model adapted from the 2023 publication, there were 133 (89%) of the total participants that were classified as PASC Zero compared to 15 (10%) classified as PASC Indeterminate. Using the model adapted from the 2024 publication, there were 126 (85%) of the total participants that were classified as PASC Zero compared to 22 (15%) classified as PASC Indeterminate and one individual classified as PASC Positive (Figure 1). Demographic data for subcohorts are listed in Table 2. The majority of participants in all subcohorts were in their third trimester at the time of COVID-19 diagnosis. For the 2023 PASC Zero subcohort, only 46% of participants declined SARS-CoV-2 vaccination or were not vaccinated until after their COVID-19 diagnosis compared to 80% for the 2023 PASC Indeterminate subcohort. Similarly, for the 2024 PASC Zero subcohort, only 46% of participants declined vaccination or were not vaccinated until after their COVID-19 diagnosis during pregnancy compared to 73% in the PASC Indeterminate subcohort (Figure 2). Based on the model adapted from the 2023 publication and 2024 publication, the same individual was classified as PASC Positive with a vaccine status of declined vaccination.

### 3.2. *Documentation of Symptoms Prior to Acute COVID-19 Diagnosis*

Eighteen participants (11%) out of the entire cohort had documentation of at least one of the 26 evaluated symptoms persisting 30 days or more following their COVID-19 diagnosis during pregnancy but also had that same symptom documented in their EHR up to a year before their COVID-19 diagnosis. Because of this previous documentation prior to their acute COVID-19 during pregnancy, these occurrences were not considered "persistent symptoms" and thus, did not result in classification within the Long COVID Present or PASC Indeterminate subcohorts; participants would have needed documentation of at least one other persisting symptom that was not present within the year prior to COVID-19 to be classified within either of these groups.

### 3.3. *Symptoms Following Acute SARS-CoV-2 Infection During Pregnancy*

Of the Long COVID symptoms documented as persisting until the latest encounter within the study window, fatigue (15%), cough (13%) and gastrointestinal symptoms (10%) are the most frequently observed symptoms seen in the 40 participants categorized in the subcohort with Symptoms Present (Figure 3): The most frequently documented symptoms that were present at least 30 days after a COVID-19 diagnosis but not persisting till the latest encounter were similar to those that persisted, with the exception of frequent documentation of resolved pain anywhere in the body. Overall, however, the majority of participants did not have documentation of many of the Long COVID symptoms that were evaluated (Figure 3). For example, 60% of the participants did not have any documentation of pain following their acute COVID-19 diagnosis and there was no recorded documentation of color changes in the skin for 99% of participants. Each of the 26 symptoms were documented as occurring following the COVID-19 diagnosis in at least one participant, however (Table 1 and Figure 3). Twenty-two of the twenty-six symptoms are documented as persisting for at least one participant, while twenty-three symptoms were documented for at least one participant, as resolving at least 30 days or more following the incident date of a SARS-CoV-2 infection during pregnancy.

### 3.4. *Pregnancy and Neonatal Outcomes*

#### 3.4.1. Outcomes Based on Overall Symptom Presence Classification

The Symptoms Absent subcohort had a greater proportion of participants for whom the incident pregnancy was their first pregnancy (19% vs. 5% for the Symptoms Present subcohort). Antithrombolytics were the most frequently prescribed medication during acute SARS-CoV-2 infection in the Symptoms Absent subcohort, whereas antivirals had been the most commonly prescribed medications in the Symptoms Present subcohort (Figure 4B and Table 3). More severe COVID-19 cases were noted in the Symptoms Absent group (8.3% in the Symptoms Absent group vs. 2.25% in the Symptoms Present group) (Figure 4C and Table 3). Both groups had relatively high rates of cesarean delivery (CS) compared to national rates; most of the cesarean deliveries were planned [34]. Cesarean deliveries trended higher in the Symptoms Present subcohort (58%) compared to the Symptoms Absent subcohort (47%). Both subcohorts had documented comorbidities (Table 3 and Figure 5).

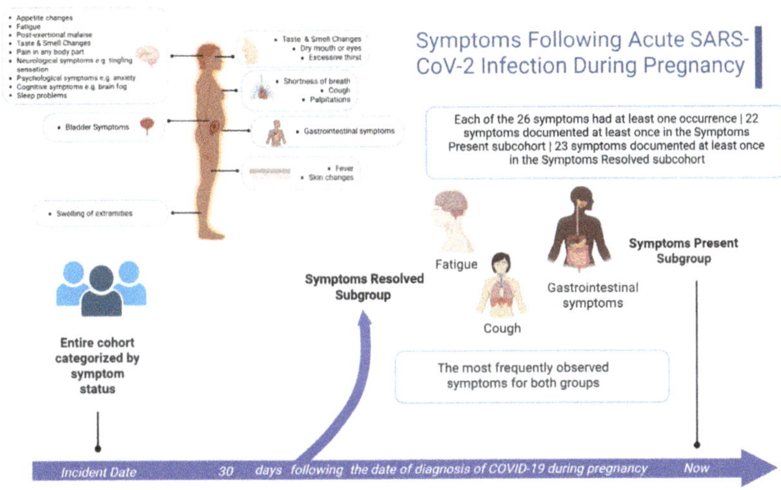


**Figure 3.** Symptoms Following Acute SARS-CoV-2 Infection During Pregnancy. Participants were classified based on overall Long COVID symptomatology based on a retrospective EHR analysis for observed documentation of 26 different symptoms. For those classified as Symptoms Present, our study design required that the symptom be present at both 30 days or morefollowing the acute COVID-19 and remain documented at the final encounter in the study period; if the symptom was no longer documented at the final encounter, the participant was classified as Symptoms Resolved. Figure created using the web-based application, BioRender. Adeyemi, C. (2025) https://BioRender.com/r8gb1n6 (accessed on 30 September 2025).

(A)

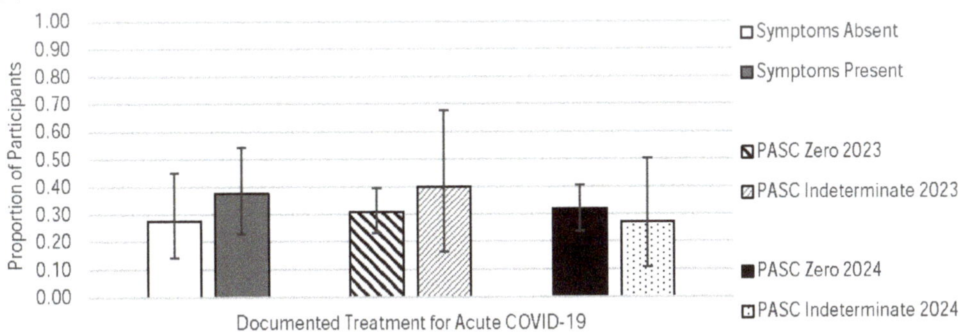


**Figure 4.** *Cont.*

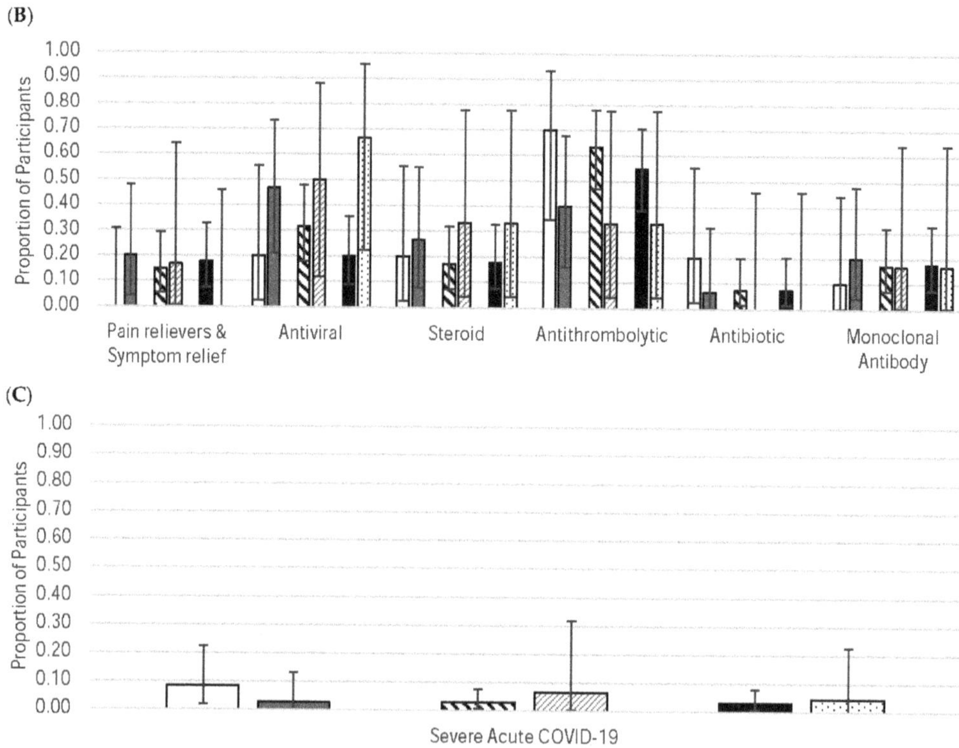


**Figure 4.** Observed Proportions of Acute COVID-19 Treatment History and Severity. (**A**) For each subgroup, the observed proportions of participants for whom treatment for acute COVID-19 was documented are reported. (**B**) Of those who had documented treatment, the observed proportion of the different treatment options given is also reported. (**C**) For each subgroup, the observed proportions of severe acute COVID-19 are reported. Corresponding 95% confidence intervals are shown to convey the precision of the estimates. The chart legend provided in panel A corresponds to all three panels. The order of the chart legend entries (listed vertically) corresponds to the order of data categories shown in the graph (left to right).

**Table 3.** Characteristics and Outcomes Associated with Pregnancy Based on Presence or Absence of Symptoms.

| | | **Symptoms Absent** | | **Symptoms Present** | |
|---|---|---|---|---|---|
| | | **(*n*)** | **(%)** | **(*n*)** | **(%)** |
| | | 36 | 47% | 40 | 53% |
| **General Characteristics of Concurrent COVID-19 and Pregnancy** | | | | | |
| Number of times pregnancy is documented in the patient's EHR (including current/recent pregnancy, previous pregnancies, live births, miscarriages, stillbirths or abortions) | 1 | 7 | 19.44% | 2 | 5.00% |
| | 2 | 11 | 30.56% | 10 | 25.00% |
| | 3 | 5 | 13.89% | 8 | 20.00% |
| | 4 | 9 | 25.00% | 6 | 15.00% |
| | 5 | 3 | 8.33% | 6 | 15.00% |
| | >5 | 1 | 2.78% | 8 | 20.00% |
| Number of multiple gestations BEFORE pregnancy during COVID-19 | | 1 | 3.45% | 1 | 2.50% |
| Prior Vaginal Birth | | 16 | 55.17% | 16 | 40.00% |

**Table 3.** *Cont.*

| | | Symptoms Absent | | Symptoms Present | |
|---|---|---|---|---|---|
| | | (*n*) | (%) | (*n*) | (%) |
| **Adverse Outcomes of Prior Pregnancies** | | | | | |
| Miscarriages | 1 | 2 | 6.90% | 9 | 23.68% |
| | 2 | 1 | 3.45% | 2 | 5.26% |
| | 3 | 0 | 0.00% | 3 | 7.89% |
| Still Birth | | 0 | 0.00% | 1 | 2.63% |
| HELLP | | 0 | 0.00% | 1 | 2.63% |
| Cesarean Section (CS) Delivery | | 7 | 24.14% | 15 | 39.47% |
| Gestational Diabetes | | 0 | 0.00% | 4 | 10.53% |
| Gestational Hypertension | | 3 | 10.34% | 6 | 15.79% |
| Preeclampsia | | 5 | 17.24% | 3 | 7.89% |
| Preterm birth | | 2 | 6.90% | 5 | 13.16% |
| **COVID-19 Experience** | | | | | |
| Stage at which acute COVID-19 was diagnosed | Pregnant | 20 | 55.56% | 31 | 77.50% |
| | In labor/at delivery | 16 | 44.44% | 9 | 22.50% |
| Treated for acute COVID-19 | | 10 | 27.78% | 15 | 37.50% |
| Acute COVID-19 treatment given | Pain relievers and symptom relief | 0 | 0.00% | 3 | 20.00% |
| | Antivirals | 2 | 20.00% | 7 | 46.67% |
| | Steroids | 2 | 20.00% | 4 | 26.67% |
| | Antithrombolytics | 7 | 70.00% | 6 | 40.00% |
| | Antibiotics | 2 | 20.00% | 1 | 6.67% |
| | Monoclonal Antibody | 1 | 10.00% | 3 | 20.00% |
| No documented treatment for acute COVID-19 | | 26 | 72.22% | 25 | 62.50% |
| Documented reasons for lack of acute COVID-19 treatment | Asymptomatic | 8 | 30.77% | 5 | 20.00% |
| | Patient declined | 1 | 3.85% | 4 | 16.00% |
| | Mild Symptoms | 4 | 15.38% | 2 | 8.00% |
| Patient hospitalized and/or given oxygen due to acute COVID-19 | | 3 | 8.33% | 1 | 2.25% |
| **Pregnancy Outcomes** | | | | | |
| Number of multiple gestations DURING pregnancy during COVID-19 | | 3 | 8.33% | 1 | 2.50% |
| Live Birth | | 32 | 89% | 40 | 100% |
| Number of babies | 1 | 30 | 93.75% | 39 | 97.50% |
| | 2 | 3 | 9.38% | 1 | 2.50% |
| Sex distribution of neonate | M | 21 | 64.00% | 20 | 50.00% |
| | F | 12 | 36.00% | 20 | 50.00% |
| Miscarriages | | 0 | 0.00% | 0 | 0.00% |
| Still Birth | | 2 | 5.56% | 0 | 0.00% |
| Preterm birth | | 11 | 30.56% | 13 | 32.50% |
| CS Delivery | | 15 | 46.88% | 23 | 57.50% |

**Table 3.** *Cont.*

| | | Symptoms Absent | | Symptoms Present | |
|---|---|---|---|---|---|
| | | (*n*) | (%) | (*n*) | (%) |
| Reason for CS Delivery | Planned cesarean delivery because of prior cesarean delivery | 6 | 40.00% | 9 | 39.13% |
| | Abnormal progress in labor | 4 | 26.67% | 4 | 17.39% |
| | Concern about baby based on the heart monitor | 2 | 13.33% | 7 | 30.43% |
| | Baby was breech | 2 | 13.33% | 2 | 8.70% |
| | Emergency due to risk to baby or participant | 3 | 20.00% | 3 | 13.04% |
| | Patient too sick with COVID-19 to be in labor | 1 | 6.67% | 0 | 0.00% |
| | Other reasons for a Cesarean | 0 | 0.00% | 3 | 13.04% |
| Forceps or Vacuum-assisted delivery | | 0 | 0.00% | 6 | 15.00% |
| Gestational diabetes | | 6 | 16.67% | 3 | 7.50% |
| Gestational hypertension | | 2 | 5.56% | 7 | 17.50% |
| Preeclampsia | | 8 | 22.22% | 8 | 20.00% |
| HELLP syndrome | | 1 | 2.78% | 2 | 5.00% |
| Seizures | | 1 | 2.78% | 0 | 0.00% |
| Placenta abruption | | 3 | 8.33% | 1 | 2.50% |
| Preterm premature rupture of membranes | | 6 | 16.67% | 5 | 12.50% |
| Oligohydramnios | | 1 | 2.78% | 1 | 2.50% |
| Hemorrhage or excessive bleeding | | 4 | 11.76% | 3 | 7.50% |
| Blood transfusion | | 1 | 2.94% | 3 | 7.50% |
| Uterine infection | | 4 | 11.76% | 3 | 7.50% |
| Blood clot in the legs of lungs requiring treatment with blood thinning medications | | 0 | 0.00% | 1 | 2.50% |
| Mechanical Ventilation | | 1 | 2.94% | 0 | 0.00% |
| Pneumonia | | 1 | 2.94% | 2 | 5.00% |
| Fetal Growth Restriction | | 0 | 0.00% | 0 | 0.00% |
| Congenital Anomalies | | 1 | 3% | 1 | 3% |
| | Before COVID-19 Diagnosis | 1 | 100% | 0 | 0% |
| | After COVID-19 Diagnosis | 0 | 0% | 1 | 100% |
| Category of Congenital Anomaly | Abdomen | 0 | 0% | 1 | 100% |
| | Brain | 0 | 0% | 0 | 0% |
| | Face or lip | 0 | 0% | 0 | 0% |
| | Cardiac | 1 | 100% | 0 | 0% |

**Table 3.** *Cont.*

| | | Symptoms Absent | | Symptoms Present | |
|---|---|---|---|---|---|
| | | (*n*) | (%) | (*n*) | (%) |
| Trimester anomaly was observed | 2nd | 1 | 100% | 0 | 0% |
| | 3rd | 0 | 0% | 0 | 0% |
| | At birth | 0 | 0% | 1 | 100% |
| Number of multiple gestations AFTER pregnancy during COVID-19 | | 0 | 0.00% | 0 | 0.00% |
| Number of participants currently pregnant | | 1 | 2.78% | 6 | 15.00% |
| **Neonatal Outcomes** | | | | | |
| Neonatal Intensive Care Unit (NICU) admittance | | 11 | 34.38% | 13 | 32.50% |
| Non-Survival at discharge | | 6 | 18.75% | 1 | 2.50% |
| Non-Survival post-partum | | 1 | 3.85% | 3 | 7.69% |
| Average Birth Weight (for those born between 37 and 41 weeks of gestation) | | 6.0 lbs 7.6 oz | | 5.8 lbs 6.2 oz | |
| Average Birth Weight (for all live births) | | 6 lbs 7.6 oz | | 5.8 lbs 6.0 oz | |

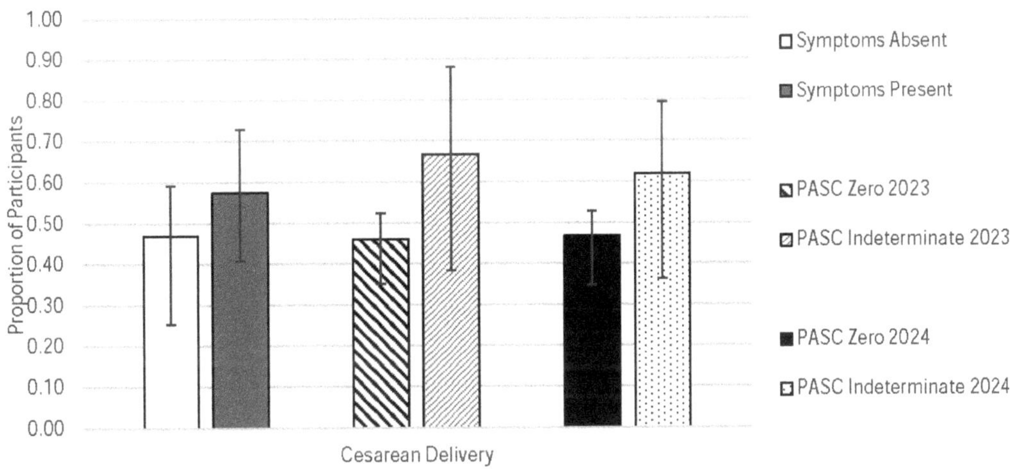


**Figure 5.** Observed Proportions of Cesarean Delivery. For each subgroup, the observed proportions of participants who underwent cesarean delivery are reported. Corresponding 95% confidence intervals are shown to convey the precision of the estimates. The order of the chart legend entries (listed vertically) corresponds to the order of data categories shown in the graph (left to right).

3.4.2. Outcomes Based on PASC Score Classification

The most frequently prescribed medication during acute SARS-CoV-2 infections for the 2023 and 2024 PASC Zero subcohorts were antithrombolytics (63% and 55%, respectively). Antivirals were the most prescribed medication for the 2023 and 2024 PASC Indeterminate subcohorts (50% and 67%, respectively) (Figure 4). Different adverse outcomes were documented in greater rates for each of the subcohorts, without a specific trend observed (Table 4 and Figure 5).

**Table 4.** Characteristics and Outcomes Associated with Pregnancy Based on PASC Score Category.

| | | PASC 2023 = 0 | | PASC Indeterminate 2023 | | PASC 2024 = 0 | | PASC Indeterminate 2024 | |
|---|---|---|---|---|---|---|---|---|---|
| | | (n) | (%) | (n) | (%) | (n) | (%) | (n) | (%) |
| | | 133 | 89% | 15 | 10% | 126 | 85% | 22 | 15% |
| **General Characteristics of Concurrent COVID-19 and Pregnancy** | | | | | | | | | |
| Number of times pregnancy is documented in the patient's EHR (including current/recent pregnancy, previous pregnancies, live births, miscarriages, stillbirths or abortions) | 1 | 17 | 12.78% | 0 | 0.00% | 15 | 11.90% | 2 | 9.090% |
| | 2 | 33 | 24.81% | 4 | 26.67% | 30 | 23.81% | 7 | 31.82% |
| | 3 | 22 | 16.54% | 3 | 20% | 19 | 15.08% | 6 | 27.27% |
| | 4 | 27 | 20.30% | 2 | 13.33% | 27 | 21.43% | 3 | 13.64% |
| | 5 | 13 | 9.77% | 3 | 20% | 13 | 10.32% | 3 | 13.64% |
| | >5 | 21 | 15.79% | 3 | 20% | 23 | 18.25% | 1 | 4.55% |
| Number of multiple gestations BEFORE pregnancy during COVID-19 | | 1 | 0.86% | 1 | 6.67% | 1 | 0.89% | 1 | 5.00% |
| Prior Vaginal Birth | | 57 | 49.14% | 5 | 33.33% | 57 | 50.89% | 5 | 25.00% |
| **Adverse Outcomes of Prior Pregnancies** | | | | | | | | | |
| Miscarriages | 1 | 29 | 25.00% | 2 | 13.33% | 29 | 25.89% | 2 | 10.00% |
| | 2 | 5 | 4.31% | 1 | 6.67% | 5 | 4.46% | 1 | 5.00% |
| | 3 | 6 | 5.17% | 1 | 6.67% | 7 | 6.25% | 0 | 0.00% |
| Still Birth | | 1 | 0.86% | 1 | 6.67% | 5 | 4.46% | 1 | 5.00% |
| HELLP | | 0 | 0.00% | 1 | 6.67% | 0 | 0.00% | 1 | 5.00% |
| Cesarean Section (CS) Delivery | | 41 | 35.34% | 5 | 33.33% | 38 | 33.93% | 8 | 40.00% |
| Gestational Diabetes | | 5 | 4.31% | 3 | 20.00% | 5 | 4.46% | 3 | 15.00% |
| Gestational Hypertension | | 12 | 10.34% | 3 | 20.00% | 11 | 9.82% | 4 | 20.00% |
| Preeclampsia | | 16 | 13.79% | 2 | 13.33% | 16 | 14.29% | 2 | 10.00% |
| Fetal Growth Restriction | | 3 | 2.59% | 0 | 0.00% | 3 | 2.68% | 0 | 0.00% |
| Preterm birth | | 13 | 11.21% | 3 | 20.00% | 37 | 33.04% | 2 | 10.00% |
| **COVID-19 Experience** | | | | | | | | | |
| Stage at which acute COVID-19 was diagnosed | Pregnant | 89 | 66.92% | 12 | 80% | 82 | 65.08% | 19 | 86.36% |
| | In labor/at delivery | 44 | 33.08% | 3 | 20% | 44 | 34.92% | 3 | 13.64% |
| Treated for acute COVID-19 | | 41 | 30.83% | 6 | 40% | 40 | 31.75 | 6 | 27.27 |
| Acute COVID-19 treatment given | Pain relievers and symptom relief | 6 | 14.63% | 1 | 16.67% | 7 | 17.50% | 0 | 0.00% |
| | Antivirals | 13 | 31.71% | 3 | 50.00% | 8 | 20.00% | 4 | 66.67% |
| | Steroids | 7 | 17.07% | 2 | 33.33% | 7 | 17.5% | 2 | 33.33% |
| | Antithrombolytics | 26 | 63.41% | 2 | 33.33% | 22 | 55.00% | 2 | 33.33% |
| | Antibiotics | 3 | 7.32% | 0 | 0.00% | 3 | 7.50% | 0 | 0.00% |
| | Monoclonal Antibody | 7 | 17.07% | 1 | 16.67% | 7 | 17.5% | 1 | 16.67% |
| Not documented treatment for acute COVID-19 | | 92 | 69.17% | 9 | 60.00% | 81 | 64.29% | 16 | 72.73% |
| Documented reasons for lack of acute COVID-19 treatment | Asymptomatic | 30 | 32.61% | 1 | 11.11% | 25 | 30.86% | 4 | 25.00% |
| | Patient declined | 7 | 7.61% | 3 | 33.33% | 6 | 7.41% | 3 | 18.75% |
| | Mild Symptoms | 10 | 10.87% | 0 | 0.00% | 9 | 11.11% | 1 | 6.25% |
| Patient hospitalized and/or given oxygen due to acute COVID-19 | | 4 | 3.00% | 1 | 6.67% | 4 | 3.17% | 1 | 4.55% |
| **Pregnancy Outcomes** | | | | | | | | | |
| Number of multiple gestations DURING pregnancy during COVID-19 | | 6 | 4.51% | 1 | 6.67% | 5 | 3.97% | 2 | 9.09% |
| Live Birth | | 126 | 95% | 15 | 100.00% | 118 | 94.00% | 21 | 95.45% |
| Number of babies | 1 | 121 | 96.03% | 14 | 93.33% | 114 | 96.61% | 20 | 95.24% |
| | 2 | 5 | 3.97% | 1 | 6.67% | 5 | 4.24% | 1 | 4.76% |
| Sex distribution of neonate | M | 64 | 51.00% | 10 | 66.67% | 61 | 50.41% | 13 | 59.09% |
| | F | 62 | 49.00% | 5 | 33.33% | 60 | 49.59% | 9 | 40.91% |
| Miscarriage | | 0 | 0.00% | 0 | 0.00% | 0 | 0.00% | 0 | 0.00% |
| Still Birth | | 3 | 2.26% | 0 | 0.00% | 3 | 2.38% | 0 | 0.00% |
| Preterm birth | | 39 | 29.32% | 2 | 13.33% | 37 | 29.37% | 4 | 8.18% |
| CS Delivery | | 58 | 46.03% | 10 | 66.67% | 55 | 46.61% | 13 | 61.90% |

**Table 4.** *Cont.*

| | | PASC 2023 = 0 | | PASC Indeterminate 2023 | | PASC 2024 = 0 | | PASC Indeterminate 2024 | |
|---|---|---|---|---|---|---|---|---|---|
| | | (*n*) | (%) | (*n*) | (%) | (*n*) | (%) | (*n*) | (%) |
| Reason for CS Delivery | Planned cesarean delivery because of prior cesarean delivery | 25 | 43.10% | 4 | 40.00% | 22 | 40.00% | 7 | 53.85% |
| | Abnormal progress in labor | 13 | 22.41% | 1 | 10.00% | 13 | 23.64% | 1 | 7.69% |
| | Concern about baby based on the heart monitor | 12 | 20.69% | 3 | 30.00% | 12 | 21.82% | 3 | 23.08% |
| | Baby was breech | 3 | 5.17% | 1 | 10.00% | 3 | 5.45% | 1 | 7.69% |
| | Uterine infection | 10 | 17.24% | 2 | 20.00% | 7 | 12.73% | 3 | 23.08% |
| | Emergency due to risk to baby or participant | 10 | 17.24% | 0 | 0.00% | 10 | 18.18% | 0 | 0.00% |
| | Patient too sick with COVID-19 to be in labor | 1 | 1.72% | 0 | 0.00% | 1 | 1.82% | 0 | 0.00% |
| | Other reason(s) | 6 | 10.34% | 0 | 0.00% | 6 | 10.91% | 0 | 0.00% |
| Forceps or Vacuum-assisted delivery | | 9 | 7.14% | 2 | 13.33% | 7 | 5.93% | 4 | 19.05% |
| Gestational diabetes | | 15 | 11.28% | 2 | 13.33% | 15 | 11.90% | 2 | 9.09% |
| Gestational hypertension | | 15 | 11.28% | 2 | 13.33% | 15 | 11.90% | 2 | 9.09% |
| Preeclampsia | | 29 | 21.80% | 1 | 6.67% | 27 | 21.43% | 3 | 13.64% |
| HELLP syndrome | | 2 | 1.50% | 1 | 6.67% | 2 | 1.59% | 1 | 4.55% |
| Seizures | | 1 | 0.75% | 0 | 0.00% | 1 | 0.79% | 0 | 0.00% |
| Placenta abruption | | 5 | 3.76% | 0 | 0.00% | 5 | 3.97% | 0 | 0.00% |
| Preterm premature rupture of membranes | | 14 | 10.53% | 1 | 6.67% | 13 | 10.32% | 2 | 9.09% |
| Oligohydramnios | | 2 | 1.50% | 1 | 6.67% | 3 | 2.38% | 0 | 0.00% |
| Hemorrhage or excessive bleeding | | 12 | 9.30% | 1 | 6.67% | 11 | 9.17% | 2 | 9.52% |
| Blood transfusion | | 4 | 3.10% | 1 | 6.67% | 2 | 1.67% | 3 | 14.29% |
| Blood clot in the legs of lungs requiring treatment with blood thinning medications | | 1 | 0.78% | 0 | 0.00% | 1 | 0.83% | 0 | 0.00% |
| Mechanical Ventilation | | 1 | 0.78% | 0 | 0.00% | 1 | 0.83% | 1 | 4.76% |
| Pneumonia | | 2 | 1.55% | 1 | 6.67% | 1 | 0.83% | 2 | 9.52% |
| Fetal Growth Restriction | | 0 | 0.00% | 0 | 0.00% | 0 | 0.00% | 0 | 0.00% |
| Congenital Anomalies | | 8 | 6.02% | 0 | 0.00% | 7 | 5.56% | 1 | 4.55% |
| Before COVID-19 diagnosis | | 7 | 87.50% | 0 | 0.00% | 6 | 85.71% | 1 | 100% |
| After COVID-19 Diagnosis | | 1 | 12.50% | 0 | 0.00% | 1 | 14.29% | 0 | 0% |
| Category of Congenital Anomaly | Abdomen | 1 | 12.50% | 0 | 0.00% | 1 | 14.29% | 0 | 0% |
| | Brain | 1 | 12.50% | 0 | 0.00% | 1 | 14.29% | 0 | 0% |
| | Face or lip | 1 | 12.50% | 0 | 0.00% | 1 | 14.29% | 0 | 0% |
| | Cardiac | 5 | 62.50% | 0 | 0.00% | 3 | 42.86% | 1 | 100% |
| | Lungs | 1 | 12.50% | 0 | 0.00% | 1 | 14.29% | 0 | 0% |
| | Limbs | 1 | 12.50% | 0 | 0.00% | 1 | 14.29% | 0 | 0% |
| Trimester anomaly was observed | 2nd | 5 | 62.50% | 0 | 0.00% | 4 | 57.14% | 1 | 100% |
| | 3rd | 0 | 0% | 0 | 0.00% | 0 | 0% | 0 | 0% |
| | At birth | 1 | 12.50% | 0 | 0.00% | 1 | 14.29% | 0 | 0% |
| Number of multiple gestations AFTER pregnancy during COVID-19 | | 1 | 0.75% | 0 | 0.00% | 1 | 0.79% | 0 | 0.00% |
| Number of participants currently pregnant | | 5 | 3.76% | 4 | 26.67% | 6 | 4.76% | 3 | 13.64% |
| **Neonatal Outcomes** | | | | | | | | | |
| Neonatal Intensive Care Unit (NICU) admittance | | 37 | 29.37% | 5 | 33.33% | 36 | 30.51% | 6 | 28.57% |
| Non-Survival at discharge | | 12 | 9.52% | 0 | 0.00% | 11 | 9.32% | 1 | 4.76% |
| Non-Survival post-partum | | 4 | 3.51% | 2 | 13.33% | 4 | 3.74% | 2 | 9.52% |
| Average Birth Weight (for those born between 37 and 41 weeks of gestation) | | 5.9 lb 8.2 oz | | 6.2 lbs 5.4 oz | | 5.8 lbs 8.2 oz | | 5.8 lbs 8.2 oz | |
| Average Birth Weight (for all live births) | | 5.8 lbs 8.9 oz | | 5.9 lbs 6.1 oz | | 5.9 lbs 7.6 oz | | 5.7 lbs 7.3 oz | |

## 4. Discussion and Conclusions

This descriptive retrospective cohort study examined the experiences of individuals diagnosed with acute COVID-19 during pregnancy, as documented in electronic health records, to advance understanding of Long COVID phenotypes in vulnerable populations. Using a manual EHR review approach encompassing clinical encounters up to one year prior to and following acute COVID-19 diagnosis, the EHRs of 149 participants that were randomly selected from an at-risk patient list at a single healthcare network serving the tri-state region of Ohio, Kentucky, and Indiana were evaluated. Participants were classified into subcohorts based on the persistence of symptoms associated with Long COVID or an adaptation of the published PASC scoring models; these two different cohort classifications were applied to reduce the risk of bias introduced by using a single classification system for a condition in an understudied population. Data was analyzed for trends related to symptom documentation and pregnancy-related outcomes to provide additional insight and an expanded scope of understanding of the complications that may occur following an acute SARS-CoV-2 infection in a pregnant individual.

A key strength of our study was the demographic diversity of the patient population. Unlike many previously published reports, our study cohort is predominantly made up of individuals who identify as Black and/or Latina. As such, it offers a perspective that is representative of the most vulnerable patient populations within the context of unacceptably high maternal morbidity and mortality rates in the United States, accounted for by racialized pregnant individuals intersecting with the disproportionate morbidity and mortality from COVID-19 reported in several racialized groups [34,35].

The documentation of persistence of at least one of the 26 symptoms previously associated with Long COVID was observed for 26.7% of the cohort. For a symptom to be considered persistent, our study design required that it be present at both 30 days or more following the acute COVID-19 and remain documented at the final encounter in the study period. This definition likely results in a conservative measure for evaluating Long COVID symptomology given the risk of both variability in symptom presentation throughout time [3], as well as bias introduced by the limitation of using symptoms documented in the EHR alone. An additional 6% of the cohort were classified as Symptoms Resolved in our study because their symptom(s) were no longer documented at the time of the final encounter. Despite the conservative nature of our estimate, however, our observed rate is higher than that reported in other reports [14,15]. This may be due to a resolution of symptoms after the 30-day time point as the other studies reported at three months or longer following a COVID-19 diagnosis in pregnancy. In contrast, other studies have reported a higher rate of up to 35% of Long COVID during pregnancy [14,15,30,31].

In our subcohort of participants experiencing persistent symptoms following acute infection, the majority of participants (78%) in the Symptoms Present subcohort had only one persisting symptom. The most frequent symptoms documented in our Symptoms Present and PASC Indeterminate subcohorts mirrored the predominant symptoms seen in adult sufferers of Long COVID, including pain and psychological symptoms [4]. Relying on EHR documentation alone, the nuances of the pain and psychological symptoms experienced are unclear. It may be interpreted as manifestation caused by the pathophysiology of Long COVID itself, or may be a reflection of the harm and the reduction in the quality of life experienced by patients who are seeking adequate care in the context of an emerging and poorly understood chronic disease [36–38]. Further study is required to gain additional qualitative insight directly from patients themselves, which would provide the necessary context for the interpretation of this finding.

The symptoms least documented in the EHR included skin color change and difficulty getting pregnant, the latter of which is explained by the fact that the study cohort was pregnant or post-partum. Skin color change may not be as apparent in individuals that are highly melanated and, thus, is perhaps a less informative symptom for the diagnosis of Long COVID in a non-White patient population. Surprisingly, one infrequently reported symptom was a loss or change in one's sense of taste or smell. The loss of these two senses is a distinct symptom of acute COVID-19 and the second highest scored symptom within the PASC determination score [4,33]. Pregnancy itself has been known to come with a change in one's sense of taste and smell [39], however, and this may have had an impact on either patient reporting or provider documentation of this symptom within the EHR.

The most notable trends between subcohorts were related to treatment patterns for acute COVID-19, vaccine status, and cesarean delivery rates. Participants in the Symptoms Absent subcohort had less frequently received treatment for their SARS-CoV-2 infections compared to those in the Symptoms Present group. Additionally, a higher proportion of participants in either the Symptoms Present, Symptoms Resolved, or PASC Indeterminate subcohorts had either declined SARS-CoV-2 vaccination or had received their vaccine following their COVID-19 diagnosis during pregnancy compared to the Long COVID Absent or PASC Zero cohorts. This finding suggests a connection between vaccination status and persistence of symptoms following acute infection in pregnant individuals. Although no inferential statistical analyses were performed in this descriptive study, including adjustments for potential confounders such as comorbidities or access to care, this observation is consistent with previous reports in the literature that support vaccination as an effective approach for reducing the risk of Long COVID [40]. Finally, overall, cesarean deliveries were unusually high in our cohort compared to national rates [41]. It is well-documented, however, that pregnant individuals of color tend to have higher rates of cesarean delivery in the United States compared to White individuals, which is a disparity that is not only a significant public health concern but also may introduce a confounding variable when evaluating the impact of Long COVID on labor and delivery outcomes in our cohort [41]. Furthermore, there are known adverse outcomes attributed to cesarean delivery, which can further confound our analysis due to the high rates observed in all cohorts, even those without persistent symptoms.

Long COVID in pregnancy is still relatively understudied. At the time of submission, this is only one of a few publications on the persistence of symptoms following acute COVID-19 during pregnancy in the United States. As such, the reported work provides important contributions to our understanding of human health, particularly because of a number of strengths in our approach. First, rather than relying on diagnosis codes or insurance claims data to identify participants, we manually reviewed EHR data, including unstructured clinical notes, to classify participants. Due to the risk of underdiagnosis or misdiagnosis of Long COVID as an emerging condition over the past five years, reliance on diagnosis codes or claims data alone would likely misidentify or fail to capture potentially undiagnosed but symptomatic Long COVID cases [11]. Of note, only 2 of the 149 patients in our cohort had any documentation of a Long COVID diagnosis in their EHR. Additionally, for further thoroughness, our manual review included analysis of symptoms up to a year before the diagnosis of COVID-19 during pregnancy and persistence of symptoms as early as three weeks following an acute SARS-CoV-2 infection. These windows of time provided us with the broadest approach to identifying symptoms that may have been present before the concurrent conditions of pregnancy and acute COVID-19, as well as allowed for a more inclusive dataset regarding persistence of symptoms.

To our knowledge, this is the first study to apply the previously published PASC scoring algorithm to an independent dataset, specifically within a pregnant population. As such, this cohort study provides important proof-of-principle evidence related to the feasibility and potential implications of such application. To date, there have been two versions of a PASC scoring algorithm published [4,33]. There have been other studies utilizing these algorithms, but they have all been within the NIH RECOVER team or do not include a pregnant population [4,18,33,42]. A limitation with the application of the scoring algorithm based on evaluation of health records alone was the inability to score certain topics that may not routinely be discussed or documented in the EHR. This included documentation regarding sexual desire, abortion, and fertility. Other symptoms might not be documented due to the area of specialty such as teeth loss. Another concern is temporality, as participants varied in the frequency of their encounters with clinicians within the healthcare system.

Limitations of our study overall include those that are well-established as being associated with any study that utilizes a retrospective EHR review [43]. EHR documentation does not reflect the entirety of a patient's health experience, particularly as the documentation is conducted by a clinician and thus, includes predominantly clinician-observed outcomes, as opposed to direct patient reported outcomes or experiences. There is also a likelihood of observer bias in the reporting of the patient's experience. Additionally, data in EHRs does not always reflect the real time experiences of the patient, in that patients do not necessarily interact with their healthcare provider every time they have a health-related incident. Underserved patient populations who have reduced healthcare access and fewer encounters with clinicians may also have less EHR documentation. As our study cohort is predominantly made up of individuals who may fall within these underserved patient populations, this bias may influence our ability to fully capture the lived experience of this cohort and this is an inherent limitation to retrospective EHR review. Further work to authentically capture and describe the lived experience of pregnant individuals who are at risk for Long COVID, particularly those from underserved communities, is critical to build upon the foundation of our descriptive study reported here. Given the limited awareness of Long COVID in many vulnerable patient populations, evaluating the Long COVID experience in pregnant individuals from their direct report has the additional benefit of increased community awareness, which can ultimately contribute to a reduction in stigma, an increase in healthcare seeking behaviors, and combat underdiagnosis [44,45]. Additionally, expanding this work to other sites and including additional variables such as socioeconomic data is critical to enhancing the generalizability of these findings. Our study contributes to a foundation upon which these future studies can build, however, by providing a description of the documented health experience for a predominantly non-White cohort of individuals who were diagnosed with an acute SARS-CoV-2 during pregnancy. The trends observed in potential risk factors and health outcomes based on presence or absence of Long COVID symptoms serve to inform future clinical studies and qualitative research designed to further delve into the nuances of Long COVID in vulnerable patient populations.

**Supplementary Materials:** The following supporting information can be downloaded at: https://www.mdpi.com/article/10.3390/jcm14217869/s1, Table S1: Details of group assignment based on symptom documentation over time. Figure S1: Long COVID Data Collection Instruments.

**Author Contributions:** Conceptualization, C.A. and M.V.P.-F.; methodology, C.A., L.B., R.K., D.M. and M.V.P.-F.; validation, C.A., L.B., R.K. and D.M.; formal analysis, C.A.; investigation, C.A., L.B., R.K. and D.M.; resources, M.V.P.-F.; data curation, C.A., L.B., R.K. and D.M.; writing—original draft preparation, C.A. and M.V.P.-F.; writing—review and editing, C.A., L.B., R.K., D.M. and M.V.P.-F.; visualization, C.A.; supervision, C.A. and M.V.P.-F.; project administration, C.A.; funding acquisition, M.V.P.-F. All authors have read and agreed to the published version of the manuscript.

**Funding:** This research received no external funding.

**Institutional Review Board Statement:** The study was conducted in accordance with the Declaration of Helsinki, and the protocol was approved by the Institutional Review Board (IRB) of the University of Cincinnati (#2020-0313) on 3 June 2020.

**Informed Consent Statement:** The IRB waived the requirement to obtain informed consent for participation due to the study being secondary research on data and the number of participants and time frame (retrospective review) would not allow for informed consent. Additionally, the IRB granted a waiver from the requirement to obtain an authorization for the use and/or disclosure of protected health information.

**Data Availability Statement:** The raw data supporting the conclusions of this article will be made available by the authors on request.

**Conflicts of Interest:** The authors declare no conflicts of interest.

## References

1. Yong, E. *COVID-19 Can Last for Several Months*; The Atlantic: Washington, DC, USA, 2020.
2. Centers for Disease Control and Prevention. *Long COVID Basics*; CDC: Atlanta, GA, USA, 2025.
3. National Academies of Sciences, Engineering, and Medicine; Health and Medicine Division; Board on Global Health; Board on Health Sciences Policy; Committee on Examining the Working Definition for Long COVID. *A Long COVID Definition: A Chronic, Systemic Disease State with Profound Consequences*; Goldowitz, I., Worku, T., Brown, L., Fineberg, H.V., Eds.; National Academies Press (US): Washington, DC, USA, 2024.
4. Thaweethai, T.; Jolley, S.E.; Karlson, E.W.; Levitan, E.B.; Levy, B.; McComsey, G.A.; McCorkell, L.; Nadkarni, G.N.; Parthasarathy, S.; Singh, U.; et al. Development of a Definition of Postacute Sequelae of SARS-CoV-2 Infection. *JAMA* **2023**, *329*, 1934–1946. [CrossRef]
5. World Health Organization (WHO). Post COVID-19 Condition (Long COVID). 2025. Available online: https://www.who.int/news-room/fact-sheets/detail/post-covid-19-condition-(long-covid) (accessed on 8 April 2025).
6. World Health Organization (WHO). Number of COVID-19 Cases Reported to WHO (Cumulative Total). Available online: https://data.who.int/dashboards/covid19/cases?n=c (accessed on 8 April 2025).
7. National Center for Health Statistics. Household Pulse Survey, 2022–2024. Long COVID. 2024. Available online: https://www.cdc.gov/nchs/covid19/pulse/long-covid.htm#print (accessed on 8 April 2025).
8. Burns, A. *As Recommendations for Isolation End, How Common is Long COVID?* Kaiser Family Foundation: San Francisco, CA, USA, 2024.
9. O'Hare, A.M.; Vig, E.K.; Iwashyna, T.J.; Fox, A.; Taylor, J.S.; Viglianti, E.M.; Butler, C.R.; Vranas, K.C.; Helfand, M.; Tuepker, A.; et al. Complexity and Challenges of the Clinical Diagnosis and Management of Long COVID. *JAMA Netw. Open* **2022**, *5*, e2240332. [CrossRef]
10. Quach, T.C.; Miglis, M.G.; Tian, L.; Bonilla, H.; Yang, P.C.; Grossman, L.; Paleru, A.; Xin, V.; Tiwari, A.; Shafer, R.W.; et al. Post-COVID-19 Vaccination and Long COVID: Insights from Patient-Reported Data. *Vaccines* **2024**, *12*, 1427. [CrossRef] [PubMed]
11. Maripuri, M.; Dey, A.; Honerlaw, J.; Hong, C.; Ho, Y.-L.; Tanukonda, V.; Chen, A.W.; Panickan, V.A.; Wang, X.; Zhang, H.G.; et al. Characterization of Post-COVID-19 Definitions and Clinical Coding Practices: Longitudinal Study. *Online J. Public Health Inform.* **2024**, *16*, e53445. [CrossRef]
12. Khullar, D.; Zhang, Y.; Zang, C.; Xu, Z.; Wang, F.; Weiner, M.G.; Carton, T.W.; Rothman, R.L.; Block, J.P.; Kaushal, R. Racial/Ethnic Disparities in Post-acute Sequelae of SARS-CoV-2 Infection in New York: An EHR-Based Cohort Study from the RECOVER Program. *J. Gen. Intern. Med.* **2023**, *38*, 1127–1136. [CrossRef]
13. Jacobs, M.M.; Evans, E.; Ellis, C. Racial, ethnic, and sex disparities in the incidence and cognitive symptomology of long COVID-19. *J. Natl. Med. Assoc.* **2023**, *115*, 233–243. [CrossRef]
14. Metz, T.D.; Reeder, H.T.; Clifton, R.G.; Flaherman, V.; Aragon, L.V.; Baucom, L.C.M.; Beamon, C.J.; Braverman, A.; Brown, J.; Cao, T.; et al. Post-Acute Sequelae of Severe Acute Respiratory Syndrome Coronavirus 2 (SARS-CoV-2) After Infection During Pregnancy. *Obstet. Gynecol.* **2024**, *144*, 411–420. [CrossRef]
15. Zang, C.; Guth, D.; Bruno, A.M.; Xu, Z.; Li, H.; Ammar, N.; Chew, R.; Guthe, N.; Hadley, E.; Kaushal, R.; et al. Long COVID after SARS-CoV-2 during pregnancy in the United States. *Nat. Commun.* **2025**, *16*, 3005. [CrossRef]
16. Woodworth, K.R.; Olsen, E.O.; Neelam, V.; Lewis, E.L.; Galang, R.R.; Oduyebo, T.; Aveni, K.; Yazdy, M.M.; Harvey, E.; Longcore, N.D.; et al. Birth and Infant Outcomes Following Laboratory-Confirmed SARS-CoV-2 Infection in Pregnancy—SET-NET, 16 Jurisdictions, March 29–October 14, 2020. *MMWR Morb. Mortal. Wkly. Rep.* **2020**, *69*, 1635–1640. [CrossRef]

17. Strid, P.; Zapata, L.B.; Tong, V.T.; Zambrano, L.D.; Woodworth, K.R.; Riser, A.P.; Galang, R.R.; Gilboa, S.M.; Ellington, S.R. Coronavirus Disease 2019 (COVID-19) Severity Among Women of Reproductive Age with Symptomatic Laboratory-Confirmed Severe Acute Respiratory Syndrome Coronavirus 2 (SARS-CoV-2) Infection by Pregnancy Status—United States, 1 January 2020–25 December 2021. *Clin. Infect. Dis.* **2022**, *75* (Suppl. S2), S317–S325. [CrossRef]
18. Boettcher, L.B.; Metz, T.D. Maternal and neonatal outcomes following SARS-CoV-2 infection. *Semin. Fetal Neonatal Med.* **2023**, *28*, 101428. [CrossRef] [PubMed]
19. Casella, C.; Giudice, M.L.; Niola, M.; DI Lorenzo, P.; Adamo, M.; Bianco, C.; Gragnano, E.; Saccone, G.; Guida, M. Need for fair inclusion of pregnant women in clinical trials: Scientific and ethical considerations about the lesson from the COVID-19 vaccines development. *Minerva Obstet. Gynecol.* **2022**, *74*, 112–113. [CrossRef] [PubMed]
20. U.S. Department of Health and Human Services; Food and Drug Administration; Center for Drug Evaluation and Research (CDER); Center for Biologics Evaluation and Research (CBER). *Pregnant Women: Scientific and Ethical Considerations for Inclusion in Clinical Trials Guidance for Industry*; U.S. Department of Health and Human Services: Washington, DC, USA, 2018. Available online: https://www.fda.gov/media/112195/download (accessed on 26 August 2025).
21. Sewell, C.A.; Sheehan, S.M.; Gill, M.S.; Henry, L.M.; Bucci-Rechtweg, C.; Gyamfi-Bannerman, C.; Lyerly, A.D.; McKinney, L.C.; Hatfield, K.P.; Baer, G.R.; et al. Scientific, ethical, and legal considerations for the inclusion of pregnant people in clinical trials. *Am. J. Obstet. Gynecol.* **2022**, *227*, 805–811. [CrossRef] [PubMed]
22. Centers for Disease Control and Prevention. Pregnancy Mortality Surveillance System. 2025. Available online: https://www.cdc.gov/maternal-mortality/php/pregnancy-mortality-surveillance-data/index.html?cove-tab=2 (accessed on 9 April 2025).
23. Mehta, N.; Chen, K.; Hardy, E.; Powrie, R. Respiratory disease in pregnancy. *Best Pr. Res. Clin. Obstet. Gynaecol.* **2015**, *29*, 598–611. [CrossRef]
24. Oseghale, O.; Vlahos, R.; O'leary, J.J.; Brooks, R.D.; Brooks, D.A.; Liong, S.; Selemidis, S. Influenza Virus Infection During Pregnancy as a Trigger of Acute and Chronic Complications. *Viruses* **2022**, *14*, 2729. [CrossRef]
25. Abu-Raya, B.; Michalski, C.; Sadarangani, M.; Lavoie, P.M. Maternal Immunological Adaptation During Normal Pregnancy. *Front. Immunol.* **2020**, *11*, 575197. [CrossRef]
26. Berumen-Lechuga, M.G.; Leaños-Miranda, A.; Molina-Pérez, C.J.; García-Cortes, L.R.; Palomo-Piñón, S. Risk Factors for Severe-Critical COVID-19 in Pregnant Women. *J. Clin. Med.* **2023**, *12*, 5812. [CrossRef]
27. Afshar, Y.; Gaw, S.L.; Flaherman, V.J.; Chambers, B.D.; Krakow, D.; Berghella, V.; A Shamshirsaz, A.; A Boatin, A.; Aldrovandi, G.; Greiner, A.; et al. Clinical Presentation of Coronavirus Disease 2019 (COVID-19) in Pregnant and Recently Pregnant People. *Obstet. Gynecol.* **2020**, *136*, 1117–1125. [CrossRef]
28. Mammaro, A.; Carrara, S.; Cavaliere, A.; Ermito, S.; Dinatale, A.; Pappalardo, E.M.; Militello, M.; Pedata, R. Hypertensive disorders of pregnancy. *J. Prenat. Med.* **2009**, *3*, 1–5.
29. Zajdenverg, L.; Negrato, C.A. Gestational diabetes mellitus and type 2 diabetes: Same disease in a different moment of life? Maybe not. *Arch. Endocrinol. Metab.* **2017**, *61*, 208–210. [CrossRef]
30. Muñoz-Chápuli Gutiérrez, M.; Prat, A.S.; Vila, A.D.; Claverol, M.B.; Martínez, P.P.; Recarte, P.P.; Benéitez, M.V.; García, C.A.; Muñoz, E.C.; Navarro, M.; et al. Post-COVID-19 condition in pregnant and postpartum women: A long-term follow-up, observational prospective study. *EClinicalMedicine* **2024**, *67*, 102398. [CrossRef] [PubMed]
31. Oliveira, A.; Carvalho, M.A.; Nacul, L.; Cabar, F.R.; Fabri, A.W.; Peres, S.V.; Zaccara, T.A.; O'boyle, S.; Alexander, N.; Takiuti, N.H.; et al. Post-Viral Fatigue Following SARS-CoV-2 Infection during Pregnancy: A Longitudinal Comparative Study. *Int. J. Environ. Res. Public Health* **2022**, *19*, 5735. [CrossRef] [PubMed]
32. Vásconez-González, J.; Fernandez-Naranjo, R.; Izquierdo-Condoy, J.S.; Delgado-Moreira, K.; Cordovez, S.; Tello-De-La-Torre, A.; Paz, C.; Castillo, D.; Izquierdo-Condoy, N.; Carrington, S.J.; et al. Comparative analysis of long-term self-reported COVID-19 symptoms among pregnant women. *J. Infect. Public Health* **2023**, *16*, 430–440. [CrossRef] [PubMed]
33. Geng, L.N.; Erlandson, K.M.; Hornig, M.; Letts, R.; Selvaggi, C.; Ashktorab, H.; Atieh, O.; Bartram, L.; Brim, H.; Brosnahan, S.B.; et al. 2024 Update of the RECOVER-Adult Long COVID Research Index. *JAMA* **2025**, *333*, 694–700. [CrossRef]
34. Ahmad, F.B.; Cisewski, J.A.; Hoyert, D.L. *Provisional Maternal Mortality Rates*; National Center for Health Statistics, Centers for Disease Control and Prevention: Atlanta, GA, USA, 2025. [CrossRef]
35. Foster, T.B.; Porter, S.R.; Pharris-Ciurej, N. *"Excess Mortality" During COVID19 Varied by Race, Ethnicity, Geography*; United States Census Burea: Suitland, MD, USA, 2024.
36. MacEwan, S.R.; Rahurkar, S.; Tarver, W.L.; Eiterman, L.P.; Melnyk, H.; Olvera, R.G.; Eramo, J.L.; Teuschler, L.; Gaughan, A.A.; Rush, L.J.; et al. The Impact of Long COVID on Employment and Well-Being: A Qualitative Study of Patient Perspectives. *J. Gen. Intern. Med.* **2025**, *40*, 1070–1077. [CrossRef]
37. Silver, S.R.; Li, J.; Ford, N.D.; Saydah, S.H. Functional disabilities and adverse well-being by COVID-19 and Long COVID history and employment status: 2022 Behavioral Risk Factor Surveillance System. *Am. J. Ind. Med.* **2024**, *67*, 1089–1107. [CrossRef]

38. Xu, Z.; Wang, W.; Zhang, D.; Tam, K.W.; Li, Y.; Chan, D.C.C.; Yang, Z.; Wong, S.Y.S. Excess risks of long COVID symptoms compared with identical symptoms in the general population: A systematic review and meta-analysis of studies with control groups. *J. Glob. Health* **2024**, *14*, 05022. [CrossRef]
39. Muluh, E.A.E.; McCormack, J.C.; Mo, Y.; Garratt, M.; Peng, M. Gustatory and olfactory shifts during pregnancy and the postpartum period: A systematic review and meta-analysis. *Physiol. Behav.* **2024**, *273*, 114388. [CrossRef]
40. Mumtaz, A.; Sheikh, A.A.E.; Khan, A.M.; Khalid, S.N.; Khan, J.; Nasrullah, A.; Sagheer, S.; Sheikh, A.B. COVID-19 Vaccine and Long COVID: A Scoping Review. *Life* **2022**, *12*, 1066. [CrossRef]
41. Hamilton, B.E.; Martin, J.A.; Osterman, M.J.K. *Births: Provisional Data for 2024*; U.S. Centers for Disease Control and Prevention: Atlanta, GA, USA, 2025; Volume 38.
42. Bello-Chavolla, O.Y.; Fermín-Martínez, C.A.; Ramírez-García, D.; Vargas-Vázquez, A.; Fernández-Chirino, L.; Basile-Alvarez, M.R.; Sánchez-Castro, P.; Núñez-Luna, A.; Antonio-Villa, N.E. Prevalence and determinants of post-acute sequelae after SARS-CoV-2 infection (Long COVID) among adults in Mexico during 2022: A retrospective analysis of nationally representative data. *Lancet Reg. Health Am.* **2024**, *30*, 100688. [CrossRef]
43. Zhang, H.G.; Honerlaw, J.P.; Maripuri, M.; Samayamuthu, M.J.; Beaulieu-Jones, B.R.; Baig, H.S.; L'yi, S.; Ho, Y.-L.; Morris, M.; Panickan, V.A.; et al. Potential pitfalls in the use of real-world data for studying long COVID. *Nat. Med.* **2023**, *29*, 1040–1043. [CrossRef]
44. Ignacio, M.; Oesterle, S.; Rodriguez-González, N.; Lopez, G.; Ayers, S.; Carver, A.; Wolfersteig, W.; Williams, J.H.; Sabo, S.; Parthasarathy, S. Limited Awareness of Long COVID Despite Common Experience of Symptoms Among African American/Black, Hispanic/Latino, and Indigenous Adults in Arizona. *J. Racial Ethn. Health Disparities* **2025**, *12*, 3013–3023. [CrossRef]
45. Sprague Martinez, L.; Sharma, N.; John, J.; Battaglia, T.A.; Linas, B.P.; Clark, C.R.; Hudson, L.B.; Lobb, R.; Betz, G.; O'nEill, S.O.O.; et al. Long COVID impacts: The voices and views of diverse Black and Latinx residents in Massachusetts. *BMC Public Health* **2024**, *24*, 2265. [CrossRef]

MDPI AG
Grosspeteranlage 5
4052 Basel
Switzerland
Tel.: +41 61 683 77 34

*Journal of Clinical Medicine* Editorial Office
E-mail: jcm@mdpi.com
www.mdpi.com/journal/jcm

www.ingramcontent.com/pod-product-compliance
Lightning Source LLC
Chambersburg PA
CBHW040316270926
51850CB00007BC/1501
* 9 7 8 3 7 2 5 8 5 9 1 1 5 *